Electrocardiography for Nurses

Physiological Correlates

Electrocardiography for Nurses
Physiological Correlates

JEANETTE G. KERNICKI, R.N., M.S.N.
Coordinator, Nurse Specialty Programs
The Methodist Hospital
Houston, Texas

KATHI M. WEILER, R.N., B.S.N.
Cardiovascular Nurse Specialist
Houston, Texas

A WILEY MEDICAL PUBLICATION
JOHN WILEY & SONS
New York • Chichester • Brisbane • Toronto

Dedicated to my mother and to my special friend, Sister M. Nazarius, O.S.F., for their encouragement and belief in me

Jeanette Kernicki

Dedicated in loving memory of my mother, Mrs. Marilyn R. Kirmer, whose strength, love, and guidance continue to be a source of inspiration for all who knew her; and to my husband, William Douglas Weiler, whose sacrifices and loving support were instrumental in the writing of this book

Kathi Weiler

Copyright © 1981 by John Wiley & Sons, Inc.

All rights reserved. Published simultaneously in Canada.

Reproduction or translation of any part of this
work beyond that permitted by Sections 107 or 108
of the 1976 United States Copyright Act without the
permission of the copyright owner is unlawful. Requests
for permission or further information should be addressed
to the Permissions Department, John Wiley & Sons, Inc.

Library of Congress Cataloging in Publication Data:

Kernicki, Jeanette.
  Electrocardiography for nurses.
  (A Wiley medical publication)
  Includes index.
  1. Electrocardiography. 2. Cardiovascular disease
nursing. I. Weiler, Kathi M., joint author. II. Title.
[DNLM: 1. Electrocardiography—Nursing texts. WY 152.5
K39e]
RC683.5.E5K47   616.1'207547'024613   80–28705
ISBN 0–471–05752–5

Printed in the United States of America

10 9 8 7 6 5 4 3 2 1

Preface

The role of the cardiovascular nurse continues to expand, and this fact has necessitated the augmentation of the nurse's basic knowledge and skill as related to electrocardiographic changes as seen on the oscilloscope and/or in the bedside detection of abnormal cardiac rhythms. Few advanced electrocardiographic books have been written with the nurse in mind. Those that are available are nonetheless devoid of concepts of the electrophysiologic-clinical relationship as reflected in rhythm and conduction disturbances.

Heretofore, knowledge of the identification of premature ectopic beats and their implication in tachyarrhythmias and bradyarrhythmias was basic to the course of study for one working with the acutely ill cardiac patient. Today, as part of nursing knowledge, we are expected to identify acute shifts in the heart's electrical axis and to recognize that extreme leftward axis deviation may indicate the presence of an anterior hemiblock, which can lead to complete heart block. In other words, it no longer suffices for nurses to have memorized certain normal and abnormal electrocardiographic patterns; they must be alert to the inherent consequences of these typical patterns. The nurse must also have a basic understanding of the hemodynamic changes produced by the rhythm and conduction problems as well as of the pathogenesis of such disturbances. This knowledge enables the nurse to have a more comprehensive understanding of what may be happening to the patient as well as of the rationale for the therapeutic plan of care.

For this reason, we have attempted to provide a nursing resource that can serve as a framework of reference for the graduate nurse (who has a basic understanding of electrophysiology), the coronary care nurse, the cardiovascular clinical specialist, and the nurse educator. The intent of this text is to provide a comprehensive overview that correlates aspects of disturbances of cardiac rate, rhythm, and conduction.

This correlative approach is applied to the chapter on the anatomy and physiology of the heart. The text also identifies the various mechanisms that act sequentially to effect ventricular depolarization and subsequent contraction.

The following questions are repeatedly addressed throughout:

1. What precipitated the rhythm/conduction disturbance?
2. How will the disturbance affect the hemodynamic aspect of the patient's clinical picture?
3. How can progressive complications be anticipated and prevented?
4. At what level of cardiac physiology is therapy directed?

Incorporated throughout the text are illustrations that comprehensively delineate sequential events associated with rhythm disturbances and/or myocardial pathology. In addition, examples of the conventional 12-lead electrocardiogram, modified chest leads, and orthogonal leads afford the nurse the advantage of considering the patterns of myocardial hypertrophy, infarction, and fascicular blocks. Cardiotonic drugs and their modes of action—a subject that has been glossed over too often—are also considered.

A set of flash cards (available from the authors upon request) complement the chapter discussions. These cards facilitate a review of the identification of atrial and ventricular rates, intervals, predominant rhythms, electrical axes, and the prodromal manifestations of cardiac disturbances.

An endeavor such as this would not be possible without the assistance and encouragement of many people. The authors are indebted to the following people, who have either critically reviewed parts of the manuscript, offered suggestions, and/or assisted in the preparation of the manuscript: Dr. James K. Alexander, Miss Betty Arnce, R.N., Mrs. Susan Davis, R.N., Mrs. Connie Doyle, Miss Doris Dumas, Dr. Mark Entman, Dr. Robert C. Fulweber, Dr. William R. Gaston, Dr. John Lewis, Mrs. Patricia Lewis, R.N., Miss Evelyn Luce, R.N., Dr. Lair Ribeiro, Dr. Frank Rickman, Dr. Jack Titus, and Miss Patricia Verbitsky, R.N.

Thanks are also due to the many authors and publishers who have granted us permission to use illustrations and tables from their work.

The authors are also grateful to Mr. Jim Simpson and Mrs. Shirley Jones, staff members of John Wiley & Sons.

J.G.K.
K.M.W.

Contents

Electrocardiography for Nurses

Physiological Correlates

1
Basic Anatomy and Physiology of the Heart

BLOOD SUPPLY TO THE HEART

For the heart to perform at its best in its role as a muscular pump, thus ensuring the effectiveness of various cellular activities, the myocardium must receive an uninterrupted supply of nutrients, such as glucose, pyruvic acid, and lactic acid, as well as oxygen (1). Such essential substrates and oxygen are carried in the bloodstream and are delivered to cardiac muscle tissue by the coronary circulatory system. In an average adult, during the basal state, the amount of blood necessary to perfuse the left ventricle (the systemic pump) is from 105 to 135 ml/min. The oxygen consumption of that same chamber per minute is 1 ml of oxygen for each gram of myocardial tissue (2). A direct relationship exists between the level of myocardial oxygen consumption and the amount of work required to meet bodily needs.

CORONARY CIRCULATION

The major branches of the coronary circulatory system supplying the myocardium originate within the coronary cusps of the aortic valve. The major coronary vessels divide and subdivide in an arborization pattern, surrounding and penetrating the wall of the heart like a crown (Figs. 1-1 and 1-2).

The right main coronary artery lies in the atrioventricular groove extending toward the extreme right margin of the heart, passes posteriorly as the posterior descending branch, and then trends in a medial direction. In most persons branches from the posterior descending coronary artery extend beyond the crux of the heart (an anatomical landmark designating the posterior junction of the atria and ventricles). The predominance of coronary circulation is thus determined by whichever artery crosses the crux of the heart. The blood supply to the anterior portion of the right atrium and ventricle is provided by means of the marginal branch, while the posterior right and left ventricular chambers are served by the posterior descending branch of the right coronary artery. The right coronary is likewise the principal source of blood supply for the sinoatrial (SA) node in 55% of the population and for the atrioventricular (AV) node in 92% (3, 4) (see p. 4).

The left main coronary artery emerges as a short trunk before bifurcating and trifurcating. Bifurcation results in a left anterior descending branch and a circumflex branch directed laterally along the atrioventricular sulcus and from there posteriorly. The lateral wall of the left ventricle derives its nourishment by way of the left circumflex coronary artery. In a number of persons it is a branch of the circumflex, rather than a branch of

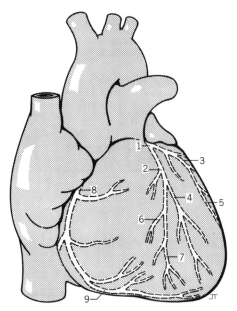

Figure 1-1. Coronary artery branches as seen on the anterior view of the heart. (*1*) Left main; (*2*) anterior descending (proximal); (*3*) circumflex; (*4*) diagonal; (*5*) left marginal; (*6*) septal; (*7*) anterior descending (distal); (*8*) right main; (*9*) right marginal.

the right coronary artery, that serves the sinoatrial node. The anterior descending branch of the left coronary artery is the parent artery of septal and diagonal branches that supply the interventricular septum, the diaphragmatic portions of the right and left ventricular apices, and the ventricular portions of the specialized conducting pathways (see the section on the conduction system in this chapter).

A vast network of intercommunicating arteries between the subendocardial layer of the heart and the extramural large vessels provides diffuse anastomoses and a secondary route

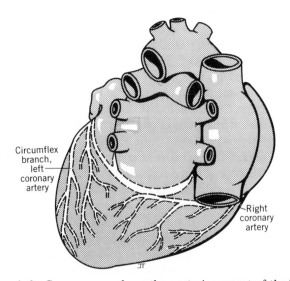

Figure 1-2. Coronary vessels on the posterior aspect of the heart.

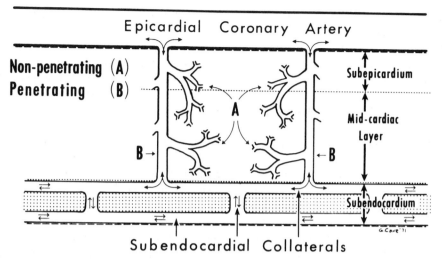

Figure 1-3. Normal myocardial circulation. (*a*) Nonpenetrating coronary arteries. (*b*) Penetrating coronary arteries. Arrows demonstrate real and potential collateral flow. (Reproduced with permission from Holsinger JW Jr, Eliot RS: The potential role of the subendocardium in the pathogenesis of myocardial infarction. *Heart Lung* 1:356-361, 1972.)

of blood flow through collateral vessels (5, 6) (Fig. 1-3). Coronary artery circulation thus cannot be considered an endarterial system. Blockage of an epicardial vessel does not necessarily preclude a transmural infarction, since collateral vessels can bypass the area of obstruction (Fig. 1-4).

Venous drainage of the right atrium and ventricle is primarily accomplished through the thebesian veins. Likewise, right ventricular myocardial drainage is maintained through the

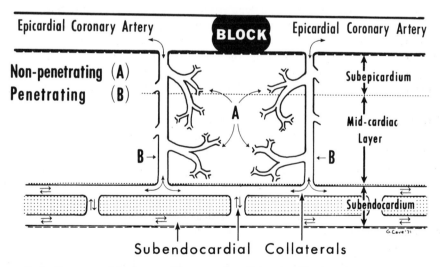

Figure 1-4. Coronary blockage with normal collaterals. Block represents new or old blockage of major epicardial coronary artery with adequate subendocardial collaterals preventing infarction. For (*a*), (*b*), and arrows, see Figure 1-3. (Reproduced with permission from Holsinger JW Jr, Eliot RS: The potential role of the pathogenesis of myocardial infarction. *Heart Lung* 1:356-361, 1972.)

anterior cardiac veins. The coronary sinus and its tributaries receive blood from the left ventricular myocardium (7).

Blood flow through the coronary vessels is cyclic. Blood flows to the left ventricle primarily during diastole since the mechanical activity associated with contraction of the cardiac muscle impedes the filling of the coronary artery. According to Resenekov (9), coronary blood flow is influenced by several factors, among the most common of which are diastolic filling time, diastolic pressure, wall tension, duration of systole, and transmural pressure. Also to be considered is the innervation of the coronary vasculature. Most of the nerve fibers located primarily in the vessels permeating the ventricles are those of the sympathetic division of the autonomic nervous system. The neurohumoral substances released upon stimulation of the fiber are epinephrine and norepinephine. These compounds can evoke either a constrictive or a dilating effect upon the vasculature, depending upon the receptor site (alpha-beta) of the neurohumoral substance (9). See the section on nervous innervation in this chapter.

Disturbances in any of the above-mentioned physical conditions, as well as those affecting the radius of the coronary vessel, can progressively lead to ischemia and/or infarction of the myocardial wall (see Chap. 10).

THE CONDUCTION SYSTEM

There is generally an orderly sequence of events occurring in the heart that ultimately leads to fiber excitation and subsequent ejection of ventricular content. The physiological properties of the heart that make this possible are automaticity, irritability (excitation), and conductivity. As a displacement pump, the heart relies upon the synchronization of muscle response with impulse formation and transmission.

Specialized cardiac muscle cells and pathways make up the conduction system (Fig. 1-5). Some cardiac cells have the potential for pacemaking, others for impulse transmission. The process of spontaneous depolarization characterizes impulse-generating cells (see the section on transmembrane action potential in Chap. 2). Although the heart is influenced by the autonomic nervous system, the origin of the cardiac impulse is myogenic. That is to say, the heart has the potential to initiate within itself the impulse. Corday and Irving (10) attribute the myogenicity of cardiac tissue to the response of the cell membrane to "rhythmic build-up and breakdown of electrical potential." See page 22 for a discussion of the action potential of cardiac tissue.

The sinoatrial (sinus) node (Keith-Flack node) with the fastest inherent rate (60 to 100 beats per minute) is normally the pacemaker of the heart throughout life. The node is elliptical and is situated in the posterior aspect of the right atrium at the junction of the superior vena cava and the body of the right atrium. The cephalad portion of the sinus node is subepicardial, whereas the caudal portion is more subendocardial (11). Because of its anatomic location, the sinoatrial node is subject to altered function resulting from disease, such as pericarditis, and/or from vascular lesions. Within the central area of the sinus node are numerous P or stellate cells. It has been postulated that the cardiac impulse originates within these cells. Blood is supplied to the sinoatrial node by means of the right coronary artery division in approximately 55% of the the population. In the remaining 45%, blood is supplied to the sinus node by way of a branch of the left circumflex artery (12).

An indistinct and poorly formed border of connective tissue appears to surround the

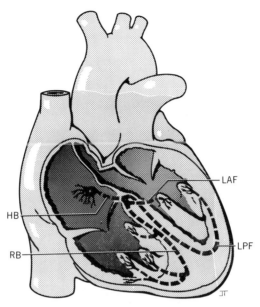

Figure 1-5. Infrajunctional conduction system. LAF: left anterior fascicle. LPF: left posterior fascicle. HB: His bundle, RB: right bundle.

sinoatrial node. This tissue is thought to function as a diffusion barrier. The significance of such a potential barrier is that it may protect the node from large changes in the composition of electrolytes such as the concentration of potassium, which among other substances is conveyed to the region of the sinus node by blood (see Chap. 2). According to Braunwald (13), nerve endings are abundant in the sinoatrial node. They originate principally from the vagus nerve as well as the three cervical ganglia (Fig. 1-6). The rate of impulse formation is modified by the influence of the nerve endings.

Stimulation of vagal fibers results in depression of sinus node discharge and, additionally, slowing of conduction through the atrioventricular node. The sympathetic stimulation and subsequent release of the neurohumoral substance norepinephrine accelerates sinoatrial node activity. The wave of excitation emerging from the sinoatrial tissue travels in orderly sequence possibly through preferential conduction pathways (Fig. 1-7). The apparent anterior internodal tract subdivides as it extends leftward and sends one branch (Bachmann's bundle) toward the left atrium and the other downward to the atrioventricular junction. The middle tract (Wenckebach's bundle) descends from the posterior aspect of the sinoatrial node to the atrioventricular node. A posterior tract (Thorel's bundle) leaves the lower border of the sinus node and merges with the other tracts in the area of the atrioventricular node (14, 15, 16). The transmission of the impulse formed in the sinus node depolarizes the atria (13). This activity is reflected electrocardiographically by the P wave. According to Wantanabe and Dreifus (12), conduction velocity is much higher in the preferential conduction tracts than in the remaining atrial musculature. Another feature of the apparent internodal, interatrial tracts is that of a lesser response to elevated concentrations of the electrolyte potassium as well as to antiarrhythmic drugs. Cholinergic nerve fibers are distributed widely in the area of the three bundle tracts.

After the cardiac impulse traverses the atria and reaches the atrioventricular junction, there is a slight delay of approximately 0.05 second in the transmission of the impulse to

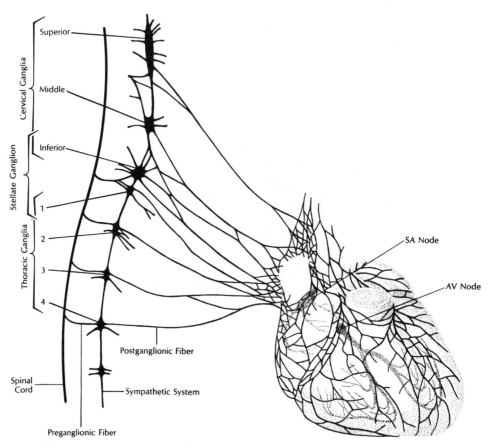

Figure 1-6. Sympathetic pathways to and in the heart. (By B Tagawa from Braunwald E, The autonomic nervous system in heart failure, in Braunwald E [ed]: *The Myocardium: Failure and Infarction.* New York, HP Publishing Co Inc, 1974. Reproduced with permission.)

the ventricles. This electrophysiological delay is associated with the mechanical advantage by which the atria complete ejection of blood before initiation of ventricular contraction, thus providing for optimal preload (increase in fiber length before ventricular contraction) (17). The delay appears to be in, or just distal to, the atrioventricular node. The atrioventricular node (node of Tawara) is located on the floor of the right atrium anterior to the coronary sinus and near the level where the septal leaflet of the tricuspid valve inserts into the annulus (17). The area surrounding the atrioventricular node is made up of two different types of tissue fiber, which may have electrophysiological implication. According to Pick and Langendorf (18) the atrioventricular node (N fibers) is void of automaticity. Its chief role is the conveyance of impulses normal and abnormal to the ventricles. The node, as was mentioned previously, offers protection to the ventricles in physiologically blocking some of the impulses conveyed to it by the sinus node or atrial tissue. It serves, so to speak, as a triage system safeguarding the ventricles. The AN fibers (lead fibers to the node) and the NH fibers (fibers adjacent to the common bundle of His), have automaticity and pacemaker potential. The AN and NH fibers are likewise

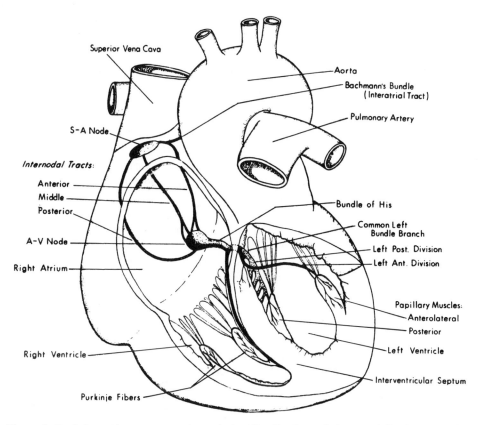

Superior Vena Cava

Aorta

Bachmann's Bundle
(Interatrial Tract)

Pulmonary Artery

S-A Node

Internodal Tracts:

Anterior

Middle

Posterior

A-V Node

Right Atrium

Bundle of His

Common Left
Bundle Branch

Left Post. Division

Left Ant. Division

Papillary Muscles:

Anterolateral

Posterior

Left Ventricle

Right Ventricle

Interventricular Septum

Purkinje Fibers

Figure 1-7. Schematic representation of the distribution of the specialized conductive tissues in the atria and ventricles, showing the impulse-forming and conducting system of the heart. The cardiac impulse normally originates in the pacemaking cells in the sinus node, located at the junction of the superior vena cava and the right atrium. Note the three specialized pathways (anterior, middle, and posterior internodal tracts) between the SA and AV nodes. Bachmann's bundle (interatrial tract) branches off the anterior internodal tract leading to the left atrium. The impulse passes from the SA node in an orderly manner through the specialized conducting tracts in the atria to activate first the right atrium and then the left atrium. The passage of the impulse is delayed at the AV node before continuing into the bundle of His, the right bundle branch, the common left bundle branch, the anterior and posterior divisions of the left bundle branch, and the Purkinje network. The right bundle branch runs along the right side of the interventricular septum to the apex of the right ventricle before it radiates significant branches. The left common bundle crosses to the left side of th septum and almost immediately divides into the anterior division (which is long and thin and descends under the aortic valve in the outflow tract to the anterolateral papillary muscle) and the posterior division (which is short and wide and passes to the posterior papillary muscle lying in the inflow tract). (Reproduced with permission from Lipman BS, Massie E, Kleiger RE: *Clinical Scalar Electrocardiography*, 6th edition. Copyright © 1972 by Year Book Medical Publishers, Inc., Chicago.)

protective. In the event that sinus impulse formation and/or conduction are impaired, the fibers will pace the ventricles at a rate of 40 to 60 beats per minute. As stated by Pick and Langendorf (18), the AV junction serves a dual purpose. According to Kennel and Titus (19), the principal source of blood supply to the atrioventricular node (junction) in many instances is the vessel that originates from the branch of the right coronary artery that tends to form a U configuration at the crux of the heart. The vessel likewise communicates with branches of the atrial arteries, subendocardial vessels of the ventricular septum, and septal branches of the anterior and posterior descending arteries.

Autonomic ganglia (predominantely cholinergic) are dispersed widely in the posterior region of the atrioventricular node (junction). These are subject to ischemic changes, particularly in association with an inferior myocardial infarction. Thus, the nausea, vomiting, diaphoretic episodes, and bradycardic rates frequently accompanying an acute inferior myocardial infarction are related to the excessive discharge of vagal fibers (4). In addition, the release of norepinephrine by adrenergic fibers acting on the AV node results in an increase in conduction velocity. Cells within the atrioventricular junction are capable of pacemaking and can either usurp the power of the normal pacemaker—the sinus node—or can become the pacemaker by default. The inherent rate of junctional tissue is within the range of 50 to 60 beats per minute.

Occasionally the cardiac impulse bypasses the atrioventricular junction and travels from the atria directly to the ventricles (Fig. 1-8). Thus, preexcitation of the ventricles occurs.

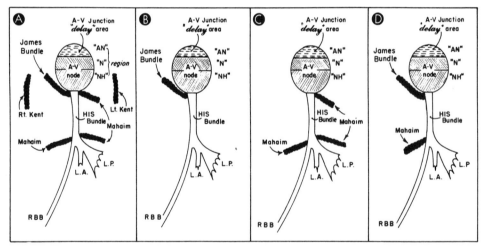

Figure 1-8. Theoretical mechanisms of conduction in the Wolff-Parkinson-White syndrome. Panel A shows normal conduction pathways as well as the anomalous bundles of Kent and Mahaim and the James fiber. Panel B shows conduction through the James fiber, producing a short PR interval and a narrow QRS complex (normal AV "delay" area bypassed). Panel C shows Mahaim bundle preexcitation with normal PR interval (normal AV node "delay") and a wide QRS with delta wave. Panel D shows a combinatin of James fiber and Mahaim bundle conduction with a short PR interval, delta wave, and a wide QRS (resembles Kent bundle preexcitation in surface electrocardiogram). (Reproduced with permission from Lipman BS, Massie E, Kleiger RE: *Clinical Scalar Electrocardiography,* 6th edition. Copyright © 1972 by Year Book Medical Publishers, Inc., Chicago.)

The Wolff-Parkinson-White syndrome is an example of such preexcitation of the ventricles (see Chap. 7).

After the delay at the atrioventricular junction, the electrical impulse proceeds rapidly down the His bundle (an extension of the lower end of the junctional tissue). Anatomically the upper segment of the His bundle lies within the vicinity of the noncoronary cusp of the aortic valve and the mitral valve ring. This then predisposes the bundle of His and its branches to inflammation and/or deposits of calcific debris, which can interfere with impulse conduction. According to Titus (20), the bundle of His is thought to extend from the terminal portion of the AV node to the area where the common bundle divides into a left and a right segment or bundle branches. In the region of the His bundle penetration of the atrioventricular junction, the left bundle branch further divides into a fascicular arrangement, the anterior superior and posterior inferior fascicles (20, 21) (see Fig. 1-5). The bundle of His is well perfused owing to the rich network of interconnecting vessels branching from the atrioventricular nodal vessel of the right coronary artery as well as the anterior descending branch of the left coronary artery. The distal right bundle branch shares its blood supply with the anterior fascicle of the left bundle branch by way of the anterior descending coronary artery. The upper segment of the right bundle likewise is perfused by branches of the right coronary artery. The posterior division of the left bundle branch has a dual blood supply, perfusion by a branch of the right coronary artery as well as by the anterior descent of the left coronary artery. The right bundle branch and the divisions of the left bundle branch terminate in an arborization network known as the Purkinje system of the ventricles. According to Braunwald (13) there is now increasing evidence that parasympathetic fibers extend beyond the region of the atrioventricular node. Heretofore, literature on the innervation of the heart limited the distribution of fibers of the parasympathetic division to the supraventricular region of the conduction system.

NERVOUS INNERVATION

The heart has primarily four properties: conductivity, excitability, contractility, and automaticity (rhythmicity) (22). All myocardial cells have the property of conductivity, which is the ability to transmit an impulse to surrounding tissues (23) and thus propagate the impulse throughout the entire myocardium. The heart will respond to external stimulation (electrical, chemical, and mechanical) as well as generate its own impulses in a rhythmic fashion. This is the property of excitability. The response is mechanical and is known as contractility (pumping of blood). Certain cardiac cells have the unique ability to initiate their own impulse, which provides automaticity; and therefore the heart does not depend upon extrinsic factors to function. However, the heart is subjected to nervous as well as humoral influences, which at times may be profound.

The autonomic nervous system with its two main subdivisions, the sympathetic and parasympathetic systems, has been found to influence heart rate (chronotropic effect) and the strength of myocardial contraction (inotropic effect) (24). Various cardiotonic agents employed produce their effects by the alteration of one or all of these influences. The sympathetic as well as the parasympathetic systems have certain features characteristic to both: (1) both have afferent fibers which transmit the impulse to the central nervous system (CNS), (2) both have efferent fibers which transmit the impulse away

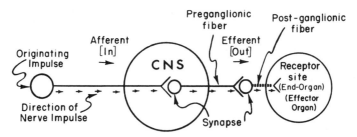

Figure 1-9. Schematic representation of the flow of a nerve impulse through afferent and efferent fibers and the involved synapses. (Reproduced with permission from White BB: *Therapy in Acute Coronary Care.* Copyright © 1971 by Year Book Medical Publishers, Inc., Chicago.)

from the CNS to the effector organ and, (*3*) both have preganglionic and postganglionic fibers (which comprise the efferent fiber) (22) (Fig. 1-9).

The nerve impulse in both sympathetic and parasympathetic systems is transmitted by a chemically mediated neurotransmitter which is then destroyed by an enzyme (22). The preganglionic neuron of the sympathetic and parasympathetic divisions as well as the postganglionic neuron of the parasympathetic division utilize acetylcholine as their neurotransmitter and thus are called cholinergic fibers. The postganglionic neuron of the sympathetic system utilizes norepinephrine as its neurotransmitter and is termed an adrenergic fiber (25).

Sympathetic preganglion fibers originate in the first four to five thoracic segments of the spinal cord (25) and extend to the sympathetic chains. The cardiac sympathetic nerves arise from the corresponding upper thoracic sympathetic ganglion and innervate all levels of the heart (26). Sympathetic fibers have their termination points in the following areas of the heart: SA node, atria, AV nodal region, bundle of His, and the ventricles. The atria have a higher concentration of sympathetic fibers than the ventricles, while the SA node contains the most dense concentration (27) (Fig. 1-10). The sympathetic nerve impulse is transmitted to the heart via the neurotransmitter norepinephrine (28). Norepinephrine is destroyed by two enzymes: (*1*) monamine oxidase and (*2*) catechol-0-methyl-transferase (1) (Fig. 1-11). Since the heart is innervated by the sympathetic system, it can easily extract norepinephrine from the circulatory system; however, this is not its only source. Recently it has been experimentally demonstrated that the heart as well as its sympathetic nerve endings can synthesize norepinephrine from its precursor amino acid, tyrosine (29).

The sympathetic system is further divided into two types of receptors, alpha and beta, as originally defined by Ahlquist in 1948 (30). Both receptors are stimulated by norepinephrine as the neurotransmitter and by epinephrine and norepinephrine, which are released from the adrenal medulla into the bloodstream upon stimulation of the sympathetic systemic (22) (Table 1-1). The beta receptors can be further divided into two groups, beta[1] and beta[2] (31). The beta[1] receptors are found primarily in the heart and produce excitatory responses when stimulated. Inhibitory responses, for example, relaxation of bronchial muscles and decreased motility of the stomach and intestines, are produced from the stimulation of beta[2] receptors (28).

Sympathetic stimulation affects the properties of conductivity, contractility, and

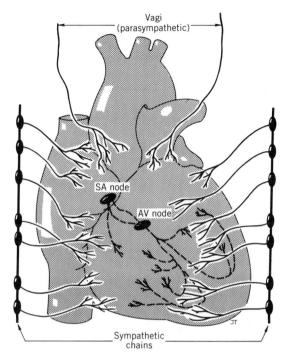

Figure 1-10. Sympathetic nerves innervate all areas of the heart while parasympathetic nerves have little if any influence in the ventricle. (Adapted with permission from Braunwald E. The autonomic nervous system in heart failure, by B. Tagawa in Braunwald E [ed] : *The Myocardium, Failure and Infarction.* New York, HP Publishing Co., Inc., 1974.)

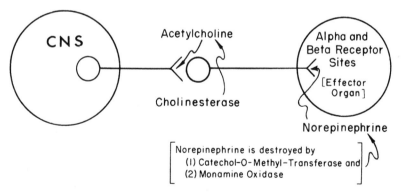

Figure 1-11. Chemical mediation of a nerve impulse in the sympathetic division of the autonomic nervous system. (Reproduced with permission from White BB: *Therapy in Acute Coronary Care.* Copyright © 1971 by Year Book Medical Publishers, Inc., Chicago.)

Table 1-1. Types of Receptors Present in Various Organs and Their Response Elicited with Sympathetic Stimulation

Effector Organ	Receptor Type	Stimulation Response
Heart	Beta$_1$	See Table 1-2
Lung (bronchial muscle)	Beta$_2$	Bronchodilatation
Coronary arteries	Alpha and Beta$_1$	Constriction and dilatation
Pulmonary arteries	Alpha	Constriction
Cerebral arteries	Alpha	Slight constriction
Skin and mucosal arteries	Alpha	Constriction
Renal arteries	Alpha and Beta$_2$	Constriction and dilatation
Skeletal muscle	Beta$_2$	Dilatation (overall effect)
Abdominal viscera	Alpha	Constriction
Liver	Beta$_2$	Glycogenolysis

Source: Adapted with permission from White, BB: *Therapy in Acute Coronary Care* (Chicago Year Book Medical Pub Inc, 1971).

automaticity (Table 1-2). When stimulated, the heart responds by increasing its sinus rate (+ chronotropic effect) as well as the force of myocardial contraction (+ inotropic effect), which produces a net increase in the cardiac output. Although sympathetic stimulation may improve the overall performance of the heart, it may lower the threshold for ventricular fibrillation (26). The lowest current intensity that is delivered during the vulnerable period (which correlates roughly with the T wave on the electrocardiogram) and that results in ventricular fibrillation is defined as the *ventricular fibrillation threshold.* Clinically, a lower ventricular fibrillation threshold may manifest itself in states of myocardial ischemia, premature ventricular contractions (PVCs), and brady-cardia (26).

Parasympathetic innervation is derived from the vagus nerves, which have their origin in the medulla oblongata. The vagus nerves terminate in the SA node, atria, and AV node (32) (Fig. 1-12). In the past, it was generally agreed that a vagal effect did not extend into the His bundle, the bundle branches, and the ventricular myocardium. However, today there is much opposition to this attitude (25, 32, 29). The right vagus nerve pre-dominantly affects the SA node, whereas the left vagus had its greatest influence on the AV node (23). The parasympathetic impulse is transmitted to the heart via the neuro-transmitter acetylcholine, which is destroyed by the enzyme cholinesterase (Fig. 1-12). The net effects of vagal stimulation are seen in Table 1-3.

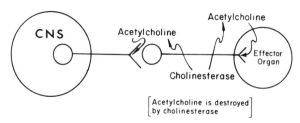

Figure 1-12. Chemical mediation of a nerve impulse in the parasympathetic division of the autonomic nervous system. (Reproduced with permission from White, BB: *Therapy in Acute Coronary Care.* Chicago Year Book Medical Pub Inc, 1971.)

Table 1-2. Effects of Alpha and Beta Adrenergic Stimulation

Effector Organ	Receptor Type	Stimulation Response	Electrophysiological	Clinical
Heart SA node	Beta₁	Increased heart rate (positive chronotropic effect)	Increases the slope of phase 4 depolarization	Sinus tachycardia (increased cardiac output and blood pressure)
AV node	Beta₁	Increased conduction velocity; decreased refractory period	Increases rate of rise of phase 0 and increases overshoot phase	Shortens PR interval (ECG) Shortens AH interval (His bundle electrogram)
Atrial myocardium	Beta₁	Small increase in contractile strength (positive inotropic effect)		Increase atrial contribution to ventricular filling (increased cardiac output)
Atrial specialized conducting fibers[a]	Beta₁	Increased atrial rate, may produce slight increase in conduction velocity	May produce phase 4 spontaneous depolarization; may increase action potential amplitude	Premature atrial beats and atrial arrhythmias
Ventricular myocardium	Beta₁	Slight increase in contractile strength (positive inotropic effect)		Slight increase in cardiac output
Ventricular specialized conducting fibers[a]	Beta₁	Increased ventricular rate	Increases the slope of phase 4 depolarization and shortens duration of action potential	Ventricular arrhythmias

Sources:
1. White BB: *Therapy in Acute Coronary Care.* Chicago, Year Book Medical Pub Inc, 1971, p 11.
2. Anderson M, del Castillo J: Cardiac innervation and synaptic transmission in heart, in De Mello WC (ed): *Electrical Phenomena in the Heart.* New York, Academic Press, 1972, p 237.
3. Reder RF, Rosen MR: The role of the sympathetic nervous system in sudden cardiac death. *Drug Therapy* 8:41, 1978.
4. Mary-Rabine L, Hordof AJ et al: Alpha and beta effects on human atrial specialized conducting fibers. *Circulation* 57:84, 1978.
5. Reuter H: Localization of beta-adrenergic receptors and effects of noradrenaline and cyclic nucleotides on action potentials, ionic currents and tension in mammalian cardiac muscle. *J Physiol* 242:429, 1974.

[a]Recent evidence has shown that there may be alpha-adrenergic effects on atrial and ventricular specialized conducting fibers in the presence of low concentrations of catecholamines (12).

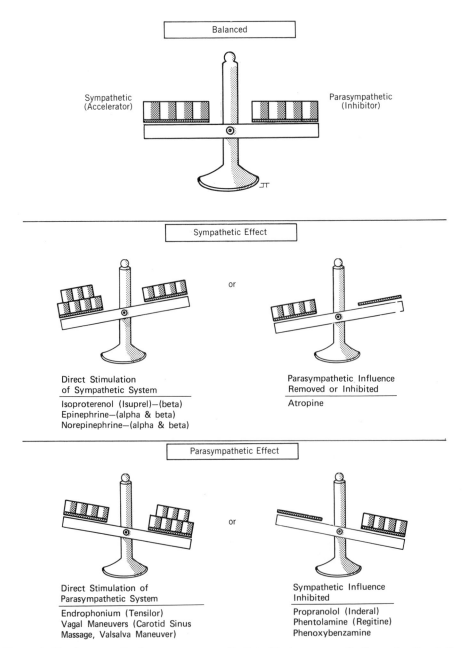

Figure 1-13. A sympathetic or parasympathetic effect may result through stimulation or inhibition of one system. Various drugs used produce their effects in this manner.

The cardiovascular system is under the influence of both sympathetic and parasympathetic divisions. These two systems are comparable to a scale in perfect balance (Fig. 1-13). A sympathetic effect results if (*1*) that system is stimulated or (*2*) the parasympathetic system is inhibited (Fig. 1-13). If these conditions are the opposite, a parasympathetic effect results (Fig. 1-13).

Table 1-3. Parasympathetic (Vagal) Stimulation

Location	Response
SA node	Decreases phase 4 spontaneous depolarization, producing sinus brady-cardia (may evoke sinus arrest) (negative chronotropic effect)
Atria	Decreases atrial contractility (negative inotropic effect); decreased excit-ability; enhances conduction velocity and may produce atrial fibrilla-tion/flutter
AV node	Decreases conduction velocity (may produce varying degrees of block)
Ventricles	No effect on contractility or intraventricular conduction

CARDIAC CYCLE

The cardiac cycle is the sequence of mechanical events required to pump blood to all parts of the body. A spontaneous action potential (normally originating from the SA node) precedes each cardiac cycle, which consists of two phases: diastole, a time of fill-ing and relaxation of the chambers, and systole, a time of contraction and emptying of the chambers (35).

Atrial filling (diastole) normally originates continually from the great veins, the pul-monary veins to the left atrium, and the vena cava to the right atrium. The AV valves (atrioventricular) are closed because the volume of blood as well as pressure in the ventri-cles exceeds that of the atria. Cardiac valves are passive and open or close only in response to pressure differences on their upper and lower surfaces (35). Gradually the atrial chambers are filled to a point at which the pressure in them exceeds that in the ventri-cles, forcing the AV valves open. This is then followed by atrial contraction (systole) (Fig. 1-14). Approximately 70% of a ventricular filling occurs passively, the remainder of

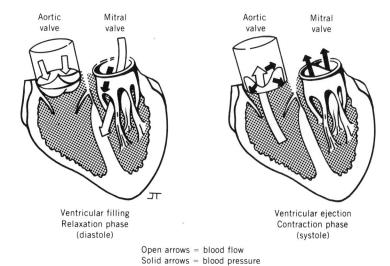

Aortic valve Mitral valve   Aortic valve Mitral valve

Ventricular filling
Relaxation phase
(diastole)

Ventricular ejection
Contraction phase
(systole)

Open arrows = blood flow
Solid arrows = blood pressure

Figure 1-14. Cardiac valves have no action of their own and are opened and closed as a result of pressure differences on their surfaces. (Reproduced with permission from Phillips RE, Feeney MK: *The Cardiac Rhythms: A Systematic Approach to Interpreta-tion.* Copyright © 1973. W. B. Saunders Co, Philadelphia.)

blood coming from atrial contraction (the atrial kick). On the electrocardiogram atrial contraction occurs after the P wave (36). A slight regurgitation of blood into the veins occurs with atrial systole.

Ventricular systole consists of two phases: (*1*) isometric contraction and (*2*) ejection. During *isometric contraction* the semilunar as well as the AV valves are closed. The intraventricular pressure is rising and the muscle tension is increasing, but there is no shortening of the muscle fibers. There is a small rise in atrial pressure during this phase because of the bulging of the AV valves into the atria (37) (Fig. 1-15).

The peak of the R wave on the electrocardiogram corresponds with the isometric contraction phase. The second phase of ventricular systole, the *ejection phase,* begins when left ventricular pressure exceeds the diastolic pressure in the aorta (80 mmHg) and the right ventricular pressure exceeds the pulmonary artery diastolic pressure (8–10 mmHg) (36). The semilunar valves are forced open, and this phase begins after the S wave and lasts until the downslope of the T wave on the electrocardiogram (Fig. 1-16).

Ventricular diastole consists of three phases: *protodiastole, isometric relaxation,* and *ventricular filling.* During protodiastole the semilunar valves close because the momentum of the ejected blood is overcome. Isometric relaxation begins with the closing of the semilunar valves and ends with the opening of the AV valves. During this phase the ventricular pressures rapidly fall and the ventricular muscle relaxes. Both the semilunar and AV valves are closed. The downslope of the T wave on the electrocardiogram corresponds with this phase. The ventricular filling phase of ventricular diastole consists of two parts: *rapid filling* and *diastasis* (retarded flow). When the atrial pressure exceeds that of the ventricular chambers, the AV valves are forced open and the ventricles fill rapidly. A period of slower filling, or diastasis, occurs after rapid filling and lasts until atrial contraction and a new cardiac cycle begins (37).

One complete cardiac cycle is approximately 0.80 second in duration at a heart rate of 75 beats per minute. Diastole contributes 0.53 second to this total, whereas the systolic component is only 0.27 second. When the heart rate increases, both systole and diastole

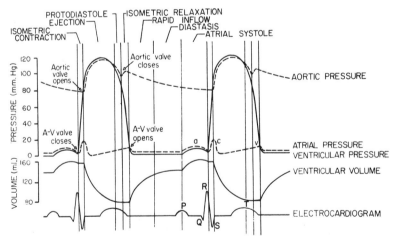

Figure 1-15. The events of the cardiac cycle showing changes in left atrial pressure, left ventricular pressure, aortic pressure, ventricular volume, and the electrocardiogram. (Reproduced with permission from Guyton AC: *Basic Human Physiology: Normal Function and Mechanisms of Disease.* Copyright © 1971, W. B. Saunders Co., Philadelphia.)

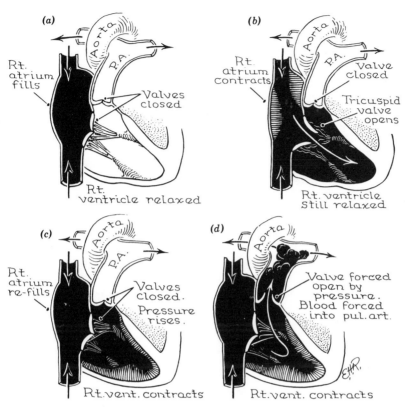

Figure 1-16. Cardiac cycle. (*a*) Period of isometric relaxation, (*b*) of rapid filling, (*c*) and (*d*) of isometric contraction. Only the right side of the heart is shown, identical events are occurring simultaneously on the left side. (Reprinted by permission of G. P. Putnam's Sons from *Basic Anatomy and Physiology* by Norman Burke Taylor, MD, and Margaret G. McPhedron, RN. Copyright © 1965 by G. P. Putnam's Sons and Macmillan Company of Canada, Ltd.)

are shortened, although diastole is shortened to a much greater degree. This feature becomes important in rapid heart rates since ventricular filling occurs primarily in diastole. Cardiac output may fall with inadequate ventricular filling when the heart rate becomes quite rapid (180 beats per minute and faster) (36). Clinically, however, one may see a decrease in cardiac output with heart rates much less than 180 beats per minute. Patients with severe heart disease (cardiomyopathy, myocardial infarction, or congestive heart failure) are often unable to tolerate a heart rate of approximately 140 to 150 beats per minute or greater for any length of time.

REVIEW QUESTIONS

1. Why are coronary arteries not considered end arteries?

2. What determines the predominance of coronary circulation?

3. What effect does mechanical contraction of the ventricle have upon coronary circulation?

4. Does the location of the sinoatrial node predispose it to injury and/or inflammation?

5. Describe the blood supply to the fascicles of the left bundle branch.

6. Correlate the phases of the cardiac cycle with the P wave, QRS complex, and T wave on the electrocardiogram.

7. In what phase of the cardiac cycle do the coronary arteries receive their blood flow?

8. Where are the beta[1] receptors located?

9. A patient with emphysema develops a tachyarrhythmia and is treated with propranolol. Shortly after the propranolol is given, bronchospasm develops. What mechanism is responsible for this bronchospasm?

REFERENCES

1. Crouch JE, McClintic JR: *Human Anatomy and Physiology.* New York, John Wiley & Sons Inc, 1971, p 319.

2. Gorlin R: Physiology of the coronary circulation, in Hurst J, Logue R (eds): *The Heart Arteries and Veins,* ed 2. New York, McGraw-Hill Book Co, 1970, p 106.

3. Corday E, Irving DW: *Disturbances of Heart Rate, Rhythm and Conduction.* Philadelphia, WB Saunders Co, 1962, p 9.

4. James TN: Arrhythmias associated with myocardial infarction. *Heart Bull* 15:90, 1966.

5. Eliot RS, Holsinger JW: The potential role of the subendocardium in the pathogenesis of myocardial infarction. *Heart Lung* 1:357, 1972.

6. Ferrans VJ: The significance of coronary collateral circulation in myocardial oxygenation. *Practical Cardiol* 4:49, 1978.

7. James TN: Anatomy of the coronary arteries and veins, in Hurst J, Logue B (eds): *The Heart Arteries and Veins,* ed 2. New York, McGraw-Hill Book Co, 1970, p 134.

8. Resenekov, L: Myocardial perfusion, in Julian DG (ed): *Angina Pectoris.* Edinburgh, Churchill Livingston, 1977, p 136.

9. Guyton AC: *Textbook of Medical Physiology.* Philadelphia, WB Saunders Co, 1976, p 323.

10. Corday E, Irving DW: *Disturbances of Heart Rate, Rhythm and Conduction.* Philadelphia, WB Saunders Co, 1962, p 4.

11. Lev M: The Conduction System, in Gould SE (ed): *Pathology of the Heart and Blood Vessels.* Springfield, Chalres C Thomas Pub, 1968, p 181.

12. Wantanabe Y, Dreifus L: *Cardiac Arrhythmias: Electrophysiologic Basis for Clinical Interpretation.* New York, Grune & Stratton Inc, 1977, p 20.

13. Braunwald E: *The Myocardium: Failure and Infarction.* New York, HP Publishing Co Inc, 1974, p 60.

14. James TN, Sherf L: Specialized tissues and preferential conduction in the atrium of the heart. *Am J Cardiol* 23:416, 1971.

15. Kulbertus HE, Demoulin JC: The conduction system: anatomical and pathological aspects, in Krikler D, Goodwin J (eds): *Arrhythmias: The Modern Electrophysiological Approach.* Philadelphia, WB Saunders Co, 1975, p 17.

16. Bilitch MG: *Manual of Cardiac Arrhythmias.* Boston, Little Brown & Co, 1971, p 2.

17. Fozzaud HA: Cardiac contractility, in Vassale M (ed): *Cardiac Physiology for the Clinician.* New York, Academic Press Inc, 1976, p 72.

18. Pick A, Langendorf R: The dual function of the A-V junction. *Am Heart J* 88:790, 1974.

19. Kennel AJ, Titus JL: The vasculature of the human atrioventricular conduction system. *Mayo Clin Proc* 47:562, 1972.

20. Titus JL: Normal anatomy of the human cardiac conduction system. *Anesth Analg Curr Res* 52:508, 1973.

21. Hackel DB: Anatomy and pathology of the cardiac conducting system, in Edwards JE, Lev M, Abell MR (eds): *The Heart.* Baltimore, Williams & Wilkins Co, 1974, p 237.

22. White BB: *Therapy in Acute Coronary Care.* Chicago, Year Book Medical Pub Inc, 1971, p 11.

23. Schamroth L: *The Disorders of Cardiac Rhythm.* Oxford, Blackwell Scientific Publications, 1971, p 5.

24. Ganong WF: *Review of Medical Physiology,* ed 6, Los Altos, Calif, Lange Medical Publications, 1973, p 415.

25. Anderson M, del Castillo J: Cardiac innervation and synaptic transmission in heart, in De Mello WC (ed): *Electrical Phenomena in the Heart.* New York, Academic Press Inc, 1972, p 237.

26. Reder RF, Rosen MR: The role of the sympathetic nervous system in sudden cardiac death. *Drug Therapy* 8:41, 1978.

27. Randall WC, Armour JA: Gross and microscopic anatomy of the cardiac innervation, in Randall WC (ed): *Neural Regulation of the Heart.* New York, Oxford University Press Inc, 1977, p 26.

28. Koelle GB: Drugs acting at synaptic and neuroeffector junctional sites, in Goodman LS, Gilman A (ed): *The Pharmacological Basis of Therapeutics,* ed 6. New York, Macmillan Inc, 1975, p 406.

29. Braunwald E: The autonomic nervous system in heart failure, in Braunwald E (ed): *The Myocardium: Failure and Infarction.* New York, HP Publishing Co Inc, 1974, p 59.

30. Ahlquist RP: A study of the adrenotropic receptors. *Am J Physiol* 153:586, 1948.

31. Lands AM, Arnold A, et al: Differentiation of receptor systems activated by sympathomimetic amines. *Nature* 214:597, 1967.

32. Chung EK: *Electrocardiography: Practical Applications with Vectorial Principles,* Hagerstown, Md, Harper & Row Pub Inc, 1974, p 35.

33. Mary-Rabine L, Hordof AJ, et al: Alpha and beta effects on human atrial specialized conducting fibers. *Circulation* 57:84, 1978.

34. Reuter H: Localization of beta-adrenergic receptors and effects of noradrenlaine and cyclic nucleotides on action potentials, ionic currents and tension in mammalian cardiac muscle. *J Physiol* 242:429, 1974.

35. Guyton AC: *Basic Human Physiology: Normal Function and Mechanisms of Disease,* Philadelphia, WB Saunders Co, 1971, p 125.

36. Ganong WF: *Review of Medical Physiology,* ed 6. Los Altos, Calif, Lange Medical Publications, 1973, p 409.

37. Selkurt EE, Bullard RW: The heart as a pump. Mechanical correlates of cardiac activity, in Selkurt EE (ed): *Physiology.* Boston, Little Brown & Co, 1971, p 288.

2
Electrophysiological Concepts

The efficiency of the heart in ejecting volumes of blood into the systemic circuit is directly related to muscle-fiber shortening. This process results from the interaction of the actin and myosin protein filaments. To better understand the concept of cardiac-muscle-fiber shortening, one must consider cardiac-fiber activity at the cellular level. In this text, only a simplified version of the depolarization-contraction coupling concept will be presented.

CARDIAC CELL STRUCTURE

As depicted in Figure 2-1, the microscopic view of a working ventricular cell resembles a maze of interconnecting structures. The matrix or sarcoplasm of the cardiac cell is enveloped by a cellular membrane, the sarcolemma, which serves as a semipermeable barrier, maintains a transport system, and activates the process of depolarization (excitation-contraction coupling). Interspersed within the matrix are mitochondria, nuclei, the sarcoplasmic reticulum, magnesium, glycogen, and calcium, as well as the myofibrils actin and myosin.

The mitochondria are considered the power plants of the working cell. It is within these structures that oxidative phosphorylation of the end products of nutrition takes place. Carbohydrates, fats, and proteins are broken down into fractional components, yielding adenosine triphosphate as a source of energy vital for the work of fiber shortening (1).

The sarcolemma invaginates the cell interior by way of the transverse system of tubules, commonly called the T tubes, which lie perpendicular to the contractile elements of cardiac muscle, the filaments. As the transverse tubules penetrate the cell interior, they are in close proximity to another system of tubules— the longitudinal, or the L, system of tubes (2, 3). The bulbous cistern, or dilated portion of the L tubules, is thought to abut the T tubules. Calcium is stored and released from the cistern. The longitudinal myofibrils actin and myosin run parallel to each other, making up the contractile unit of a cardiac cell. Myosin, the thicker of the two activating filaments, has ATPase properties. That is, through the action of enzymes, it has the potential for linkage with the actin filament by way of cross bridges (lateral projections). The thin filament of the contracting mechanism is composed of actin, troponin, and tropomyosin. Tropomyosin plays an inhibitory role in the linkage of the actin filament to myosin (4, 5). The role of sarcoplasmic magnesium is thought to be myosin inhibitory.

20

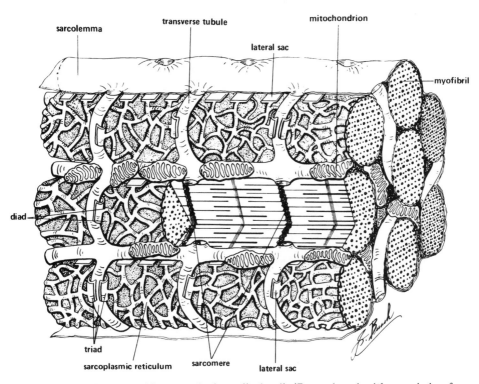

Figure 2-1. Ordinary working ventricular cell: detail. (Reproduced with permission from Legato MJ: *The Myocardial Cell for the Clinical Cardiologist.* Mount Kisco, NY, Futura Pub Co Inc, 1973.)

Physiological Basis for Myofibril Shortening

Depolarization of the cell membrane (sarcolemma) causes the electrical impulse (action potential) to travel to the interior of the cell by way of the T tubular system (Fig. 2-2). The abutting arrangement of the T tubes with the L tubes triggers the release of calcium from the cistern as the impulse arrives at the level of the bulb (1). The release of calcium inactivates the inhibitory effect of tropomyosin, which acts as a shield over the site where calcium binds to troponin. As the site is exposed, calcium binds to the troponin complex (4). Simultaneously, the cross bridges of the myosin filament become activated and attach themselves to the actin filament (3, 4). The electromagnetic attraction of the thick and thin protein filaments initiates phosphorylation of adenosine triphosphate found on the H-meromysin spine of the myosin filament by the enzyme ATPase (adenosine triphosphatase). This process results in the release of energy and subsequently initiates the interdigitation process of the actin and myosin filaments (5). This activity is in accordance with the Huxley-Hanson sliding filament hypothesis. As soon as the interdigitation takes place and shortening of the fibers occurs, calcium is pumped back into the longitudinal tubules and the muscle fiber relaxes. In addition to that stored within the lateral sacs, calcium is likewise found in the binding sites on the sarcolemma and enters the cell during the process of depolarization. Thus the excitation-contraction coupling is related to the effects of four protein molecules—actin and myosin, which

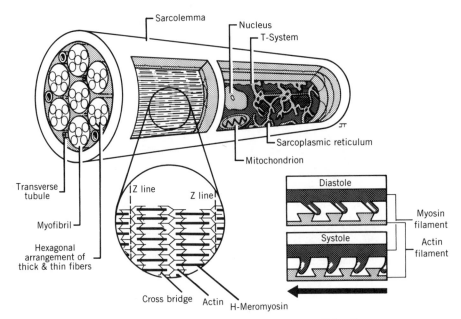

Figure 2-2. Ultrastructure of the myocardial cell.

take an active part in the interaction, and troponin and tropomyosin, which influence or regulate the primary interaction (6).

Microscopic View of Cardiac Fiber

The longitudinal arrangement of the actin and myosin protein filaments show up as striation of cardiac muscle fiber. Through electron microscopy, various hues of color are identified within the scheme of the striations (7).

The Z line is the point of junction of one cardiac fiber with another. Adjacent to the Z line are the thin filaments, actin thus constituting the I band or that part of the muscle fiber isotropic to light. A rather dense area, which corresponds to the overlapping of actin and myosin filaments is then identified. This band is anistropic to light; thus the term A band. The A band includes the overlapping actin and myosin filaments. A less dense area of the H zone corresponds to the isolated myosin filament. The overlapping of the thick and thin protein filaments is then repeated (8). Thus the area from Z line to Z line is the contractile unit of the myocardial cell, the sarcomere (Fig. 2-2). Upon contraction or shortening of the muscle fiber, there is greater density of the A band as there is greater interdigitation of actin and myosin filaments (1, 9).

TRANSMEMBRANE ACTION POTENTIAL

All mechanical (contracting/relaxing) activity of the heart is preceded by an electrical event easily recorded with the use of an electrocardiogram (ECG). Changes in the permeability of selective membranes to ions govern all electrophysiological events in the heart as well as what is recorded on the electrocardiogram. These changes are responsible for the production of the normal action potential and greatly influence impulse formation and conduction. Arrhythmias are produced from some alteration of the normal action potential, and consequently all therapeutic interventions attempt to restore normal action potential.

Studies (10) have been carried out on single cells to determine the characteristics of the ionic permeability of sodium (Na^+), potassium (K^+), chloride (Cl^-), and calcium (Ca^{2+}). Intracellular microelectrodes have shown that the inside of a ventricular muscle cell is more negative than the outside. This potential difference has been recorded to be approximately -80 to -95 mV (11) at rest and thus is termed the *resting membrane potential* (RMP). Because the permeability of the cell membrane to potassium is many times that to sodium, the intracellular concentration of potassium is approximately 30 times greater than the extracellular, accounting for this -90 mV RMP (12). In contrast, sodium concentration is found to be approximately 30 times greater extracellularly than intracellularly (Fig. 2-3). Several anions, including proteins are not able to cross the cell membrane owing to its selective permeability, and these help account for the difference in negative charge intracellularly at rest (13). This large difference in concentration of sodium and potassium across the cell membrane is also the result of an active transport system, the sodium-potassium pump, which is located in the cell membrane. This pump, activated by the enzyme ATPase, actively pumps sodium out and potassium into cells (14) (Fig. 2-3).

When a stimulus is applied to the cell, its membrane permeability to sodium increases markedly, resulting in a positive shift in transmembrane potential. If the stimulus is strong enough to reach a critical level known as *threshold potential* (approximately -60 to -70 mV) (15), the cell responds entirely and depolarization occurs. This is known as phase 0 or the upstroke of the action potential curve (16) (Fig. 2-4). When the stimulus is of such character that the threshold point is not reached, there is no depolarization response by the cell to that stimulus, hence the "all or none law of the heart" (17). The spike of phase 0 usually peaks at approximately +25 to +35 mV. (11), and this accounts for a slight overshoot (above zero value). Immediately after depolarization are three phases of repolarization: phase 1, initial rapid repolarization; phase 2, plateau phase;

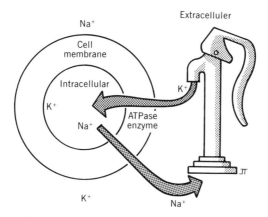

Figure 2-3. Diagrammatic representation of the sodium-potassium pump, located in the cell membrane. The concentration ratio of potassium intracellularly to extracellularly is 30:1. (Reproduced with permission from Gould SE: *Pathology of the Heart and Blood Vessels.* Copyright © 1968. Courtesy of Charles C Thomas, Publisher, Springfield, Ill.)

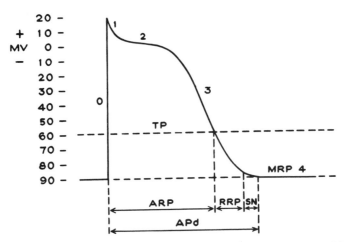

Figure 2-4. Diagram of the action potential of a ventricular muscle cell. MRP: membrane resting potential; 0: depolarization; 1, 2, 3: phases of repolarization; 4: diastolic phase, MRP; APd: duration of action potential; TP: threshold potential; ARP: absolute refractory period; RRP: relative refractory period; SN: supernormal period. (Reproduced with permission from Goldman MJ: *Principles of Clinical Electrocardiography,* 10th ed. Copyright © 1979, Los Altos, California, Lange Medical Publications.)

and phase 3, final repolarization or terminal repolarization (18). Phase 0 is thought to be due to the fast channels which permit small amounts of sodium to quickly enter (fast inward current) (11). Depolarization of the ventricles is then depicted at the beginning of the QRS on the electrocardiogram. Phase 1 of the curve shows a slight but abrupt downward trend thought to be due to the inward flow of a small amount of negatively charged chloride ions (16). After phase 1 is the plateau phase, or phase 2. During this phase there is a slow inward current for sodium and calcium while there is a small outward current for potassium, thus producing the plateau effect (19) (Fig. 2-5). From the beginning of depolarization with phase 0 and including phases 1 and 2 of repolarization, the heart is said to be in a state of *absolute refractoriness*. Once a cell has been depolarized it cannot respond to another stimulus regardless of its strength until the cell is repolarized to a value of approximately -50 mV (12). This period is referred to as the *absolute or effective refractory period* (16) and protects the heart from reaching a state of tetany (20). The absolute refractory period correlates with the beginning of the QRS complex, includes the ST segment, and terminates just before the beginning of the T wave on the electrocardiogram. During phase 3 repolarization, the cell again becomes increasingly permeable to potassium, producing a sharp return of transmembrane potential to negative values intracellulary (16). Phase 3 is known as the *relative refractory period* and correlates with the T wave on the electrocardiogram. A relatively strong stimulus may evoke a response if applied during this phase. If an ectopic focus fires during this vulnerable period (R on T phenomenon), then lethal arrhythmias may occur, that is, ventricular fibrillation. The fact that cells are being repolarized at different times accounts for the vulnerability during this phase (21).

The period before the cell returns to phase 4 is known as the *supernormal phase,* which corresponds to the terminal portion of the T wave and the U wave (22) (Fig. 2-6). The supernormal phase occurs only when conduction is depressed; thus it is absent in

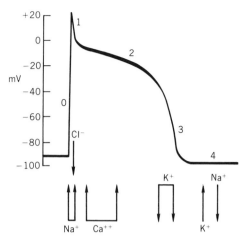

Figure 2-5. Schematic representation of the net movement of ions during the action potential. The arrows pointing downward indicate movement out of the cell, and those pointing upward indicate movement into the cell. A small amount of Cl^- ions leave the cell during phase 1, whereas Ca^{2+} is the major ion entering the cell during phase 2. Sodium enters the cell primarily during phase 0, and potassium leaves rapidly during phase 3. The sodium-potassium pump is employed during phase 4 to pump sodium out of and potassium into the cells. (Reproduced with permission from Fozzard HA, Gibbons WR: Action potential and contraction of heart muscle. *Am J Cardiol* 31:182, 1973.)

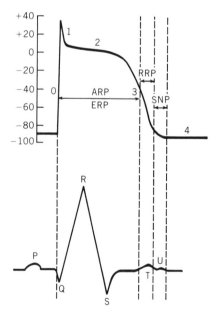

Figure 2-6. Correlation of the action potential curve with an ECG complex. Phases 0, 1, and 2 correspond the QRS complex and include the ST segment. This period is known as the absolute refractory period (ARP) or the effective refractory period (ERP). The relative refractory period (RRP) occurs during phase 3 and corresponds to the T wave. The supernormal phase of conduction (SN) occurs during the terminal portion of the T wave as well as the U wave. (Reproduced with permission from Hoffman BF, Cranefield PF: *Electrophysiology of the Heart.* Copyright © 1960, Futura Publishing Co., Inc., Mount Kisco, New York.)

Table 2-1. Comparison of Properties of Rapid and Slow Inward Currents

	Rapid	Slow
Activation and inactivation kinetics		
Dependent on extracellular ion concentration of	Sodium	Calcium
Threshold of activation	–60 to –70 mV	–30 to –40 mV
Resting membrane potential	–80 to –95 mV	–40 to –70 mV
Conduction velocity	0.5 to 3.0 M/sec	0.01 to 0.1 M/sec
Overshoot	+20 to +35 mV	0 to +15 mV
Rate of rise (dV/dt) of action potential upstroke	200 to 1000 V/sec	1 to 10 V/sec
Action potential amplitude	100 to 130 mV	35 to 75 mV
Safety factor for conduction	High	Low

Source: Zipes, DP: *Circulation* 51:761, 1975. With permission from the American Heart Association.

normal hearts. During this short critical period, conduction is temporarily improved (23). Finally the cell returns to its phase 4 resting state and the sodium-potassium pump actively pumps potassium into and sodium out of the cell.

The action potential curve just discussed is known as the *fast response* and is present in atrial and ventricular fibers as well as specialized conducting fibers of the atria and ventricles. The fast response is characterized (Table 2-1) by a rapid rate of rise during depolarization (phase 0), which is primarily due to the changes in sodium conductance. Fibers of the heart with a fast response are capable of conducting electrical activity at relatively rapid rates (0.5-5.0 M/sec) (24), thus providing them a high safety factor for conduction (Table 2-1). A second depolarizing current, the calcium current, is thought to be present in the fast fibers as well. This current, which is carried by calcium, enters the cell through slow membrane channels. When the membrane potential reaches ap-

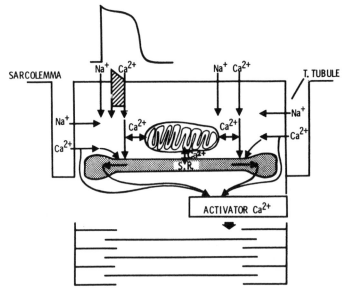

Figure 2-7. Schematic representation of the relationship between Ca^{2+} influx associated with the rising and plateau phases of the action potential, and the supply of activator Ca^{2+} which mediates the mechanical response. (Reproduced with permission from Krikler DM, and Goodwin JF [eds]: *Cardiac Arrhythmias: The Modern Electrophysiologic Approach.* Copyright © 1975, W. B. Saunders Co., Ltd., London.)

proximately –55 mV, the calcium current is activated (24) and is primarily responsible for phase 2 or the plateau phase of the action potential curve. This slow current does not contribute significantly to depolarization under normal conditions; its primary role in normal atrial and ventricular cells is the entrance of calcium during systole. The key role that calcium plays in the excitation-contraction mechanism was previously discussed in this chapter, and the reader is referred back to it for review. It is believed that calcium enters the cell during phase 2 (Fig. 2-7) and that this inward calcium current is enhanced by such catecholamines as epinephrine and norepinephrine (13), accounting at least in part for their stimulating affect on contraction. The slow response may be the primary mode of depolarization in abnormal conditions such as an elevated potassium level (13). During states of hyperkalemia, the fast channels for sodium conductance markedly diminish to a point at which only the slow channels for the inward conductance of calcium remain available (Fig. 2-8).

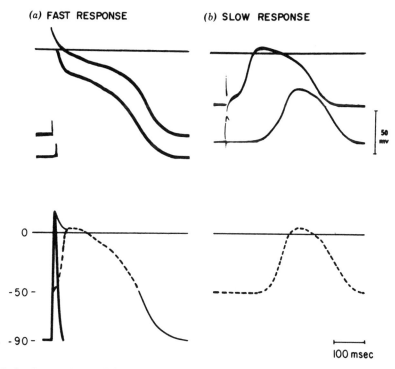

Figure 2-8. Comparison of fast and slow responses. Panel A (top) shows two transmembrane action potentials recorded from different cells in bundle of canine Purkinje fibers (fast fibers) perfused with normal Tyrode solution [K⁺] (4 mmol). Reference line 0 is for top action potential only. Microelectrodes are located 15 mm apart at either end of unbranched bundle, and the Purkinje fiber bundle is stimulated at one end. Action potentials shown in panel A are examples of fast response. Panel B (top) shows transmembrane action potentials recorded from same two cells while the Purkinje fiber bundle is being perfused with Tyrode solution containing high [K⁺] (16 mmol) and epinephrine levels. Stimulation of the Purkinje fiber bundle now results in slow response action potentials. Diagrams at bottom of each panel indicate relative time course of Na⁺ (dark trace) and Ca²⁺ (dashed trace) currents. (Reproduced with permission from Wit AL, Friedman PL: Basis for ventricular arrhythmias accompanying myocardial infarction. *Arch Intern Med.* 135:459, 1975. Copyright © 1975 American Medical Association.)

The *slow response* is the other type of electrical activity present in cardiac fibers and is normally found in the SA and AV nodes, the fibers in the mitral and triscupid valve leafelets and coronary sinus (11). The slow fibers conduct electrical activity at relatively slow rates (0.01 to 0.1 M/sec) (11) and thus have a low safety factor for conduction and are prone to being blocked. These fibers have an RMP between –40 and –70 mV, and their threshold potential is between –30 and –40 mV (15) (see Table 2-1). When a stimulus is applied, there is a slow regenerative depolarization phase, which is thought to be carried by calcium through slow membrane channels. The peak of depolarization is between 0 and +15 mV, and since this channel is inactivated slowly, cardiac arrhythmias are likely to occur, owing to its prolonged phase of repolarization (11) (see Table 2-1).

Conduction velocity in all cells is largely determined by three factors: (*1*) amplitude of action potential, (*2*) rate of change of the potential during phase 0, and (*3*) the value of the membrane potential at rest (12). The amplitude of the action potential is the difference in the potential when the cell is fully depolarized and when it is fully polarized, or approximately 130 mV in a working ventricular cell. The rapid rate of change during phase 0 is referred to as V_{max} or *dV/dt*, and it corresponds to the steepest part of the upstroke (18). The less negative the resting membrane potential becomes (from –90 to –70 mV), the slower the conduction velocity also becomes. This slowing of the rate of depolarization and relatively low amplitude of the action potential is the producer of slow conduction and the formation of *reentry arrhythmias* (24) (see Chap. 6). It may be present in fast fibers when disease processes alter their normal ionic mechanisms; (11) slow response action potentials are found in tissues that are experimentally infarcted, that are bathed with high concentrations of potassium, and that are subjected to toxic levels of digitalis (Fig. 2-9). Atria which are found to be markedly dilated or hypertrophied also exhibit characteristics of the slow response action potential (12).

Cardiac cells (both myocardial and specialized conducting fibers), when adequately stimulated, are capable of initiating an action potential. This gives the heart its property of excitabiilty (12), and certain cardiac cells have the unique property of automaticity, whereby spontaneously they gradually depolarize themselves up to threshold potential to initiate an action potential (12). The action potential curve for pacemaking cells is very different from that for cells previously described. This type of action potential is present in the SA node and lower or NH region (AV node–His bundle region) of the AV

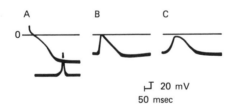

Figure 2-9. Fast and slow response action potentials. Panel A shows a normal or fast response Purkinje fiber action potential. The upper trace is the action potential, the lower, a 200 V/sec calibration wave followed by the electronically differentiated maximum upstroke velocity of phase 0 (V_{max}). Panels B and C are records taken from the same fiber 30 and 40 minutes after exposure to a toxic concentration of ouabain. These are slow responses. Note that resting membrane potential has decreased, as have action potential overshoot and the rate of rise of phase 0. (Reproduced with permission from Rosen MR: Cellular electrophysiologic basis of cardiac arrhythmias. *Angiology* 28:289, 1977.)

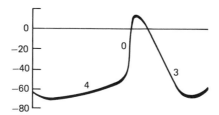

Figure 2-10. Diagram of the action potential of the SA node. Note the absence of a plateau phase and the presence of phase 4 diastolic depolarization. All cells capable of acting as pacemakers possess phase 4 spontaneous depolarization. (Reproduced with permission from Hoffman BF, Cranefield PF: *Electrophysiology of the Heart.* Copyright © 1960, Futura Publishing Co., Inc., Mount Kisco, New York.)

node, the specialized fibers of the atria, and His-Purkinje system (16). The characteristics of pacemaking cells include: (*1*) a gradual slope during phase 0 rather than a steep up-stroke, (*2*) absence of an overshoot phase, (*3*) a small or absent plateau phase, and (*4*) spontaneous diastolic depolarization during phase 4. The possession of phase 4 *spontaneous diastolic depolarization* is unique to the pacemaker cell and is responsible for its automaticity (Fig. 2-10). The actual mechanisms responsible for phase 4 diastolic depolarization are poorly understood. It is believed that the permeability of the cell to potassium is high immediately after repolarization, which accounts for a large efflux of potassium (19). During phase 4 this high permeability to potassium as well as its rapid efflux gradually decline. A small sodium influx during phase 4, which does not decline with time, is also present (16). It is the combination of a decreasing outward current of potassium and a steady inward current of sodium that shifts the membrane potential gradually to less negative values (25) (Fig. 2-11). A steady inward calcium current may also play a role in phase 4 spontaneous diastolic depolarization (13). Gradually the membrane potential reaches threshold potential and produces phase 0 depolarization. The faster the resting membrane potential reaches threshold potential, the faster the heart rate becomes. The pacemaker of the heart then is that which reaches threshold potential most quickly and is normally the SA node (Fig. 2-12). Pacemakers other than the SA node (atria, ventricles, AV junction) are generally considered ectopic pacemakers. One of these ectopic pacemakers may become the dominant pacemaker when (*1*) the SA node or

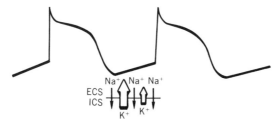

Figure 2-11. Diagrammatic representation of the ionic events thought to be responsible for phase 4 depolarization. ECS: extracellular space; ICS: intracellular space. A small and relatively constant inward sodium current (Na+) occurs throughout phase 4. A larger outward current for potassium (K+), which decreases in magnitude with time, occurs during phase 4 also. (Reproduced with permission from Rosen MR: Cellular electrophysiologic basis of cardiac arrhythmias. *Angiology* 28:289, 1977.)

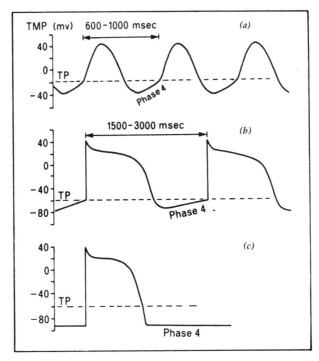

Figure 2-12. Transmembrane action potentials of three different types of isolated cardiac cells are schematized. (*a*) Cells of the sinus node demonstrate spontaneous phase 4 diastolic depolarization, until threshold potential (TP) is reached and depolarization occurs. This spontaneous diastolic depolarization toward threshold is the critical characteristic of automatic cells that enables them to self-excite. (*b*) Cells of the Purkinje network also develop phase 4 diastolic depolarization, but their rate of spontaneous action potential production is slower than that of the sinus node. Thus, in the intact heart, a conducted impulse from a higher, faster automatic site will depolarize these cells before their intrinsic mechanism. (*c*) Ventricular muscle cells have a constant resting potential and do not have spontaneous phase 4 diastolic depolarization. They are not automatic under normal conditions. TMP: transmembrane potential (in millivolts). (Reproduced with permission from Sherrid M, Goldschlager N: Escape rhythms. *Practical Cardiol* 4:130, 1978.)

other ectopic pacemaker's automaticity becomes depressed; (*2*) when the ectopic pacemaker's automaticity becomes enhanced above the SA node's activating capacity, and (*3*) if all the conduction paths are blocked between the ectopic pacemaker and the pacemaker with a faster rate of activation (13). The rate of pacemaker discharge depends on three variables: (*1*) rate of spontaneous diastolic depolarization (steepness of the curve), (*2*) value of maximum diastolic potential, and (*3*) threshold potential (26) (Fig. 2-13).

When the slope of phase 4 depolarization is increased, threshold potential is reached more quickly. Agents such as atropine and epinephrine increase the heart rate by this action at phase 4 (Fig. 2-14). A low extracellular potassium concentration likewise increases the slope of phase 4 diastolic depolarization. Vagal intensification (acetylcholine) and a high extracellular potassium concentration have the opposite effect and decrease the slope, thus producing a slower heart rate (27).

(a)

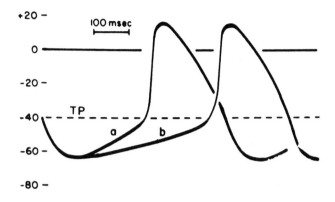

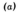
(a)

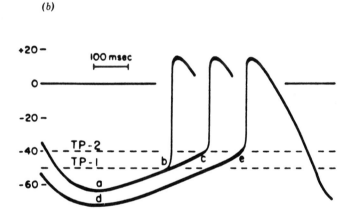
(b)

Figure 2-13. Transmembrane action potentials typical of those recorded from fibers of the sinoatrial node showing the expected effects of changing the slope of phase 4 depolarization, the magnitude of the maximum diastolic potential, and the level of the threshold potential. In (a), when the slope of phase 4 is decreased from a to b, more time is required to reach threshold potential and the cycle length is increased. In (b), under control conditions (TP-1) the fiber depolarizes from a maximum diastolic potential of a and attains threshold at b. If threshold potential shifts to a less negative value (TP-2), the phase 4 depolarization will not attain threshold until c. If maximum diastolic potential is increased to d, phase 4 depolarization will not attain threshold until e. Opposite changes in the slope of phase 4, the value of TP, or the value of MDP would have the opposite effect on cycle length and rate. (Reproduced with permission from Hoffman B, Cranefield P: *Electrophysiology of the Heart.* Copyright © 1960, Futura Publishing Co, Inc, Mount Kisko, NY, 1960.)

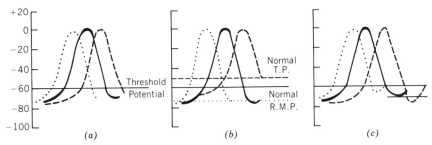

Figure 2-14. (*a*) Increasing the slope of phase 4 is depicted by the dotted line. Atropine increases the heart rate by this alteration of the action potential. Vagal maneuvers slow the heart rate by decreasing the slope of phase 4 as seen in the dashed line. The solid lines represent the normal action potential in all three panels. (*b*) As the threshold potential is shifted closer (dotted line) to resting potential the heart rate increases. (*c*) The heart rate slows when the resting membrane potential is increased as indicated by the dashed line. (Reproduced with permission from Rakita L, and Broder MI: *Cardiac Arrhythmias: Basic Concepts and an Approach to Self-Instruction,* Copyright © 1973, Year Book Medical Publishers, Inc., Chicago.)

Shifts in threshold potential to more positive values (toward zero) depress automaticity, and this is seen in states of elevated extracellular calcium levels (Fig. 2-14). A low concentration of calcium has the opposite effect of shifting threshold potential to more negative values and thus closer to resting membrane potential (28).

An increase in resting membrane potential (making it more negative) moves it further away from threshold potential and produces a slower heart rate. Acetylcholine also affects the action potential by this mechanism (primarily on supraventricular fibers) (28). A decrease in resting membrane potential will make it more positive and thus closer to threshold potential (Fig. 2-14).

DIPOLE CONCEPT THEORY

The conduction mechanism and the generation of electrical action is thought to be related to an "ionic theory," whereby the cellular membrane potential builds up and breaks down. This is accomplished by the selective intracellular passage of certain ions and the rejection of others. A bioelectric potential thus exists as a result fo the transmembrane concentration gradient, which is a result of the uneven distribution or concentration of two major electrolytes, potassium and sodium (29). Potassium is found predominantly within the cell and sodium is the major electrolyte surrounding the cellular compartment.

The ratio of intracellular potassium to the extracellular concentration is 30:1, whereas the concentration of sodium within and outside the cell is 1:10. It has been postulated that the uneven concentration of potassium and sodium ions due to transmembrane selectivity results in a -90 mV resting membrane potential characteristic of a ventricular muscle cell (30). Contributing to the inner cellular negativity are anions—phosphate and sulphate—as well as proteins that are unable to cross the cell membrane. A resting cell (polarized) may be seen to have positive charges bordering the outer parameter of the membrane and negative charges lining the interior (31) (Fig. 2-15). This arrangement produces a dipole affect (a potential source for activity). As long as an electrical gradient

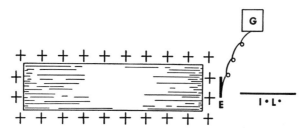

Figure 2-15. Inactive resting cell. E: electrode. G: galvanometer (EKG machine). I.L.: isoelectric line. In a resting muscle all the positive ions are on the outside of the cell membrane. There is no difference in electric potential, and no electric current is flowing. Electrode E, facing the right side of the resting muscle and connected to a galvanometer (G), will record no current, and the isoelectric line (I.L.) remains undisturbed. (Reproduced with permission from Bernreiter M: *Electrocardiography,* ed 2. Philadelphia, JB Lippincott Co, 1963.)

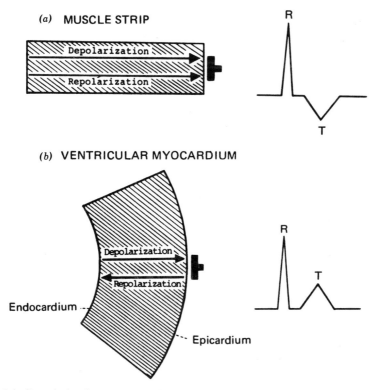

Figure 2-16. Depolarization and repolarization of a muscle strip (diagram A) and a ventricular myocardium (diagram B). Note that the direction of depolarization and repolarization processes is the same in a muscle strip. In contrast to this, depolarization and repolarization processes are opposite in direction in a ventricular myocardium. As a result the T wave is inverted in a muscle strip, whereas the T wave is upright in the ventricular myocardium. (Reproduced with permission from Chung EK: *Electrocardiography: Practical Applications with Vectorial Principles.* Hagerstown, Md, Harper & Row Pub Inc, 1974.) (See text on next page.)

33

exists across the cell membrane (all like charges on the exterior or interior), no intermingling takes place and no electrical activity can be identified on the oscilloscope. However, a stimulus (chemical and/or mechanical) can alter the membrane permeability and initiate an ionic exchange (32). The process of ionic displacement known as depolarization precedes the physical activity of muscle contraction and is inscribed as the R wave on the electrocardiogram. This occurs as a result of the current that flows with negative and positive charges appearing on each side of the membrane. Repolarization follows the process of depolarization (Fig. 2-16). During this phase, there is an exchange of ions across the cellular membrane, that is, the positive charges return to the exterior while the negative particles penetrate the interior surface. The activity restores the state of the cell to a resting state. Electrocardiographically, the T wave is representative of this activity. Hence, before ventricular ejection of blood, a series of events occurs: (1) stimulation of cell membrane, (2) process of depolarization, and (3) subsequent contraction.

REVIEW QUESTIONS

1. Under electron microscopy, the cardiac muscle fiber appears to be striated. What is responsible for the striations?
2. The contractile unit of the myocardium is the sarcomere. What makes up the sarcomere?
3. Describe the concept of the sliding filament hypothesis.
4. What role does calcium play in myocardial fiber shortening?
5. Describe what is meant by the term dipole.
6. What initiates the linkage of the myosin spine to the actin filament?
7. The R wave as depicted on the electrocardiogram is representative of ventricular depolarization and subsequent contraction. Identify what is occurring at the precise moment in regards to the following:
   a. at the level of actin and myosin filaments
   b. in the conduction system
   c. at the entrance of the electrical potential into the cell interior by way of the T tubule system
   d. on the action potential curve
   e. in the cardiac cycle
8. The "fast response" of cardiac fibers have a high safety factor for conduction of the impulse. Which features of this fast response protect the impulse from being blocked?
9. Describe the sequence of events (ionic exchange) that occurs during phase 0, phase 1, phase 2, phase 3, and phase 4 of the action potential curve.

REFERENCES

1. Warner HF, Russel MW, Spann JF: Heart muscle: clinical applications of basic physiology and cellular anatomy. *Heart Lung* 1:495, 1972.
2. Kelman GR: *Applied Cardiovascular Physiology.* Boston, Butterworth & Co, 1977, p 23.
3. Guyton AC: *Textbook of Medical Physiology,* ed 5. Philadelphia, WB Saunders Co, 1976, p 132.
4. Katz AM: Biochemical basis for cardiac contraction, in Mirsky I (ed): *Cardiac Mechanics.* New York, John Wiley & Sons Inc, 1974, p 70.

5. Shine, KI: Ionic basis of excitation and of excitation-contraction coupling, in Robers N and Gelband H (eds): *Cardiac Arrhythmias in the Neonate Infant and Child*. New York, Appleton-Century-Crofts, 1977, p 102.

6. Katz AM: Contractile proteins in normal and failing myocardium, in Braunwald (ed): *The Myocardium: Failure and Infarction*. New York, PH Publishing Co Inc, 1975, p 57.

7. Keele CA, Neil E: *Samson Wrights, Applied Physiology*, ed 12. New York, Oxford University Press Inc, 1971, p 212.

8. Katz AM: Congestive heart failure. *N Eng J Med* 293:1184, 1975.

9. Cooksey JD, Dunn M, Massie E: *Clinical Vectorcardiography and Electrocardiography*, ed 2. Chicago, Year Book Medical Pub Inc, 1977, pp 4, 5.

10. Brady AJ, Woodbury JW: The sodium-potassium hypothesis as the basis of electrical activity frog ventricle. *J Physiol (London)* 154:385, 1960.

11. Wit AL, Rosen MR, Hoffman BF: Electrophysiology and pharmacology of cardiac arrhythmias. II. Relationship of normal and abnormal electrical activity of cardiac fibers to the genesis of arrhythmias. *Am Heart J* 88:515, 1974.

12. Rosen MR: Cellular electrophysiological basis of cardiac arrhythmias. *Angiology* 28:289, 1977.

13. Berne RM, Levy MN: Electrical activity of the heart, in: *Cardiovascular Physiology*. St. Louis, CV Mosby Co, 1977, p 8.

14. Guyton AC: *Basic Human Physiology: Normal Function and Mechanisms of Disease*. Philadelphia, WB Saunders Co, 1971, p 45.

15. Zipes DP, Besch HR, Watanabe AM: Role of the slow current in cardiac electrophysiology. *Circulation* 51:761, 1975.

16. Rosen MR, Wit AL, Hoffman BF: Electrophysiology and pharmacology of cardiac arrhythmias. I. Cellular electrophysiology of the mammalian heart. *Am Heart J* 88:380, 1974.

17. Ganong WF: *Review of Medical Physiology,* ed 6. Los Altos, Calif, Lange Medical Publications, 1973, p 25.

18. Hoffman BF, Cranefield PF: *Electrophysiology of the Heart*. Mount Kisco, Futura Pub Co Inc, 1960, p 8.

19. Fozzard HA, Gibbons WR: Action potential and contraction of heart muscle. *Am J Cardiol* 31:183, 1973.

20. Taylor NB, McPhedron MG: *Basic Physiology and Anatomy*. New York, GP Putnam's Sons, 1965, p 11.

21. Krikler DM: Cardiac electrophysiology. *Lancet* 1:852, 1974.

22. Scherf D, Bornemann C: The supernormal phase of conductivity. *Dis Chest* 53:356, 1968.

23. Schamroth L: *The Disroders of Cardiac Rhythm*. Oxford, Blackwell Scientific Publications, 1971, p 893.

24. Wit AL, Friedman PL: Basis for ventricular arrhythmias accompanying myocardial infarction. *Arch Intern Med* 135:459, 1975.

25. Vassalle M: Automaticity and automatic rhythms. *Am J. Cardiol* 28:245, 1971.

26. Greenspan K, Thies WH: Slow currents and the genesis of cardiac dysrhythmias. *Practical Cardiol* 4:48, 1978.

27. Rakita L, Broder MI: Normal membrane function as it relates to arrhythmias, in: *Cardiac arrhythmias: Basic Concepts and an Approach to Self Instruction*. Chicago, Press of Case Western Reserve Univ, 1973, p 7.

28. Hoffman BF, Rosen MR, Wit AL: Electrophysiology and pharmacology of cardiac arrhythmias. III. The causes and treatment of cardiac arrhythmias. Part A. *Am Heart J* 89:115, 1975.

29. Strong P: *Biophysical Measurements*. Beaverton, Ore, Tektronix Inc, 1970, p 6.

30. Lipman BS, Massie E, Kleiger RE: *Clinical Scalar Electrocardiography,* ed 6. Chicago, Year Book Medical Pub Inc, 1972, p 33.

31. Bernreiter M: *Electrocardiography,* ed 2. Philadelphia, JB Lippincott, Co, 1963, p 2.

32. Kelman GR: *Applied Cardiovascular Physiology,* ed 2. Boston, Butterworth & Co, 1977, p 27.

3
Lead Reference System and Calculation of the Heart's Electrical Axis

A routine ECG normally includes 12 leads (6 extremity leads and 6 chest leads), and some institutions record 15 leads (12 leads plus the X, Y, and Z leads). For better understanding of the orientation of the 12 leads, the body may be compared to a cylinder. Like the body, a cylinder may be divided into three planes (dimensions): frontal, horizontal, and sagittal (Fig. 3-1).

STANDARD LIMB LEADS

The standard limb leads, I, II, and III (bipolar leads), as well as leads aV_R, aV_L, and aV_F (unipolar limb leads), record the heart's electrical activity in the frontal plane. The six chest (precordial) leads record the electrical activity in the horizontal plane. The three standard limb leads (I, II, and III) were originally devised by Einthoven and include electrodes applied to the right arm, left arm, and left leg. Although the electrodes are normally placed at the wrists and ankles, the same recording will be obtained if the arm electrodes are placed anywhere from the wrists to the shoulders and the left leg electrode between the ankle and groin (1, 2, 3). The bipolar leads represent a difference of electrical potential between two sites (positive and negative electrodes) (Fig. 3-2). Lead I records the difference in electrical potential between the negative electrode on the right arm and the positive electrode on the left arm. Lead II records the difference between the negative electrode on the right arm and the positive electrode on the left leg. Lead III records the difference between the positive pole on the left leg and the negative pole on the left arm. Application of the electrodes and leads becomes easy if one remembers that the right arm is always negative and the left leg is always positive. The left arm then changes charge appropriately. These three leads theoretically form an electrically equilateral triangle, known as the Einthoven triangle. The heart is the center or zero point of this triangle. Einthoven's law algebraically explains the relationship between these three leads in the following equation: Lead II = lead I + lead III. This rule is important to recall when the leads have been incorrectly labeled, since the P wave in lead II must be the tallest P wave if it is upright in all three leads (2).

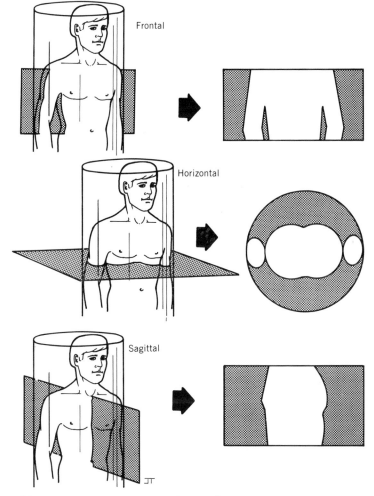

Figure 3-1. Shaded areas represent the planes of the body and their resemblance to a cylinder.

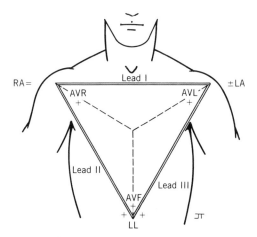

Figure 3-2. The bipolar limb leads I, II, and III form the Einthoven's triangle. The augmented unipolar limb leads include aV_R, aV_L, and aV_F.

UNIPOLAR LIMB LEADS

The unipolar limb leads consist of aV_R, aV_L, and aV_F and record electrical activity in the frontal plane like the standard limb leads (Fig. 3-2). These leads were originally devised by Wilson in 1932 and include positive electrodes (poles) attached to the right arm, left arm, and left leg (3). The letter V indicates that the lead is unipolar while the letter "d" signifies that the amplitude of the recorded voltage is augmented for easier reading (4). These unipolar limb leads record the same information as the standard bipolar leads, but their deflections are different since their axes are from slightly different directions in the frontal plane (5).

The Einthoven triangle can be modified by rearranging all three limb leads to intersect with each other at a common reference point (zero reference point) without alteration of their axis (Fig. 3-3). This forms the triaxial reference system of Bayley. If the unipolar

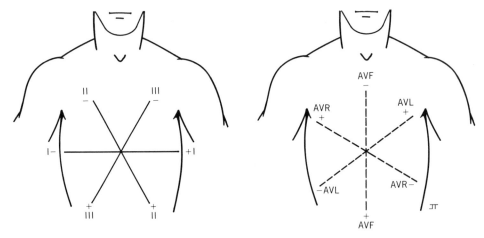

Figure 3-3. The three bipolar limb leads are moved in a manner causing intersection of each other at a common reference point. (*b*) In a similar fashion, the augmented limb leads interesect each other at the same common point.

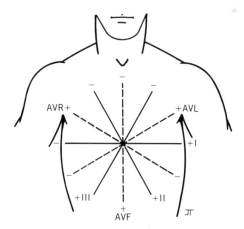

Figure 3-4. The hexaxial reference system consists of all six limb leads intersecting each other at a common reference point.

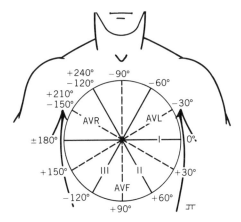

Figure 3-5. The hexaxial reference system with the appropriate degrees assigned to each lead.

limb leads are added to the triaxial reference system, the figure now consists of six bisecting lines referred to as the hexaxial system, which is essential in the determination of the electrical axis (4) (Fig. 3-4). The hexaxial system is then enclosed by a circle whose center overlies the electrical center of the heart. By convention, lead I has its positive pole at $0°$ and its negative pole at $±180°$, lead II has its positive pole at $+60°$ and its negative pole at $-120°$, and lead III has its positive pole at $+120°$ and its negative pole at $-60°$ (Fig. 3-5). It becomes obvious that the standard limb leads are separated by $60°$ (3).

Improper placement of the ECG leads is one of the most common errors made in the recording of the electrocardiogram. The reversal of the left-arm and right-arm leads produces a right-axis deviation along with an inverted P wave in lead I (6) (Fig. 3-6). Different body positions can also alter the ECG recording, as illustrated in the tracings in Figure 3-7—one taken from a recumbent patient and the other with the patient at a $45°$ angle.

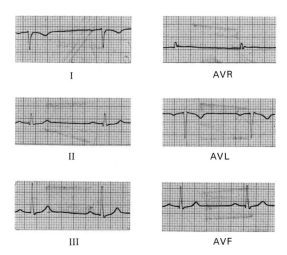

Figure 3-6. Arm electrodes (lead I) are reversed. Lead II is actually lead III and lead III is actually lead II. Lead I is a mirror image of lead I. Lead aV_R is actually lead aV_L and lead aV_L is actually lead aV_R.

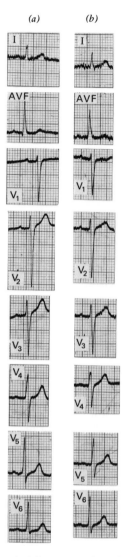

Figure 3-7. (*a*) Tracing was recorded from a patient in a recumbent position. (*b*) Tracing from the same patient now at a 45° angle. Note the loss of R wave amplitude in leads V_{4-5} and increase in S wave depth in V_6. The decrease in R wave amplitude may include all the precordial leads, which then mimics an anterior myocardial infarction. (Artifact is present in both tracings.)

PRECORDIAL (UNIPOLAR CHEST) LEADS

The six precordial leads record electrical activity in the horizontal plane. The American Heart Association recommends the following positions for the leads commonly used today (3): (*1*) V_1, fourth intercostal space to the right of the sternum; (*2*) V_2, fourth intercostal space to the left of the sternum; (*3*) V_3, placed equally between leads V_2 and V_4; (*4*) V_4, fifth intercostal space in the left midclavicular line; (*5*) V_5, fifth intercostal space in the left anterior axillary line; and (*6*) V_6, fifth intercostal space in the left medaxillary line (Fig. 3-8). Additional precordial leads may be necessary in certain

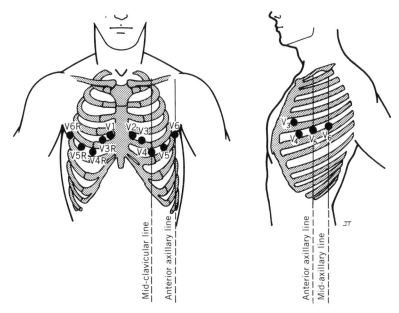

Figure 3-8. Proper positioning of the six precordial leads. The leads with the letter R are those recorded from the right side of the chest and are especially helpful in the tracings recorded from infants and children.

situations; for example, leads V_{3R} to V_{6R} provide valuable information in congenital heart disease. These leads correspond to the location of the leads on the left side of the chest (1). The limb leads provide more detailed information since they are closer to the heart, and lead V_1 is a valuable lead in identifying P waves (1).

Any lead may be used for monitoring purposes; however, a modified version of V_1 (MCL_1) is useful. MCL_1 (modified chest lead of V_1) is derived by placing the positive electrode in the conventional V_1 location and the negative electrode on the left arm, the right-arm electrode acting as the grounding electrode (Fig. 3-9). This lead is useful

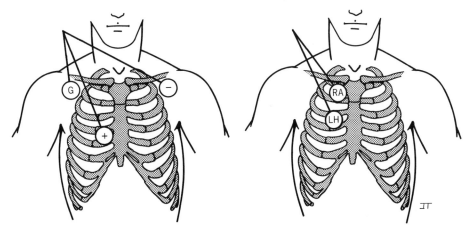

Figure 3-9. (*Left*) Proper lead placement of the MCl_1 lead. All six precordial leads can be modified in a similar fashion by moving the positive electrode in the correct location, that is MCl_2, MCl_3, MCl_4, MCl_5, and MCl_6. (*Right*) The Lewis lead is useful in the recognition of P wave activity.

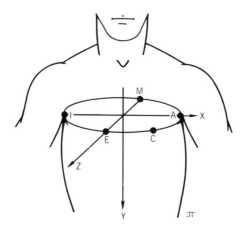

Figure 3-10. The Frank lead system is the most commonly used method for recording the orthogonal leads X, Y, and Z.

in differentiating aberrancy from ectopy (Chap. 6) and also provides good visualization of P wave activity. Another lead that gives a good view of P wave activity is the Lewis lead. This lead is composed of a right-arm electrode placed in the intercostal space to the right of the sternum and the left-arm electrode placed in the V_1 position. The recording is made on lead I (3) (Fig. 3-9).

X, Y, Z (ORTHOGONAL) LEADS

It will be recalled that the three planes of the body are the horizontal, the sagittal, and the frontal. These are referred to as orthogonal planes, each plane being perpendicular to the other two. The X lead (right to left axis) corresponds to lead I; Y lead (head to foot axis) corresponds to lead aV_F; and Z lead (anteroposterior axis) corresponds to an inverted V_1 recording (3). The Frank system (7) is the most popular method for recording the orthogonal leads because it requires fewer electrodes than other systems (3, 8) do.

Five electrodes are placed at certain points around the chest at the level of the fourth or fifth intercostal space (Fig. 3-10). Electrodes I and A are positioned in the left and right midaxillary lines, E and M are positioned in the midline over the sternum and vertebral column, and C is positioned in a line bisecting the angle formed by the axes of leads A and E. Electrodes are then placed on the left leg, F, and on the back of the neck, H (9).

ELECTRICAL AXIS

As previously described in Chapter 2, many dipoles contribute their effect to the electrical potential (force) developed during depolarization and repolarization. This force can be measured with regard to its magnitude and direction and is referred to as a *vector*. The vector has magnitude, direction, and sense (polarity) and is symbolically depicted as an arrow. A single vector (dipole) is known as the *instantaneous vector* and represents the net electrical force at a given instant (Fig. 3-11). The average of all the instantaneous vectors results in a *mean vector* for any part of the cardiac cycle (depolarization and repolarization) and is synonymous with the term *mean electrical axis* (see Fig. 3-11).

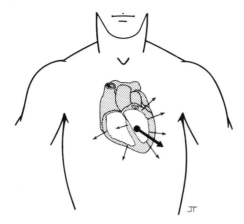

Figure 3-11. Many instantaneous vectors (small arrows) are averaged to provide a mean vector (large arrow) of the ventricles.

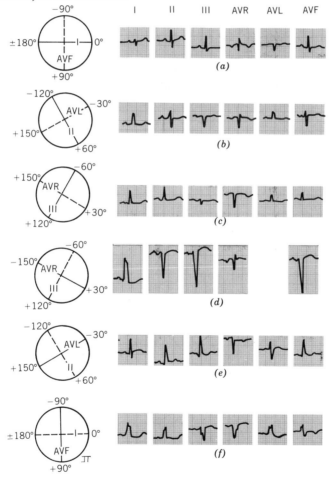

Figure 3-12. The determination of the mean QRS axis utilizing the lead with an isoelectric QRS complex. The axis in parenthesis is calculated by another means for comparison. (*a*) Axis is perpendicular to lead I (calculated axis is $+90°$). (*b*) Axis is perpendicular to lead II (calculated axis is $-30°$). (*c*) Axis is perpendicular to lead III (calculated axis is $+32°$). (*d*) Axis is perpendicular to lead aV_R (calculated axis is $-59°$). (*e*) Axis is perpendicular to lead aV_L (calculated axis is $+60°$). (*f*) Axis is perpendicular to lead aV_F (calculated axis is $0°$). (See text on next page.)

A mean QRS vector (ventricular depolarization) can be easily calculated (8). The electrical axis can be determined from the frontal plane (extremity leads) and in the horizontal plane (precordial leads), but for convenience the axis is usually determined from the frontal plane.

The mean P, QRS, and T axes are determined by using the hexaxial reference system. Two methods for obtaining the axis may be used. The easiest method is to find a lead with an isoelectric QRS complex (algebraic sum of the deflection of the QRS complex equals zero). The QRS axis is perpendicular to that lead (9). A lead with the smallest QRS complex can be used if no lead with an isoelectric complex can be found (2) (Fig. 3-12). The longest QRS deflection will produce an axis parallel to that lead (8). The other method is to use the algebraic sum of the deflections in any two leads to plot the axis, leads I and III being the most commonly used (Fig. 3-13). A variance of up to ±35° may be obtained in the same person if the axis is calculated with different pairs of leads (10), and the mean axis derived from these two described methods may also differ (9). The normal QRS axis falls between -30° and +110°; left-axis deviation (superior axis) is between -30° and -90° and right-axis deviation between +110° and ±180° (3). The area between -180° and -90° is sometimes referred to as indeterminate axis (8) (Fig. 3-14). The same principle and method used to calculate the QRS axis is used for the T wave and P axes, the mean P wave axis normally varying between 0° to +90° (8). Normally the mean QRS and T axes are similar and do not differ by more than 60° from each other. If these two axes do differ by more than 60°, a myocardial abnormality is usually present (1).

Relationship of the Heart Position and the Electrocardiogram

The heart may rotate on either its anteroposterior axis (frontal plane) or its longitudinal axis (horizintal plane). There are five categories included in the anteroposterior axis;

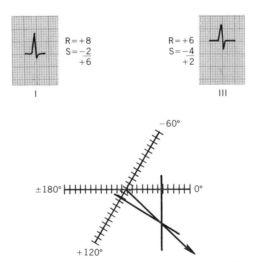

Figure 3-13. Calculation of the mean QRS axis by the use of the algebraic sums of the QRS complex in two limb leads. The hexaxial reference system with the appropriate degrees of each lead is then superimposed on these two leads. The axis of these two leads is approximately +45°.

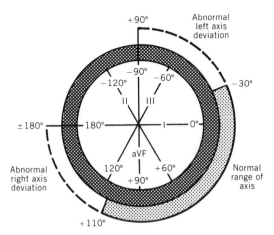

Figure 3-14. The normal range of axis is from +110° to –30°. Indeterminate axis ranges from ±180° to –90°.

vertical, semivertical, intermediate, semihorizontal, and horizontal (3) (Fig. 3-15). Rotation of the heart on its longitudinal axis is either counterclockwise or clockwise This rotation is from a reference point looking upward frontally at the heart from below the diaphragm. The precordial leads are used for the diagnosis of clockwise and counter-clockwise rotation. The normal transition zone (diphasic QRS complex) is around V_4 (9); in counterclockwise rotation this is shifted to the right. The left ventricle rotates anteriorly and the right ventricle rotates posteriorly to account for the presence of a left ventricular epicardial complex (QR) in V_2 or V_3 (8) (Fig. 3-16). Commonly, the ST segment is elevated in V_{2-4} in counterclockwise rotation (3). Clockwise rotation produces a transi-tion zone displaced to the left, because the right ventricle becomes more anterior and the

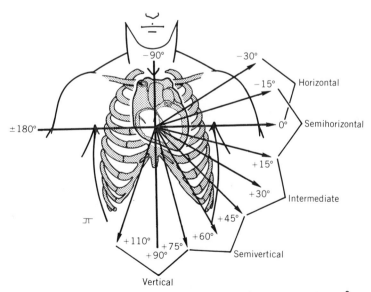

Figure 3-15. Five categories of the anteroposterior axis include vertical (+110° to +75°), semivertical (+75° to +45°), intermediate (+45° to +15°), semihorizontal (+15° to –15°), and horizontal (0° to –30°).

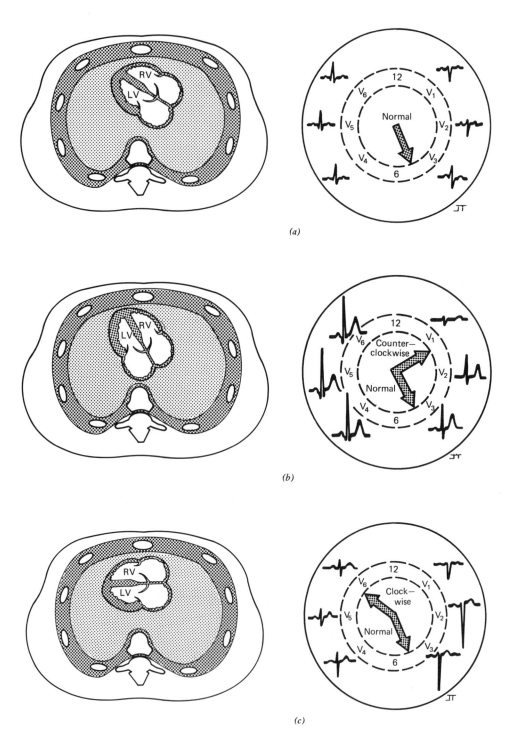

Figure 3-16. (*a*) Normal location of the heart in the chest and the normal QRS complexes as seen in each of the precordial leads with reference to a clock. (*b*) In counterclockwise rotation the transition zone occurs in V_1 or V_2. (*c*) In clockwise rotation the transition zone occurs in V_5 or V_6.

Table 3-1. Lead Reference System

QRS Axis	Age
$+90°$ to $+150°$	Birth to 1 year
$+45°$ to $+105°$	1–8 years
(Same as adult)	8 years and older

left ventricle more posterior. This shift produces a right ventricular epicardial complex (RS) as far left as V_5 or V_6 (Fig. 3-16). Clockwise and counterclockwise rotation are older terms and are gradually being replaced by posterior and anterior axis deviation (1).

QRS and T Axes in Childhood

The fetal right ventricle works harder than the left ventricle, which accounts for the ECG appearance of right ventricular hypertrophy at birth. This also explains the presence of an axis that is shifted to the right and a mean QRS axis commonly near $+120°$ (11). As the child becomes older, the left ventricle becomes larger than the right and a gradual shift in axis to the left is seen (Table 3-1). The mean T wave axis at birth is between $+60°$ and $-90°$ in the frontal plane but changes quite drastically over the course of a week (11) (Fig. 3-17).

Significance of the Electrical Axes

The mean QRS axis varies with body build, age, and anatomic positions, to account for a wide range in the normal axis. Clinical conditions producing abnormal shifts in the QRS axis are seen in Table 3-2. The presence of left axis deviation alone on the ECG of apparently healthy men has been show to be associated with latent diabetes and development of coronary artery disease (12). The T wave axis likewise changes with age and usually with a diseased myocardium. An abnormal P wave axis is seen in chronic obstructive lung disease as well as conditions producing left and right atrial enlargement (see Chap. 10).

Table 3-2. Lead Reference System: Clinical Conditions Producing Axis Deviation

Right Axis	Left Axis
Right ventricular hypertrophy	High diaphragm (pregnancy, ascites,
Right bundle branch block	obesity, abdominal tumors)
Left posterior fascicular block	Left anterior fascicular block
Dextrocardia	Inferior myocardial infarction
Lateral myocardial infarction	(pseudo)
(pseudo)	Wolff-Parkinson-White syndrome
Pulmonary embolism and/or	Hyperkalemia
infarction	Right ventricular ectopic rhythms
Emphysema	Endocardial cushion defect
Left ventricular Ectopic rhythms	Pulmonary disease

Source: Modified from Marriott, HJL: *Practical Electrocardiography,* ed 6. Copyright © 1977 by Williams & Wilkins Co, Baltimore.

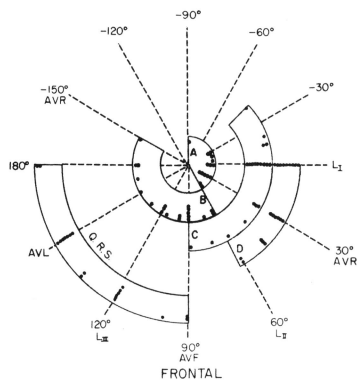

FRONTAL

Figure 3-17. The mean T axis of electrocardiograms of 20 normal newborns in the frontal plane (shaded area). (A) at birth; (B) at the end of the transient phase; (C) restitution phase at age 3 days; and (D) restitution phase at age 7 days. Note the distribution of the mean QRS axis at birth in the nonshaded area with a mean QRS axis of 125.3°. (Reproduced with permission from Hait G, Gasul BM: The evolution and significance of T wave changes during the first seven days of life. *Am J Cardiol* 12:494, 1963.)

ACTIVATION OF THE HEART AS VIEWED
BY EACH OF THE TWELVE LEADS

As previously described in Chapter 1, the activation of the heart normally originates from the SA node and passes through the atria via three pathways (anterior, middle, and posterior) to the AV node, on to the bundle of His, to the right and left bundle (left anterior-superior division and posterior inferior division) branches, and finally into the Purkinje system of both ventricles. The impulse travels in an orientation from head to foot (superior to inferior). Activation of the ventricles occurs initially in the middle of the interventricular septum in a left to right fashion. The anteroseptal area of the ventricles is activated next and is followed by activation of both right and left ventricles. The posterobasal portion of the left ventricle, the pulmonary conus, and the upper part of the interventricular septum are activated last (3) (Fig. 3-18). The myocardium is activated (depolarized) from the endocardium to the epicardium, and repolarization occurs in the opposite direction, epicardium to endocardium. Atrial depolarization is recorded as the P wave on the ECG, and its configuration is seen in Figure 3-19.

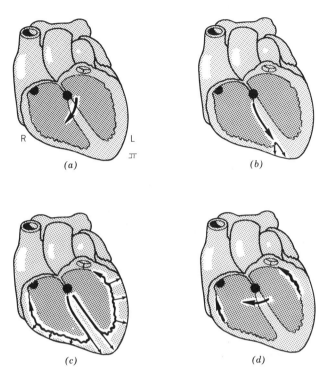

Figure 3-18. (*a*) Septal activtion across the ventricular system from left to right. (*b*) The anterior part of the ventricular septem is activated next. (*c*) Activation of both left and right ventricles proceeds from the endocardium to the epicardium. (*d*) The last part to be activated is the pulmonary conus, the posterobasal part of the left ventricle, and the upper part of the ventricular septum.

The P wave is negative in aV_R because the spread of the impulse is away from the positive pole of that particular lead. Leads aV_F, I, II, and V_{3-6} normally sense the impulse traveling toward their positive poles and inscribe an upright P wave. Leads III, aV_L, and V_{1-2} may record upright or inverted P waves, since the P vector is oriented to the left, inferiorly and anteriorly (3). The initial QRS vector is oriented to the right anteriorly and usually superiorly because the activation of midportion of the interventricular septum occurs in a left-to-right fashion. The right precordial leads (V_{1-2}) and lead aV_R sense this vector traveling toward them and inscribe a small R wave. The left precordial leads (V_{4-6}), the standard limb leads (I, II, and III), and aV_F and aV_L see this impulse traveling away from their positive poles and initially inscribe a small Q wave (Fig. 3-20).

The right and left ventricles are then activated with a greater electrical potential spreading through the left ventricle because of its larger size. The major QRS vector is oriented to the left inferiorly and posteriorly, accounting for the R waves in leads V_{4-6}, I, II, III, and aV_F. Lead aV_L will record a QS deflection if the mean axis is vertical ($+110°$ to $+75°$) or semivertical ($+75°$ to $+45°$), but will record an R wave if the mean axis is $+45°$ or less. A negative deflection (deep S wave) is recorded in leads aV_R and V_{1-2} (Fig. 3-21). The last portions of the myocardium to be activated include the posterobasal portion of the left ventricle, the pulmonary conus area, and the uppermost part of the

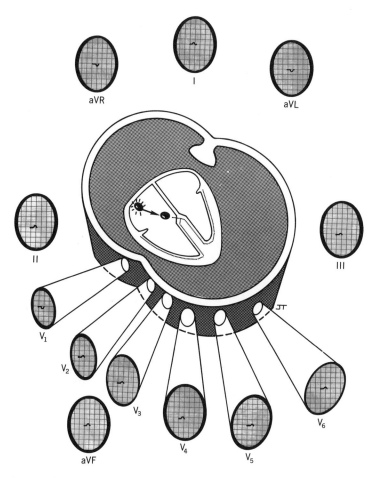

Figure 3-19. Development of the P wave (atrial activation) as seen in each of the 12 leads.

interventricular septum. This part of the QRS vector is oriented to the right and superiorly. A negative deflection (small S wave) is recorded in leads aV_F and V_{4-6}, and a small second positive deflection (r') may be recorded in leads aV_R and V_1 (3) (Fig. 3-22). Repolarization occurs after depolarization in a direction of epicardium to endocardium, the mean T vector oriented to the left, inferiorly and anteriorly. The T wave will then be upright in leads V_{3-6}, I, and II; inverted in aV_R; and variable leads in III, aV_L, aV_F, and V_{1-2} (2) (Fig. 3-23). Normal electrocardiograms of a young child, teenager, and adult are seen in Figures 3-24, 3-25, 3-26 respectively.

(Text continued on page 58.)

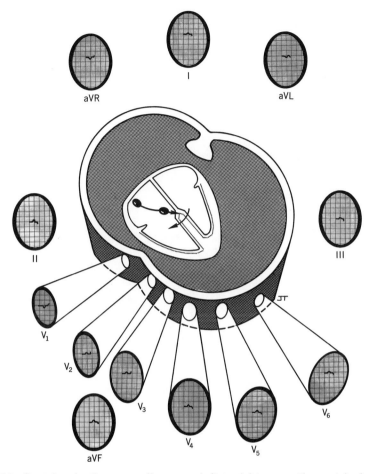

Figure 3-20. Septal activation normally occurs left to right across the ventricular septum. This is responsible for the initial part of the QRS complex.

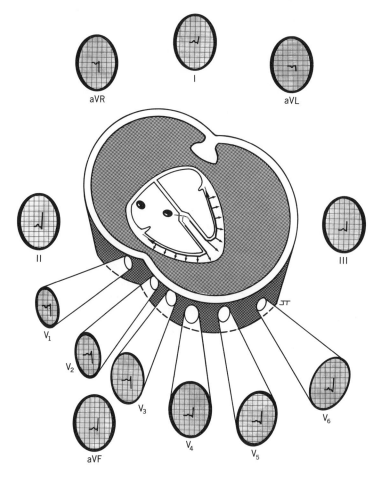

Figure 3-21. The majority of the right and left ventricles have been activated, accounting for the QRS complex.

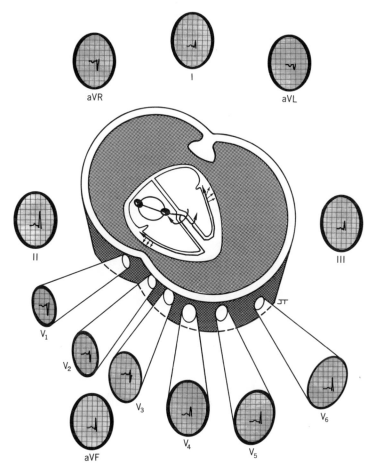

Figure 3-22. The last part of the QRS complex reflects activation of the pulmonary conus, the posterobasal part of the left ventricle and the upper part of the interventricular septum.

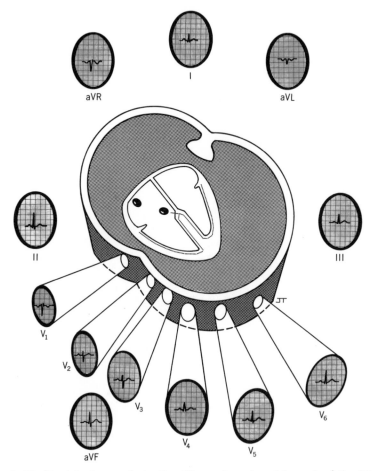

Figure 3-23. Ventricular repolarization (T wave) as viewed in each of the 12 leads.

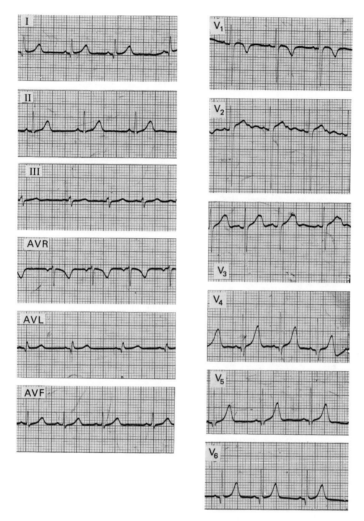

Figure 3-24. Rate: (atrial) <u>100</u> (ventricular) <u>100</u> Rhythm: sinus (sinus arrhythmia present)
PR interval: <u>0.10</u> sec QRS duration: <u>0.06</u> sec $\overline{QT}$c: <u>0.31</u> sec
P wave: (amplitude) <u>0.5</u> mm (duration) <u>0.04</u> sec
QRS: (amplitude) <u>12 mm in V_5</u> (Axis) <u>+49°</u> (pathologic Q waves) <u>none</u>
ST segment: (elevated) <u>none</u> (depressed) <u>none</u>
T wave: (amplitude) <u>6 mm in V_5</u> (axis) <u>+47°</u>
U wave: <u>$V_3 - V_4$</u> VAT: (V_1) <u>0.01</u> sec (V_6) <u>0.02 sec</u>
Impressions: Normal ECG tracing from a healthy 5-year-old boy. Note the prominent
sinus arrhythmia typically seen in young children.

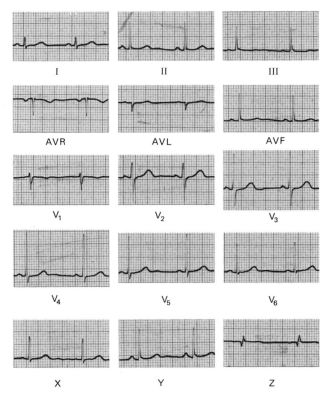

Figure 3-25. Rate: (atrial) <u>65</u> (ventricular) <u>65</u>. Rhythm: <u>sinus</u>
PR inteval: <u>0.16 sec</u> QRS duration: <u>0.06 sec</u> QTc: <u>0.37 sec</u>
P wave: (amplitude) <u>normal</u> (duration <u>0.10 sec</u>
QRS: (amplitude) <u>normal</u> (axis) <u>+79°</u> (pathologic Q waves) <u>none</u>
ST segment: (elevated) none (depressed) <u>none</u>
T wave: (amplitude <u>normal</u> (axis) <u>+53°</u>
U wave: none VAT: (V_1) <u>0.01 sec</u> (V_6) <u>0.01 sec</u>
Impressions: Normal ECG. (This is a tracing from a 15-year-old girl.)

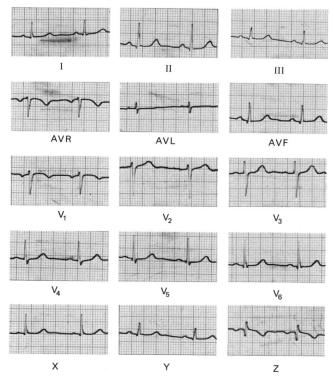

Figure 3-26. Rate: (atrial) <u>68</u> (ventricular) <u>68</u> Rhythm: <u>sinus</u>
PR interval: <u>0.16 sec</u> QRS duration: <u>0.09 sec</u> QTc duration: <u>0.40 sec</u>
P wave: (amplitude) <u>1 mm</u> (duration) <u>0.11 sec</u>
QRS: (amplitude) <u>normal</u> (axis) <u>+58°</u> (pathologic Q waves) <u>none</u>
ST segment: (elevated) <u>none</u> (depressed) <u>none</u>
T wave: (amplitude) <u>normal</u> (axis) <u>+65°</u>
U Wave: <u>none</u> VAT: (V$_1$) <u>0.01 sec</u> (V$_6$) <u>0.01 sec</u>
Impressions: Normal ECG. (This is a tracing from a 52-year-old
woman admitted for evaluation of severe chest pain.)

REVIEW QUESTIONS

1. Identify the proper positions for the placement of the six precordial (chest) leads.
2. How does a clockwise rotation differ from a counterclockwise rotation of the heart?
3. List four clinical conditions that can produce an abnormal left-axis deviation.

REFERENCES

1. Chung EK: *Electrocardiography: Practical Applications with Vectorial Principles.* Hagerstown, Md, Harper & Row Pub Inc, 1974, p 28.
2. Marriott HJL: *Practical Electrocardiography,* ed 6. Baltimore, Williams & Wilkins Co, 1977, p 2.
3. Goldman MJ: *Principles of Clinical Electrocardiography,* ed 10. Los Altos, Calif, Lange Medical Publications, 1979, p 3.
4. Arbeit SR, Rubin IL, Gross H: *Differential Diagnosis of the Electrocardiogram*, ed 2. Philadelphia, FA Davis Co, 1975, p 2.
5. Beckwith JR: *Grant's Clinical Electrocardiography: The Spatial Vector Approach.* New York, McGraw-Hill Book Co, 1970, p 17.
6. Waxman, HL, Castellanos A: Common Errors in electrocardiographic diagnosis. *Practical Cardiol* 5:25, 1979.
7. Frank E: An accurate, clinically practical system for spatial vectorcardiography. *Circulation* 13:737, 1956.
8. Lipman BS, Massie E. Kleiger RE: *Clinical Scalar Electrocardiography*, ed 6. Chicago, Year Book Medical Pub Inc, 1972, p 356.
9. Chou TC: *Electrocardiography in Clinical Practice*. New York, Grune & Stratton Inc, 1979, p 7.
10. Okomoto N, Kaneko K, et al: Reliability of individual frontal plane axis determination. *Circulation* 44:213, 1971.
11. Hait G, Gasul BM: The evolution and significance of T wave changes in the normal newborn during the first seven days of life. *Am J Cardiol* 12:494, 1963, p 494.
12. Eliot RS, Millhoun WA, Millhoun J: The clinical significance of uncomplicated marked left axis deviation in men without known heard disease. *Am J Cardiol* 12:767, 1963, p 770.

4
Systematic Analysis
of the
Electrocardiogram

The electrocardiogram is recorded on a graphlike paper, normally at a speed of 25 mm/sec. The paper has both vertical and horizontal lines at 1 mm intervals. Voltage or amplitude is measured along the vertical lines in millimeters (mm), and time is recorded along the horizontal lines in seconds. The distance between two darker lines on the electrocardiographic paper is 0.2 second in time and 5 mm in voltage; likewise, the distance between two lighter lines is 0.04 second and 1 mm respectively (Fig. 4-1). Most ECG paper is marked with vertical lines at the top at 3 second intervals, a convenient way for counting heart rate. Heart rate may be counted in a number of ways. The easiest method is to count the number of P-QRS complexes in a 6-second interval and multiply by 10. Another method is to count the number of small squares between R waves and divide this number into 1500. This gives the ventricular rate and the atrial rate to be obtained in a similar fashion using the P waves. The number 1500 is used because normal ECG paper speed is 25 mm/sec, which gives 1500 small squares (1500 mm) per minute. The heart rate may be roughly estimated by counting the number of large squares between R waves (or P waves) and divide into 300 (Fig. 4-1). If the heart rate varies considerably, then the slowest and fastest rates should be calculated or an average given.

Complexes are characterized as being upright (positive), inverted (negative), or diphasic with respect to the isoelectric line. The isoelectric line is a flat line used as a reference point for the measurement and configuration of all ECG complexes. It usually is considered to be level with that portion of the base line between the termination of the T wave and the beginning of the P wave or the TP segment. If the baseline is continued on through the ECG complex, the PR interval is usually level with the TP segment, and therefore for convenience it is often referred to as the isoelectric line (Fig. 4-2). The components of an ECG complex include P wave, PR interval, QRS complex, ST segment, T wave, QT interval, U wave, and the ID (intrinsicoid deflection). The latter component is also referred to as VAT (ventricular activation time) (1) (Fig. 4-3).

P WAVE

The P wave is the first component of the ECG and represents atrial depolarization or the spread of the electrical impulse through the atria. The ECG does not record SA node activity even though it normally precedes atrial activation (Fig. 4-4). The P wave does

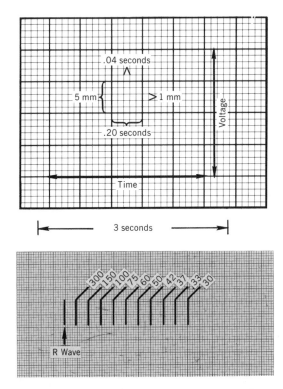

Figure 4-1. ECG paper consists of small and large squares that measure voltage and time. The heart rate may be calculated in the manner shown in this figure.

not represent atrial contraction that occurs after the P wave is recorded. It is normally upright in lead II and inverted in lead aV_R and may be variable in the other leads, depending on the P axis (normal P axis is $0°$ to $+90°$) (2) (Fig. 4-5) (see Chap. 4 for axis calculation). Comparison of the configurations of the P waves with a P wave axis of $0°$ and one of $+90°$ is seen in Table 4-1. The P waves in leads V_{1-2} are usually biphasic, the remainder of the precordial leads showing upright P waves; however, the mean P wave axis also influences this. A rule of thumb is that the P wave must be upright in lead II and inverted in lead aV_R to be considered normal. The normal P wave is rounded gently and not notched or pointed. It is not taller than 2.5 mm and does not have a duration longer than 0.11 second (1, 2). Clinical conditions producing an increased amplitude of the P wave include tricuspid valve disease, cor pulmonale, pulmonary hypertension, and various forms of congential heart disease. Left atrial enlargement of diseased atrial muscle usually produces an increased width of the P wave. An additional finding in the left

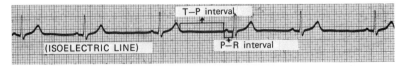

Figure 4-2. The isoelectric line (baseline) is a reference point used to determine whether complexes are negative (below baseline) or positive (above baseline).

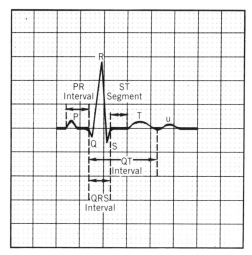

Figure 4-3. Components of the ECG complex.

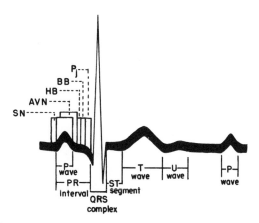

Figure 4-4. Normal sequence of activation in the surface electrocardiogram: from SA node through internodal and interatrial tracts to right atrium, left atrium, and AV node; from AV node through bundle of His, trifascicular system (right bundle, left anterior division, and left posterior division of left bundle) to Purkinje network and ventricles. Note that surface electrocardiogram records only atrial and ventricular activation. The sinus node activation is not recorded. The PR interval includes atrial conduction as well as the activation through the AV junction, AV node, His bundle, bundle branches, and Purkinje network. Intracardiac His bundle electrograms as well as bundle branch electrograms are recordable and permit localization of the site of any delay or block on the specialized conducting system. SN: sinus node activation; P wave: right and left atrial activation; AVN: atrioventricular node activation; HB: bundle of His activation; BB: right and left bundle branch activation; and P_j: Purkinje network activation. (Reproduced with permission from Lipman BS, Massie E, Kleiger RE: *Clinical Scalar Electrocardiography,* 6th edition. Copyright © 1972 by Year Book Medical Publishers, Inc., Chicago.)

Table 4-1. Systematic Analysis of the Electrocardiogram

P AXIS of 0°		*P AXIS of +90°*	
Lead	*Configuration*	*Lead*	*Configuration*
I, II, aV$_L$	Upright	II, III, aV$_F$	Upright
III, aV$_R$	Inverted	aV$_L$, aV$_R$	Inverted
aV$_F$	Isoelectric or biphasic	I	Isoelectric or biphasic

atrial enlargement is that the second half of the P wave is significantly negative in lead V$_1$ or lead III (3). Left atrial enlargement often becomes notched in the presence of mitral valve disease, and this M-shaped appearance has been termed the P mitrale wave (Fig. 4-6). In contrast, the right atrial enlargement is often characterized by tall, peaked (pointed) P waves in leads II, III, and aV$_F$ (2) (Fig. 4-7). The presence of upright P waves in lead aV$_R$ usually indicates an ectopic atrial or junctional rhythm. (Fig. 4-8). The Ta

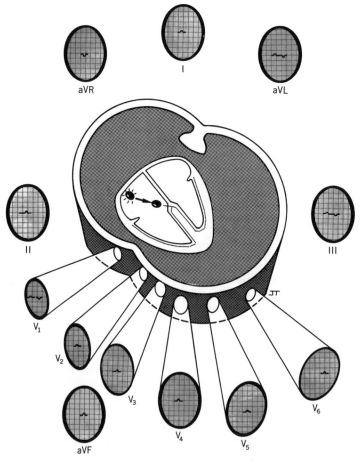

Figure 4-5. The direction of the normal frontal plane P vectors as seen by each of the six frontal plane leads.

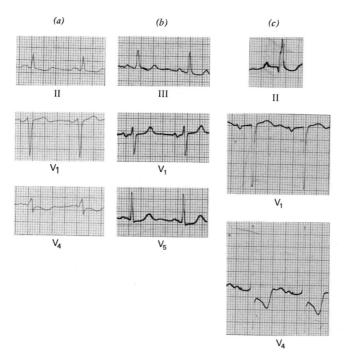

Figure 4-6. Three examples of left atrial enlargement with the typical features of broad, M-shaped P waves and the deep negative component of the P wave in V_1. (*a*) The P wave is quite broad, measuring 0.13 second. (*b*) Recorded from a 66-year-old woman with severe mitral stenosis. (*c*) Recorded from a man with long-standing systemic hypertension and congestive heart failure.

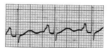

Figure 4-7. Tall, peaked P waves recorded in lead II. The P wave measures 3 mm tall.

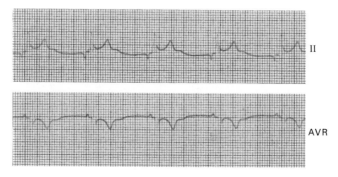

Figure 4-8. Junctional rhythm with the typical appearance of inverted P waves in lead II and upright P waves in lead aV_R.

wave represents atrial depolarization and is normally obscured from view because it coincides with the QRS complex. The Ta wave is normally in a direction opposite to the P wave and therefore is inverted in lead II and upright in lead aV_R (2).

PR INTERVAL

The PR interval or PQ interval represents the time it takes the impulse to travel from the SA node through the atria to the ventricular fibers and includes the normal 0.05-second delay at the AV node. This delay permits the atria to complete their systole and optimizes ventricular filling before the ventricles are activated (2). The PR interval is measured from the beginning of the QRS (Q or R wave) complex and is normally from 0.12 to 0.20 second in duration (see Fig. 4-3). The PR interval varies with heart rate and may become shorter with faster rates. Children also have shorter PR intervals, the average being 0.11 second at 1 year and 0.14 second at age 12. Prolonged PR intervals are seen in patients with conducting system disease, coronary artery disease, and rheumatic heart disease and who take digitalis (3). Normal persons with no evidence of heart disease have also been found to have a prolonged PR interval (4).

QRS COMPLEX

The QRS complex represents depolarization of the ventricles and is measured from the beginning of the Q wave to the end of the S wave. Normal QRS duration is 0.06 to 0.10 second, and frequently a slightly longer QRS interval (0.07-0.12 second) is present in the precordial leads (3). The first deflection, if it is negative (below the baseline), is called the Q wave. The presence of Q waves is one criterion used in the diagnosis of myocardial infarction. However, the mere presence of Q waves does not imply necrosis of the myocardium since certain criteria must be met to make them *diagnositc Q waves*. If the Q wave is 0.04 second (or greater) in duration and/or 25% (or greater) of the amplitude of the R wave, it is considered abnormal (2) (Fig. 4-9). Normal, small Q waves are seen in leads I, II, III, aV_L, aV_F, and V_{5-6} (1). The first positive deflection (above the baseline) is an R wave, which is normally less than 20 mm tall in the limb leads (may reach 30 mm) and less than 25 mm in the precordial leads (3). Normally, small R waves are seen in the

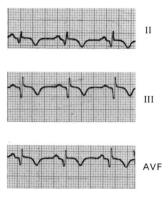

Figure 4-9. Pathologic Q waves seen with an acute inferior myocardial infarction. Note the depth and amplitude of these Q waves.

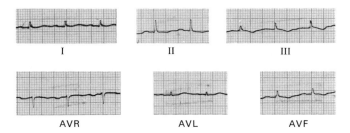

Figure 4-10. Low voltage seen in all six limb leads in a tracing from a patient with a pericardial effusion.

right precordial leads (V_{1-3}). The R wave is considered abnormal in these leads if the R:S (R wave to S wave) ratio exceeds 1.0. The total amplitude of the QRS (above and below the isoelectric line) must be 5 mm or greater in all three standard limb leads to be considered normal. Clinical conditions producing low voltage include pericardial effusion, obesity, emphysema, myxedema, primary amylidosis, cardiac failure, and diffuse myocardial damage (3) (Fig. 4-10).

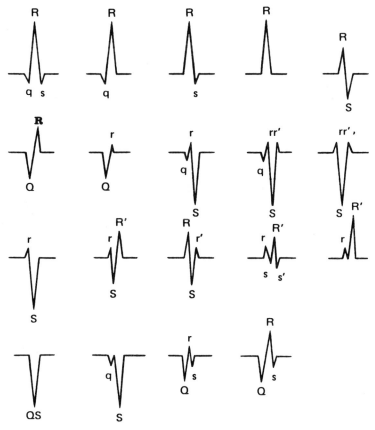

Figure 4-11. Various configurations of the QRS complex. (Reproduced with permission from Chung EK: *Electrocardiography: Practical Applications with Vectorial Principles.* Copyright © 1974 by Harper and Row, Pub., Inc. Hagerstown, Maryland.) (See text on next page.)

The negative deflection following the R wave is an S wave and is normally quite small except in the right precordial leads, but it becomes deep and wide in abnormal conditions, that is, ventricular hypertrophy and bundle branch blocks. Various configurations of the QRS complex may occur, and the term QRS complex may be used to describe the ventricular complex regardless of the deflections present (Fig. 4-11).

ST SEGMENT

The ST segment is that portion of the tracing that immediately follows the QRS complex. The J point is the point at which the ST segment departs form the main body of the QRS complex (3) (Fig. 4-12). Rather than forming a sharp angle with it, the ST segment

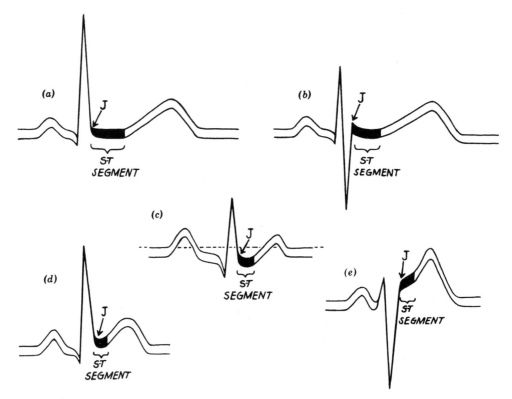

Figure 4-12. (a) The junction (J) between the QRS complex and the ST segment is isolectric, as is the ST segment. (b) The J is slightly elevated; the ST segment is isolectric. This is a normal variant. (c) The J and ST segment are slightly depressed; the PR segment is also depressed. This ST segment depression is within normal limits and is due to the repolarization wave of P (T_a wave). (d) The J and the ST segments are slightly elevated. Note that the ST segment is concave. The shift of J and ST is usually within normal limits. (e) The J and ST segments are elevated. The ST segment is slightly concave. Note the deep S wave and tall upright T associated with the shift of J and ST. This type of ST segment displacement is normal in right precordial leads. (Reproduced with permission from Arbeit SR, Rubin IL, Gross H: *Differential Diagnosis of the Electrocardiogram,* ed 2. Philadelphia, FA Davis Co, 1975.)

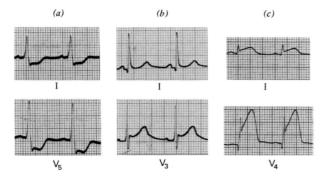

Figure 4-13. Abnormalities of the ST segment. (*a*) ST segment depression seen in states of myocardial ischemia. (*b*) ST segment elevation in a patient with pericarditis. (*c*) Marked ST segment elevation in a patient with an acute myocardial infarction (myocardial injury pattern).

normally curves gently into the T wave. The ST segment is isoelectric (level with the TP line) and may be elevated 2 mm or depressed 0.5 mm or less and still be considered normal (1) (Fig. 4-13). A deviation from this is found in about 2% of healthy adults, more commonly in young black persons (5, 6). The ST segment may be elevated as much as 4 mm in the anterolateral precordial and/or inferior limb leads. Upright T waves are usually associated with the concave appearance of the ST segment. This ST segment change is hypothesized to be related to an enhanced activity of the right sympathetic nerves (7) and is called the *early repolarization syndrome* (8) (Fig. 4-14).

T WAVE

Repolarization of the ventricles is manifested on the electrocardiogram in the T wave. Normally T waves are slightly rounded and slightly asymmetrical, the upstroke being longer than the downstroke. They are usually less than 5 mm tall in any standard lead and less then 10 mm tall in the precordial leads. An excess of potassium or myocardial infarction are two common conditions producing tall T waves (Fig. 4-15). Additional clinical settings in which tall T waves may be seen include: myocardial ischemia, ventricular overloading, psychosis, and cerebrovascular accidents (3). The direction of the T wave normally in the adult is upright in leads I, II, and V_{3-6}; inverted in lead aV_R; and variable in other leads, III, aV_L, aV_F, and V_{1-2} (3). However, before an abnormal T wave is implicated as reflecting myocardial ischemia, one must remember how sensitive the repolarization process is. The T wave is recorded during the mechanical systole of the ventricles and therefore it is subjected to a higher pressure gradient across the ventricular wall as well as to mechanical forces. Repolarization (T wave) requires metabolic work at the cellular level, whereas depolarization (QRS) does not; therefore any factor that affects cellular metabolism affects the T wave (9). A few of the factors affecting the T wave include drugs, acidosis, alkalosis, ice water, fever, exercise, eating, infections, anoxia, shock, hormones, and tilting (9).

There are two major groups of T wave changes, primary and secondary. The T wave

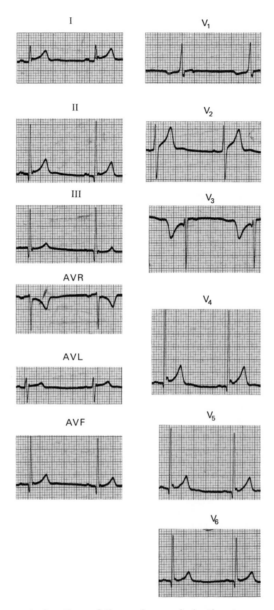

Figure 4-14. ST segment elevation of the early repolarization type recorded from a 22-year-old black male.

change is considered to be primary if it occurs independently of depolarization (QRS), and it is a secondary change if it occurs because of an abnormality of depolarization (QRS) (2). Primary T wave changes may be seen as a result of the following conditions: the presence of drugs (digitalis), tachycardia, cooling, ischemia, electrolyte imbalance, and increased stroke volume (9) [Fig. 4-16 (*a*)]. Secondary T wave changes may be seen with the left or right ventricular hypertrophy, Wolff-Parkinson-White syndrome, ventricular ectopic beats, left or right bundle branch block, and paced beats [Fig. 4-16 (*b*)].

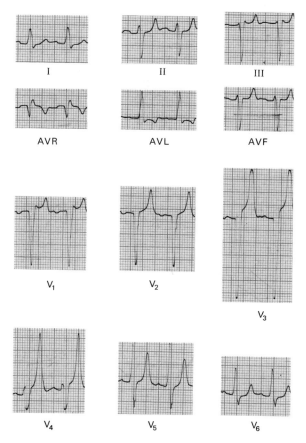

Figure 4-15. Tall tent-shaped T wave recorded from a patient with hyperkalemia.

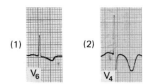

Figure 4-16. (a) Primary T wave changes: (1) digitalis (therapeutic levels) and (2) myocardial ischemia.

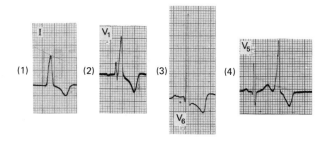

Figure 4-16. (b) Secondary T wave changes: (1) paced beat, (2) bundle branch block of the right bundle, (3) hypertrophy of the left ventricle, and (4) premature ventricular contraction.

69

QT INTERVAL

The QT interval is measured from the beginning of the QRS to the end of the T wave and varies with heart rate, sex, and age. This interval reflects the total time of ventricular (mechanical) systole. The QTc (corrected QT) intervals are usually determined by referring to a prepared table based on Ashman's (10) calculations (Table 4-2). An easy measurement for the calculation of the QT interval is the comparison of the RR interval with the QT interval. A general rule of thumb is: Normal QT interval = one-half preceding RR interval. This roughly holds true for a heart rate of approximately 65 to 90 beats per minute (3). Quinidine, procainamide (Pronestyl), hypocalcemia, and congestive heart failure may prolong the QT interval; and digitalis, hypercalcemia, and hyperpotassemia may shorten it (3). The significance of a prolonged QT interval is greater than a shortened one because of its effect of prolonging the relative refractory period. This sets the environment for the production of lethal ventricular arrhythmias. The relative refractory period (Chap. 2) includes the T wave, which is the ECG correlate of the vulnerable period of the ventricles. The ventricular vulnerable period is that period of the cardiac cycle in which the ventricles are thought to be susceptible to ventricular fibrillation if a PVC falls within that period. This is commonly referred to as the R-on-T phenomenon, in which a PVC falls on the upstroke or peak of the preceding T wave. The vulnerable period can be calculated from the ECG by measuring the QT intervals of the patient's

Table 4-2. Normal QT Intervals and the Upper Limits of the Normal

Cycle Lengths (sec)	Heart Rate (min)	Men and Children (sec)	Women (sec)	Upper Limits of the Normal Men and Children (sec)	Women (sec)
1.50	40	0.449	0.461	0.491	0.501
1.40	43	0.438	0.450	0.479	0.491
1.30	46	0.426	0.438	0.466	0.478
1.25	48	0.420	0.432	0.460	0.471
1.20	50	0.414	0.425	0.453	0.464
1.15	52	0.407	0.418	0.445	0.456
1.10	54.5	0.400	0.411	0.438	0.449
1.05	57	0.393	0.404	0.430	0.441
1.00	60	0.386	0.396	0.422	0.432
0.95	63	0.378	0.388	0.413	0.423
0.90	66.5	0.370	0.380	0.404	0.414
0.85	70.5	0.361	0.371	0.395	0.405
0.80	75	0.352	0.362	0.384	0.394
0.75	80	0.342	0.352	0.374	0.384
0.70	86	0.332	0.341	0.363	0.372
0.65	92.5	0.321	0.330	0.351	0.360
0.60	100	0.310	0.318	0.338	0.347
0.55	109	0.297	0.305	0.325	0.333
0.45	133	0.268	0.276	0.294	0.301
0.40	150	0.252	0.258	0.275	0.282
0.35	172	0.234	0.240	0.255	0.262

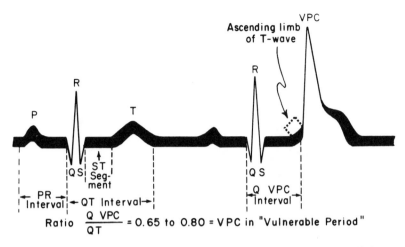

Figure 4-17. Representation of VPC falling in the "vulnerable period" of the preceding heart beat as seen on the ECG: R-on-T phenomenon. (Reproduced with permission from White, BB: *Therapy in Acute Coronary Care.* Copyright © 1971 by Year Book Medical Publishers, Inc., Chicago.)

normal beat and of the PVC (12) (Fig. 4-17). The PVC is considered to fall during the vulnerable period if the ratio of Q-PVC/QT intervals is from 0.65 to 0.80 second (12).

The long QT syndrome includes two primary syndromes: (*1*) Jervell and Lange Nielsen syndrome and (*2*) Romano-Ward syndrome, which are considered to be contributors to sudden death in children (13). The former syndrome is characterized by prolonged QT interval, congenital deafness, and syncope from ventricular fibrillation following physical or emotional stress (14). The Romano-Ward syndrome (15) is similar, but congenital deafness is absent (16).

U WAVE

The U wave is a small deflection sometimes seen following the T wave. There is little agreement about the cause of the U wave. Slow repolarization of the Purkinje system, stretch of the ventricles in diastole, and the result of "after potentials" have been implicated (11).

The U wave is normally 0.02 to 0.03 mV tall and normally has the same polarity as the preceding T wave (Fig. 4-18). Clinical conditions of hyperthyroidism, hypokalemia, and left ventricular hypertrophy may produce prominent U waves (11).

THE INTRINSICOID DEFLECTION

The intrinsicoid deflection (ID) is synonymous with ventricular activation time (VAT) and is measured from the beginning of the Q wave to the peak of the R wave. This interval reflects the time it takes the impulse to travel from endocardium to epicardium and is measured in the precordial leads (Fig. 4-19). The normal limits are 0.03 second or less in V_{1-2} and 0.05 second or less in V_{5-6} (1). This measurement is one criterion used by Estes in the diagnosis of LVH (Chap. 9).

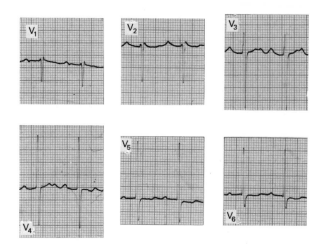

Figure 4-18. U waves are seen best in V_3 and V_4 in this tracing recorded from a patient wth hypokalemia. The U waves are upright and immediately follow the T waves.

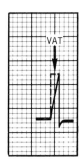

Figure 4-19. VAT is measured from the beginning of the QRS complex to the peak of the R wave (or S wave if the complex is negative).

Rate: (atrial) _____ (ventricular) _____ Rhythm _____

PR interval:_____ QRS duration _____ QT duration _____

P wave: (amplitude) _____ (duration) _____ (axis)_____

QRS: (amplitude)_____ (axis)_____ (pathologic Q waves)_____

ST segment: (elevated) _____ (depressed) _____

T wave: (amplitude) _____ (axis) _____

U wave: _____

VAT: V_{1-2} _____ V_{5-6} _____

Impressions: _____

_____

_____

Figure 4-20. Analysis of the electrocardiographic tracing.

A uniform approach should be adapted in the analysis of an electrocardiogram to avoid overlooking certain subtle abnormalities. Normally the heart rate and rhythm are evaluated first. The following is one approach to use in the analysis (Fig. 4-20).

LADDERGRAMS

Ladder diagrams were used by Sir Thomas Lewis and are therefore sometimes called Lewis lines. They are especially helpful in the analysis of complex arrhythmias. Although five tiers are used in the laddergram (Fig. 4-21), the SA and E tiers may be omitted for simple rhythms. The site of the impulse formation is usually indicated by a black dot, and the lines representing atrial and ventricular depolarization are drawn under the tracing. The A line begins at the beginning of the P wave and ends at the end of that wave. The QRS complex is drawn next, the line beginning at the Q wave and terminating at the end of the S wave in the V tier (Fig. 4-22). The lines are drawn in a superior-

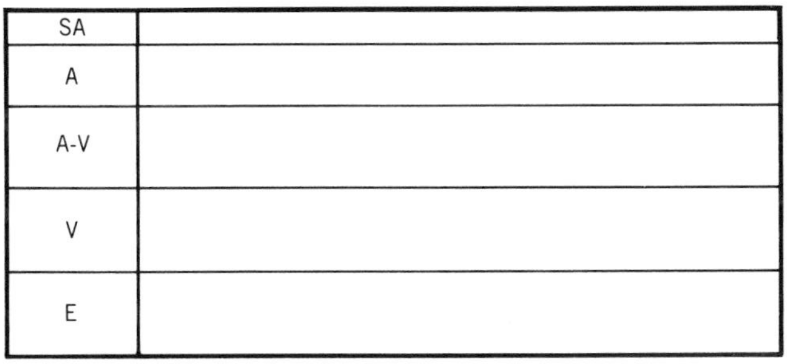

SA	
A	
A-V	
V	
E	

Figure 4-21. Five tiers may be used in the construction of a laddergram; however, three tiers (A, AV, and V) are most commonly used. SA: sinoatrial node; A: atrial; AV: atrioventricular; V: ventricular; and E: ectopic.

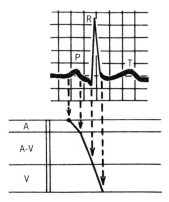

Figure 4-22. The construction of a ladder diagram during normal sinus rhythm. (Reproduced with permission from Lipman BS, Massie E, and Kleiger RE: *Clinical Scalar Electrocardiography,* 6th edition. Copyright © 1972 by Year Book Medical Publishers, Inc., Chicago.)

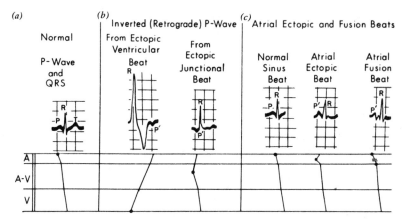

Figure 4-23. (*a*) Normal conduction through atria, specialized conducting system, and ventricles with normal laddergram. (*b*) Ectopic ventricular and ectopic junctional beats with retrograde P waves (P′). (*c*) Normal atrial, ectopic atrial, and atrial fusion beats with laddergrams. Note contour of P′ waves. (Reproduced with permission from Lipman BS, Massie E, Kleiger RE: *Clinical Scalar Electrocardiography*, 6th edition. Copyright © 1972 by Year Book Medical Publishers, Inc., Chicago.)

inferior direction (left to right), indicating normal antegrade spread of the electrical impulse. Arrows may be used to show the direction of the impulse as well. After the A and V tiers are drawn, the AV tier is then drawn in to connect all three tiers. A pair of slightly divergent lines has been used to indicate that conduction through the ventricles is aberrant (9) (see Chap. 6). A short line drawn perpendicular (horizontally) to the line depicting conduction indicates that the impulse is blocked. Retrograde conduction is

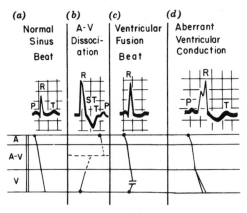

Figure 4-24. (*a*) Normal sinus conduction with laddergram. (*b*) AV dissociation with independent ventricular and atrial rhythms delayed (as represented by dashed line) and blocked (as shown by horizontal dashed line) at the AV level. (*c*) Ventricular fusion beat with merging at the ventricular level of two impulses, one originating in the sinus node and the other originating in an ectopic ventricular focus. (*d*) Aberrant ventricular conduction from a supraventricular origin, showing the aberration of the ventricular level by the two divergent lines. (Reproduced with permission from Lipman BS, Massie E, Kleiger RE: *Clinical Scalar Electrocardiography*, 6th edition. Copyright © 1972 by Year Book Medical Publishers, Inc. Chicago.)

depicted as a line sloping upward from right to left. A dotted line is used to represent the His bundle area and is commonly drawn in the middle of the AV tier to depict AV dissociation (9) (Fig. 4-23). Ectopic beats and fusion beats may be associated with retrograde conduction, which is graphically displayed as a line drawn left to right in an upward fashion (Fig. 4-24).

REVIEW QUESTIONS

1. List the normal values for the following components of the ECG:
   a. P wave width and amplitude
   b. QRS width and amplitude
   c. PR interval
   d. T wave amplitude
2. Myocardial infarctions are in part based on the presence of pathologic Q waves on the ECG. What is a pathologic Q wave and in what leads may a small Q wave normally be seen?
3. Abnormalities of the ST segment may be present without signifying organic heart disease. Explain the ECG appearance of the early repolarization syndrome. What is the J point and what purpose does it serve?

REFERENCES

1. Goldman MJ: *Principles of Clinical Electrocardiography,* ed 10, Los Altos, Calif, Lange Medical Publications, 1979, p 25.
2. Chung EK: *Electrocardiography: Practical Applications with Vectorial Principles.* Hagerstown, Md, Harper & Row Pub Inc, 1974, p 51.
3. Marriott HJL: *Practical Electrocardiography*, ed 6. Baltimore, Williams & Wilkins Co, 1977, p 16.
4. Johnson, RL: Electrocardiographic findings in 67,375 asymptomatic individuals. Part VII. AV block. *Am J Cardiol* 6:153, 1960.
5. Parisi AF, Beckman CH, Lancaster MC: The spectrum of ST segment elevation in the electrocardiograms of healthy adult men. *Electrocardiol* 4:137, 1971.
6. Seriki O, Smith AJ: The electrocardiograms of young Nigerians. *Am Heart J* 72:153, 1966.
7. Morace G, Padeletti L: Effect of isoproterenol on the "early repolarization" syndrome. *Am Heart J* 97:343, 1979.
8. Grant RP, Estes EH, Doyle JT: Spatial vector electrocardiography. The clinical characteristics of ST and T vectors. *Circulation* 3:182, 1951.
9. Lipman BS, Massie E, Kleiger RE: *Clinical Scalar Electrocardiography*, ed 6. Chicago, Year Book Medical Pub Inc, 1972, p 60.
10. Ashman R, Hull E: *Essentials of Electrocardiography*. New York, Macmillan Inc, 1944, p 344.
11. Kossman CE: The U Wave, in Kossman CE (ed): *Advances in Electrocardiography*. New York, New York, Grune & Stratton Inc, 1958, p 186.
12. White BB: *Therapy in Acute Coronary Care*, Chicago, Year Book Medical Pub Inc, 1971, p 28.
13. Fraser G, Froggatt P: Unexpected cot deaths. *Lancet* 2:56, 1966.
14. Jervell A, Lange-Nielsen F: Congenital deaf-mutism, functional heart disease with prolongation of the QT interval, and sudden death. *Am Heart J* 54:59, 1957.
15. Romano C, Gemme G, et al: Aritmie cardiache rare dell'età pediatrica. *Clin Pediatr* 45:656, 1963.
16. Ward O: New familial cardiac syndrome in children. *J Ir Med Assoc* 54:103, 1964.

5
Sinus Disturbances

SINUS TACHYCARDIA

According to Myerburg and El-Sherif (1), sinus tachycardia may be defined as a sinus rhythm with a rate in excess of 100 beats per minute in the average adult population. It is said to be present in children when the heart rate is greater than 150 beats per minute and in the newborn when the rate is up to 300 beats per minute (2).

The mechanisms related to the onset of sinus tachycardia are multifactorial (Table 5-1). Any condition that permits the pacemaking cells of the sinoatrial node to reach threshold potential more rapidly can initiate sinus tachycardia. The sinus node has the ability to gradually depolarize until the threshold potential is reached and complete electrical discharge takes place. When diastolic depolarization occurs, it produces the characteristic upward slope of the action potential curve termed *phase 4*. The extent to which certain physiological conditions produce sinus tachycardia is related to their direct action on phase 4.

Pathogenesis

As the slope of phase 4 is increased, the cycle length is shortened and the rate increases (3). Hence, it is not uncommon to see sinus tachycardia in association with the following conditions:

1. As a physiological mechanism in response to an increase in metabolic activity of the body resulting in greater demand for oxygenation (4, 5)
2. As a compensatory mechanism in an effort to increase cardiac output
3. In response to pharmacological agents
4. As a consequence of underlying pathology

Sinus tachycardia may be related to various physiological mechanisms. In the presence of a fall in blood pressure, baroreceptors located in the arch of the aorta as well as in the carotid sinus are stimulated and evoke the sympathetic response of a rapid heart rate.

An increase in right atrial volume associated with an augmented venous return, secondary to increased body activity and/or heart failure, are accompanied by sinus tachycardia mediated by the Bainbridge reflex. Exercise produces tachycardia through the mechanism of sympathetic stimulation and catecholamine release (6). Body temperature elevation is accompanied by an increase in heart rate. For every degree of temperature rise, the cardiac rate increases from eight to ten beats. A decrease of oxygen content associated with high altitude or in association with congenital heart defects, is accompanied by tachycardia (7). During periods of hypoxia or anxiety, catecholamines are released through adrenal and sympathetic stimulation.

Table 5-1. Mechanism of Sinus Tachycardia

Compensatory Mechanism (to increase cardiac output for)	Physiological Mechanism (in response to)	Drug-Related	Pathological Mechanism
Hemorrhage	Maximal exercise	Atropine	Infection (febrile illness)
Shock	Pain	Amphetamines	Sepsis
Anemia	Emotion	Isoproteronol	Fluid depletion
Congestive heart failure	Psychic trauma	Ephedrine	Embolic phenomenon
	Respiration (end-inspiration)		Fever
	Application of heat to body		Hyperthyroidism
	Ingestion of food		Myocardial infarction (impaired cardiac reserve)
	Excessive use of coffee, tea, alcohol		Neurosis
	Increase in sympathetic tone		
	Decrease in vagal tone		

Electrocardiographic Features

The discharge sequence of sinus tachycardia in the adult is within the range of 100 to 160 beats per minute (8) (Fig. 5-1). Occasionally, the rate may be as rapid as 180 beats per minute, especially in the presence of electrolyte imbalance, fluid depletion, sepsis, and/or maximal exertion (2). The remaining diagnostic criteria for normal sinus rhythm are not altered.

P wave	Clearly identifiable in heart rates less than 150 beats per minute
PR interval	Constant and within normal range, 0.12–0.20 msec
QRS complex	Normal in duration and configuration
ST segment and T wave	Changes may be seen with exercise
QT interval	May shorten as the cycle length decreases
PP or RR intervals	Regular or slightly irregular

Clinical Spectrum

Generally, the average rate of sinus tachycardia does not of itself produce such adverse hemodynamic effects as to be responsible for the production of symptoms (8). However,

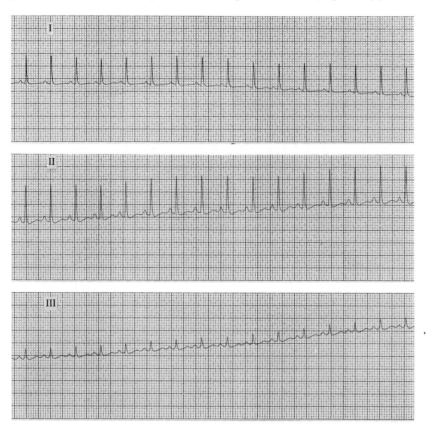

Figure 5-1. Sinus tachycardia.

with extremely rapid heart rates, the person may experience palpitations, breathlessness, and/or chest discomfort.

Palpitations are usually a result of the rapid action of the heart and may be described by the patient as a pounding or racing heart. Consequently the patient may become apprehensive, restless, or anxious.

Chest discomfort may be attributed to the shortening of the diastolic phase of the cardiac cycle as well as to the increase of metabolic needs of the myocardium. Since the coronary arteries fill primarily during diastole, encroachment upon this particular phase of the cardiac cycle generally shortens the filling time during which coronary blood flow occurs. Consequently an imbalance develops between blood supply and myocardial demand.

Breathlessness as experienced by the patient may be attributed to pooling of the blood in the lungs secondary to the decrease in filling time of the ventricles. The accumulation of blood can account for the labored breathing (9). The onset of sinus tachycardia in the presence of mitral valvular disease imposes a burden on the left atrium and subsequent pulmonary vasculature. Since an impediment to the free flow of blood exists with stenosis of the valve, an increase in cardiac rate further encroaches on the time in which atrial emptying can occur. This then predisposes the pulmonary vasculature to a state of congestion. Pulmonary plethora can also occur when the mitral valve is incompetent, and reflux of blood takes place during the isometric contraction phase of the cardiac cycle.

Sinus tachycardia, when sustained in the presence of an extensively damaged myocardium, is of graver prognostic significance than in the absence of myocardial infarction (10). The rapid sinus rate, by increasing the workload of the heart, can likewise extend the area of infarction. Sustained sinus tachycardia in the presence of a myocardial infarction may imply that the efficiency of the heart as a pump has become compromised. Thus in the presence of sinus tachycardia, the clinical spectrum may range from a total absence of manifestations to symptomology of minor significance.

Therapy

Intervention when necessary is usually directed at the cause of the tachycardia. Frequently when the rate of sinus tachycardia exceeds 150 beats per minute, it may be somewhat difficult to differentiate this rhythm from that of other paroxysmal tachycardias. Carotid sinus pressure during sinus tachycardia may have no effect or only a slight slowing of cardiac activity. However, when the maneuver of carotid sinus pressure is terminated, heart rate will gradually return to the premaneuver rate. In contrast, if atrial or junctional tachycardias are responsive to carotid sinus pressure, termination of the pressure will restore the heart rate to a normal sinus rhythm (11).

SINUS BRADYCARDIA

Sinus bradycardia, a subgroup of the classification bradyarrhythmias, may be defined as a heart rate of less than 60 beats per minute in the average adult (12), less than 100 beats in infants, and less than 80 beats in children (2). The sequence of conduction from the sinus node through atrioventricular pathways is otherwise normal.

Pathogenesis

Sinus bradycardia reflects a slow discharge of the sinus node which may be secondary to a variety of conditions (Table 5-2). The mechanisms related to the bradycardia differ (13).

Table 5-2. Mechanism of Sinus Bradycardia

Physiological Responses	Increase in Vagal Tone	Pathology-Related	Drug-Related
Increase in aortic pressure and carotid sinus pressure	Emotional trauma	Obstructive jaundice	Narcotics Demerol Morphine
Vagal maneuvers	Eyeball compression (patients secondary to surgery; compression bandage in patients previously digitalized)	Myxedema	Cardiotonic Digitalis
Decreased metabolic needs (during sleep) (aging process)	Carotid massage	Hyperthyroidism Increased intracranial pressure Myocardial infarction Hypothermia	Beta blockage Agents
Conditioned training	Valsalva maneuver Endotracheal suctioning Manipulation of viscera, gall bladder tugging Mushroom poisoning		

Myerburg and El-Sherif (1) consider sinus bradycardia to be a normal physiological event during sleep and during the time a trained athlete is resting.

The bradycardia commonly found in athletes who train for a long period of time is attributed to the mechanism of slowing of the intrinsic rate of the sinoatrial node and depression of tonic influence upon the sympathetic nerves. In the nonathlete, greater body activity is met by an increase in heart rate, whereas in the long distance runner or cross country skier, for example, there is a greater utilization of stroke volume (14).

In association with obstructive jaundice, sinus bradycardia is thought to be related to the depressant effect of bile salts upon the sinoatrial node. A decrease in sympathetic stimulation as a result of a decrease in metabolic activity may be the mechanism of sinus bradycardia in myxedema and hypopituitrism (7). According to Sokolow (15) sinus bradycardia in the presence of hypothyroidism results from a decrease in the phase 4 depolarization slope of the action potential curve (see page 30). Digitalis has a vagal stimulatory effect upon the heart. Since vagal fibers are predominant within the sinoatrial and atrioventricular nodes, the action of digitalis increases the refractoriness of the junctional tissue (2). Chung (16) emphasizes the fact that the sudden onset of sinus bradycardia in a patient treated with digitalis could reflect toxicity of the drug. Morphine sulfate, a drug commonly used for the relief of pain, likewise has vagomimetic properties. Deaths attributed to mushroom poisoning occur as a result of inhibition of sinoatrial activity by muscarine, the principle ingredient of certain mushrooms (17). Sinus bradycardia is frequently a secondary event in the occurrence of an inferior myocardial infarction (see Chap. 10).

Electrocardiographic Features

Rate	Less than 60 beats per minute in the average adult population (Fig. 5-2).
	Less than 80 beats per minute in children.
P wave	Normal in configuration (shape, amplitude, duration).
	Indicative of sinus origin.
PR interval	Normal range (0.12–0.20) constant.
	May be associated with first-degree block.
	The mechanism causing increased vagatonic effect on the sinus node can also affect the junctional area.
QRS duration	Normal (0.10 upper limits).
	The impulse upon reaching first the interventricular septum and then the free wall of the ventricles is conducted normally; hence the QRS complex is undisturbed.
QT interval	An increase in the cycle length results in prolongation of the QT interval (13).

QT Interval
Associated with Heart Rate

Heart Rate	Men and Children	Women
60	0.386 sec	0.396 sec
50	0.414 sec	0.425 sec
40	0.449 sec	0.461 sec

Rhythm	Usually regular but may be associated with sinus arrhythmia.

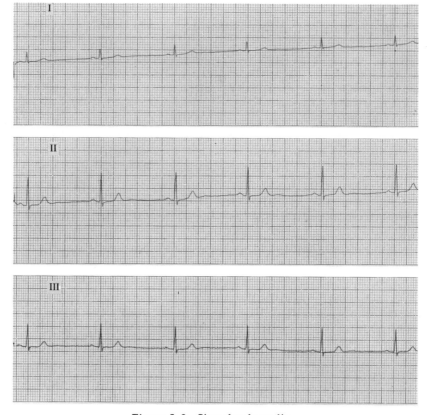

Figure 5-2. Sinus bradycardia.

Clinical Spectrum

Usually there are no symptoms associated with sinus bradycardia unless the heart rate is extremely slow. Rates below 40 beats per minute are known to produce hemodynamic alterations, especially in the presence of a myocardial infarction (13). Symptoms, when present, occur as a result of a decrease in cardiac output. Lightheadedness, dizziness, fatigability, hypotension, and syncope thus become evident (11). Dyspnea too may occur and is usually a response to reflex stimulation of the ventilatory apparatus in the medulla. Exercise intolerance may be a finding in the individual who is taking Inderal.

The significance of extreme sinus bradycardia lies in its effect upon cardiac output and/or the predisposition to heart ectopy, either as active rhythms (usurpation) or by passive rhythms (escape).

Therapy

Usually sinus bradycardia requires no treatment unless the sinus rate is extremely slow and the patient has symptoms of disease. This may be especially true in the presence of a compromised cardiac output, which cannot be increased in response to the metabolic needs of the body. Atropine is a drug of choice in sinus bradycardia because of its anti-cholinergic effects. Other sympathomimetic agents used, although less frequently are isoproterenol and epinephrine. The insertion of an electronic or artificial pacemaker may be considered if the sinus node discharge is extremely slow and cardiac output is diminished. A maneuver employed during the angiocardiography process is that of asking the patient to cough. This maneuver tends to break the vagal tone. The monitoring of vital measurements for indices of compromised circulation and/or dysrhythmias is an important aspect of nursing care, particularly when the sinus bradycardis is associated with myocardial infarction (see Chap. 10).

SINUS ARRHYTHMIA

Sinus arrhythmia is a cyclic variation in heart rate that can be associated with either respiratory or nonrespiratory factors. The more common type, respiratory or phasic sinus arrhythmia, is a response to vagal stimulation and/or suppression. On inspiration, the heart rate tends to increase, while on exhalation, the rate slows. One of the mechanisms involved in the cyclic influence upon the sinus node is thought to be related to an increase in pressure in the right atrium and great veins.

Mechanisms

During inspiration, as the chest cavity enlarges, the thoracic, vena caval, and atrial pressures decrease (18). This is thought to create a vacuum effect, which enhances a greater venous return to the right atrium. With greater filling of the right atrium, the pressure-sensitive receptors reflexly accelerate the heart rate (Bainbridge reflex) (19). As the volume in the chamber is lost, the pressure and stretch of the atrium decreases, thus abolishing the accelerating effect on the heart. According to Cooksey (20), the inhibitory effect of vagal stimulation associated with expiration is limited primarily to the head of the sinus node, thus allowing the lower segment, or tail, which has a slower rate of impulse formation to control the heart rate momentarily. The cycle variant is then repeated with the beginning of inspiration. Another reflex influencing heart rate during respiration is the Hering-Breuer reflex. Pleural stretching secondary to inspiration influences receptors, which initiate a vagal inhibitory response on the heart, permitting the rate to increase. Sinus arrhythmia is intensified by exaggerated breathing and is detensified by breath holding. Iriuchijima (21), after much experimental work, believes that the major problem associated with respiratory sinus arrhythmia is the lack of response of the cardioinhibitory center to baroreceptor impulses. He further contends that in addition to the cardiorespiratory center two other factors are implicated in the mechanism of respiratory sinus arrhythmia. These are an intact respiratory center and functional baroreceptor impulses.

A less common form of sinus arrhythmia is the ventriculophasic type, which is thought to be induced by mechanical and/or hemodynamic mechanisms. This is the type of sinus arrhythmia that occurs in approximately 30% to 40% of persons who have complete heart block (see p. 127). Several mechanisms have been postulated to cause nonrespiratory (ventriculophasic) sinus arrhythmia. According to Chung (16) and Schamroth (7), the following must be considered:

1. A rise in intra-atrial pressure after ventricular contraction. As the right atrial pressure rises, afferent nerve fibers within atrial muscle are stimulated and evoke the Bainbridge reflex. The result is an increase in heart rate resulting from vagal inhibition.

2. Augmented blood supply to the sinoatrial node following contraction. The sinus node responds to the increased perfusion by more rapid discharge.
3. Traction on the atria resulting from the tension and pressure buildup associated with ventricular contraction.

Schamroth (7) identifies still another type of nonrespiratory sinus arrhythmia, *the prematurity induced sinus arrhythmia*. An ectopic focus in the atria can suppress the activity of the sinoatrial node and alter its rhythmicity. This then results in the irregularity of sinus discharge.

Electrocardiographic Features

The electrocardiographic criterion for sinus arrhythmia is the time interval between the longest and shortest cycle, which must exceed 0.16 second (13) (Fig. 5-3). In the respiratory form, the tracing will depict a cycle length (PP interval) that gradually increases and shortens in association with the phase of respiration. The P wave at times may appear more peaked than a preceding P wave. This suggests that the pacemaking site within the sinoatrial node may be variable. The PR interval usually is constant and within the normal range. However, it can be shorter than normal, depending upon the effect the phase or respiration has upon vagal tone. Since the transmission of the impulse through the ventricles is unaltered, the QRS-T complex is normal in configuration and duration.

Significance

Phasic sinus arrhythmia is a normal physiological response to respiration and in some instances to the mechanical effect of ventricular contraction. It is commonly seen in children, young adults, and occasionally older persons. With increasing age, however, respiratory sinus arrhythmia is less marked. Usually the individual is unaware of the fact that changes in the electrocardiogram occur concomitantly with the respiratory phases of breathing or with the mechanical activity of the heart; therefore intervention is not indicated. Although nonrespiratory sinus arrhythmia is frequently seen in healthy individuals, it is nonetheless found in association with cardiac disease. Therefore there may be graver implications associated with it.

There are usually no symptoms associated with sinus arrhythmia. However, if an extremely slow heart rate is associated with the disturbance, the individual may experience palpitations or presyncopal attacks. Therapy therefore is directed toward the causative factor, particularly in the nonrespiratory type.

SINOATRIAL BLOCK; SINUS PAUSE

As mentioned in Chapter 1 under "The Conduction System," the sinus node has the fastest inherent rate and thus sets the "tempo" of the cardiac rate. Occasionally, the sinoatrial node may fail to discharge an impulse; it may take longer for the impulse to activate the atrial myocardium, or an exit block may prevent the discharged impulses from reaching the atrial muscle. Dysfunction of this type results in what is commonly termed *sinoatrial block*, which, according to Ferrer (22), may be subdivided into three forms: first-degree, second-degree, and third-degree. First-degree sinoatrial block implies that the sinus node has discharged an impulse, but there is a delay in reaching the atrial myocardium. The most common form of second-degree sinoatrial block may be identified electrocardiographically by the absence of one or more P-QRS-T complexes. In third-

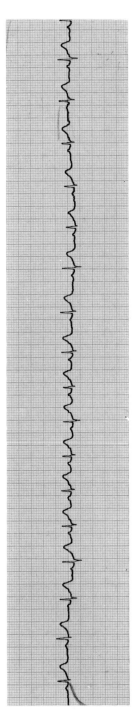

Figure 5-3. Normal ECG. There is a prominent sinus arrhythmia.

degree sinoatrial block, there is a complete absence of impulses leaving the pacemaker site, resulting in an escape beat-rhythm or cardiac arrest with asystole (23).

The term *sinus pause* has likewise been used to designate the failure of the sinus node to discharge an impulse for one or more beats (20). The difference between the two is reflected electrocardiographically.

Pathogenesis

Failure of the sinus node to discharge or relay its impulse to the atrial myocardium may be a result of digitalis or quinidine therapy, slowing of the atrial rate, vagotonia (gagging, vomiting), hypersensitivity of the carotid sinus, infectious processes such as myocarditis, or electrolyte imbalance such as hyperkalemia, or as a secondary event to myocardial infarction and/or a degenerative process of the sinus node (22, 23). In the presence of an inferior myocardial infarction, Hatle and associates (24) believe that the sinus node dysfunction is most frequently a temporary event. Dhingra and associates have found a high incidence of sinus and atrial dysrhythmias in subjects who had prolongation of sino-atrial conduction time (25). Occasionally sinoatrial activation can likewise be prolonged as a result of sinus node depression by an ectopic pacemaker which prematurely de-polarizes the sinus node.

Electrocardiographic Features

First- and third-degree sinoatrial block cannot be detected on the electrocardiographic tracing. A sinus pause equal to two or three times the cycle length may suggest second-degree sinoatrial block. Owing to the absence of atrial activation, the P-QRS-T complex is missing for one or more beats. Sinus pause has been distinguished from sinoatrial block by the time of the pause between two sinus beats. In sinoatrial block, the RR interval contains a pause equal to twice or another multiple of the duration between two sinus beats (22) (see Fig. 7-1). The term *sinus pause* has been reserved for that part of the electrocardiographic tracing depicting absence of sinoatrial activation, as evidenced by a pause less than twice the normal RR interval (20).

Clinical Spectrum

In itself, sinoatrial block may not be accompanied by symptoms. If, however, they are present, they are usually associated with irregularity of pulse. Other manifestations are dizziness and syncope. Dhingra (25) found that in the presence of sinus and atrial dys-rhythmias associated with prolonged sinoatrial conduction time, syncope had been related to the bradyarrhythmias and in one instance to ventricular tachycardia. Dizziness was related to atrial tachycardia. Exertional angina, dyspnea, and palpitation occurred secondary to underlying cardiovascular disease.

Palpation of the radial pulse may reveal a normal but occasionally slower heart rate that is regular in rhythm but periodically interrupted by a pause. This finding may suggest the presence of a premature ventricular beat with a complete compensatory pause. The distinction is made upon auscultation of the heart. Absence of both apical and radial beats is more suggestive of sinoatrial block than premature ventricular beat (26).

Therapy

The mode of therapy is directed to the elimination of the cause. If it is drug-initiated, the agent should be withdrawn and a sinoatrial stimulant such as isoproterenol should be administered. Vagotonia may respond to atropine. Isoproterenol is a positive iono-tropic and chronotropic agent. It stimulates pacemaker cells, dilates coronary vessels, and increases stroke volume and cardiac output. Atropine, when given in moderate to large doses, has an accelerating effect upon the heart rate by interfering with vagal stimuli of the heart (27). In the presence of frequent and prolonged pauses accompanying sino-atrial block, the insertion of an electronic, artificial, or mechanical pacemaker may be indicated (22).

SICK SINUS SYNDROME

The sick sinus syndrome, often referred to as the bradycardia-tachycardia syndrome, encompasses symptoms of syncope or presyncope resulting from sinus nodal and/or atrial disturbances in which cardiac output is compromised (28). Included in the entity are episodes of inappropriate sinus bradycardia, sinoatrial block, sinus arrest with alternate periods of tachyarrhythmias in the form of paroxysmal atrial and junctional tachycardia, atrial fibrillation, and atrial flutter (12). (Fig. 5-4). The mechanism implicated in the bradyarrhythmias and tachyarrhythmias has been attributed to several factors. According to Fruehan (29), the following mechanisms must be considered:

1. The functional ineffectiveness of the sinus node to initiate and conduct the impulse. This may be attributed to sinus node dysfunction and/or replacement of sinus nodal tissue by fibrous strands.
2. The presence of sinoatrial block.
3. The reactivation of the sinus node by the process of reentry.

Pathogenesis

According to Cooksey and associates (20), a wide etiology can be implicated in the genesis of the sick sinus syndrome. Ischemic lesions and/or infiltrative processes of the sino-atrial node, atrial myocardium, and junctional tissue can interfere with impulse formation and conduction. Patients experiencing an inferior myocardial infarction may likewise develop the sick sinus syndrome (see Chap. 10). Jordan and colleagues (30) have likewise

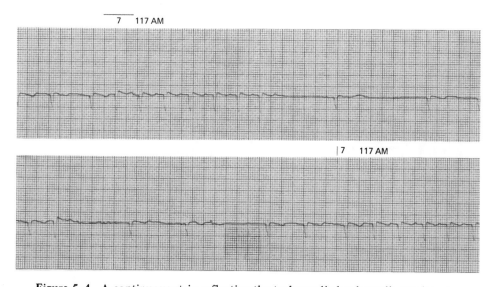

Figure 5-4. A continuous strip reflecting the tachycardia-bradycardia syndrome.

Table 5-3. Sequelae of Bradyarrhythmia (See text on page 90.)

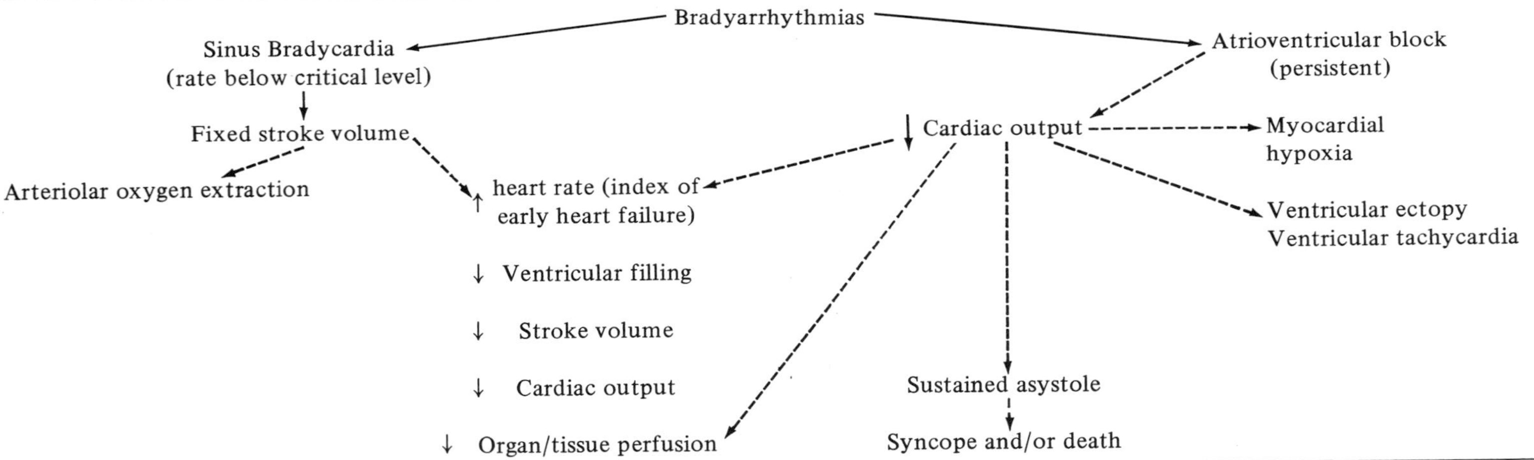

Bradyarrhythmias

Sinus Bradycardia (rate below critical level)

Fixed stroke volume

Arteriolar oxygen extraction

↑ heart rate (index of early heart failure)

→ Ventricular filling

→ Stroke volume

→ Cardiac output

↓ Organ/tissue perfusion

Cardiac output

Atrioventricular block (persistent)

Myocardial hypoxia

Ventricular ectopy
Ventricular tachycardia

Sustained asystole

Syncope and/or death

Cardiovascular Effects

Asynchronous atrial systolic thrust
Precordial pain due to—↑O_2 extraction
Compensatory tachycardia
  ↓Ventricular filling
  ↓Cardiac output
Thumping in chest, head
  (Result of prolonged diastole)
Varying intensity of 1st heart sound
  (seen in association with complete heart block)
Split 2nd sound with **RBB** block or **LBB** block

CSN Effects

Behavioral change
↓Responsiveness
Restlessness
Apprehension
Syncopal attacks
Vertigo, Dizziness
  (on sudden exertion)
Unsteadiness
Lightheadedness
Swimming feeling
Fatigue, weakness

Mesenteric Effects

Secondary to angiospasm

Abdominal distention,
Pain
Diarrhea
Flatulence
Paralytic ileus

88

Peripheral Effects	Pulmonary Effects	Renal Effects
Neck vein pulsation	Dyspnea due to:	No change or if bradycardia
Diastolic pressure (prolonged diastolic phase)	1. Inability to increase cardiac output with exercise	and/heart block is prolonged
Skin: pale, cold, clammy, diaphoresis (Compensatory mechanism of vasoconstriction)	2. Anxiety	↓Blood flow
Pulse initially fast then decreasing with bradycardia, 50–60/min	3. Left ventricular failure	→ Oliguria →
Complete heart block, 30–40/min		Proteinuria
Pulse volume bounding (second to stroke volume)		
"Waterhammer pulse" (rapid rise and fall) Secondary to ejection of large amount of blood into the low resistance vessels		

89

considered the possibility of an increase in the resting parasympathetic tone attributable to the aging process as a possible mechanism for the sick sinus syndrome. According to Winslow and Powell (31), bradycardic rates, sinus arrest, and atrial fibrillation can possibly be related to impairment of impulse formation and/or conduction. Tachycardia may be precipitated by an escape mechanism. Although one would expect a junctional escape beat to occur in the presence of a sick sinus, Kleinfeld and Boal (32) have found that dysfunction of the junctional mechanism can also occur simultaneously. The diagnosis of sick sinus syndrome is rarely made on the basis of a single electrocardiograph tracing, for it may reveal only one aspect of the syndrome, such as an isolated sinus bradycardia or a sinus tachycardia. It is generally made in the context of presenting symptomology such as syncope, palpitations, worsening congestive heart failure, and/or angina pectoris in association with the electrocardiogram (33). Much information has been gained from continuous monitoring using the Holter monitoring technique. Other diagnostic tools available in assessing impulse conductance are the His bundle recording and atrial pacing. (See Chapter 7 for a discussion of His bundle studies.)

Electrocardiographic Features
Various rhythm and conduction disturbances may be reflected on the electrocardiogram. Marked sinus bradycardia with a cardiac rate of less than 40 beats per minute may be identified as well as rhythms by default (escape). These may be interspersed with a sequence of atrial tachyarrhythmias or by second-degree sinoatrial block (20).

Clinical Spectrum
The clinical manifestations if present are referrable to the reduction in cardiac output. This may be related to excessively long periods of electrical inactivity due to the failure of subsidiary pacemakers to control heart rate; to tachyarrhythmias; or, as outlined by Winslow and Powell (31), to the failure of the heart to increase its stroke volume during periods of excessively slow heart rates (Table 5-3).

The patient may experience episodes of lightheadedness and syncope, reflecting inadequate perfusion of the cerebral hemispheres, or anginal pain, an indication of compromised coronary circulation. Palpitations and heart failure, as well as generalized weakness, are likewise indications that the heart is unable to expel its normal volume of blood per minute.

Therapy
Therapy for the sick sinus syndrome in the symptomatic patient is directed to effecting an adequate cardiac output to meet the metabolic needs of the body. This may be accomplished through the use of drugs such as atropine or isoproterenol to diminish vagal tone, the insertion of a pacemaker, and the use of digoxin if needed to treat the heart failure or tachyarrhythmias.

REVIEW QUESTIONS

1. What is the mechanism involved when sinus tachycardia accompanies gastrointestinal hemorrhage?
2. What effect if any does hypothermia have upon the sinus node?
3. In extreme sinus bradycardia, what are the associated clinical features?
4. What dysrhythmias are included in the concept of the sick sinus syndrome?

5. Mr. Jones is a 48-year-old construction worker who has sustained a lacerating injury to the upper left leg and was transported to the hospital by the local ambulance service. On admission to the unit, the physician's order read, "place in Trendelenberg position." From your knowledge of the Trendelenberg position

a. How would the position affect cardiac output?

b. Identify the cardiovascular reflex initiated by the position.

c. How would the physician's order affect vital measurements of body function?

REFERENCES

1. Myerburg RJ, El-Sherif N: Electrocardiographic diagnosis of sinus rhythm variations and sino-atrial block, in Schlart RC, Hurst JW (eds): *Advances in Electrocardiography*, vol 2. New York, Grune & Stratton Inc, 1976, p 61.

2. Lipman BS, Massie E. Kleiger RE: *Clinical Scalar Electrocardiography*, ed 6. Chicago, Year Book Medical Pub Inc, 1972, p 413.

3. Pollock, GH: Cardiac pacemaking: an obligatory role of catecholamines? *Science* 196:73, 1977.

4. Rothe CF: Cardiodynamics, in Selkurt (ed): *Physiology*. Boston, Little Brown & Co, 1962, p 296.

5. Reder R, Rosen MR: The role of sympathetic nervous system in sudden cardiac death. *Drug Therapy,* July 1978.

6. Fowler NO: *Cardiac Arrhythmia,* ed 2. Hagerstown, Md, Harper & Row Pub Inc, 1977, p 35.

7. Schamroth L: *The Disorders of Cardiac Rhythm.* Oxford, Blackwell Scientific Publications, 1973, p 29.

8. Goldman MJ: *Principles of Clinical Electrocardiography*, ed 10. Los Altos, Calif, Lange Medical Publications, 1979, p 206.

9. Langley LL, Cheraskin E. Skoper R: *Dynamic Anatomy and Physiology*. New York, McGraw-Hill Book Co, 1958, p 375.

10. Bigger JT, Dresdale RJ, Heissenbuttel RH, Weld FM, Wit AL: Ventricular arrhythmias in ischemic heart disease: mechanism, prevalence, significance, and management. *Progress in Cardiovas Diseases* 14:270, 1977.

11. Fowler NO: *Cardiac Diagnosis and Treatment,* ed 2. Hagerstown, Md, Harper & Row Pub Inc, 1976, p 891.

12. Fowler NO, Fenton JC, Conway GF: Syncope caused by bradycardia without atrioventricular block. *Am Heart J* 80:303, 1970.

13. Lipman BS. Massie E, Kleiger RE: *Clinical Scalar Electrocardiography*, ed 6. Chicago, Year Book Medical Pub, 1972, p 303.

14. Badeer HS: Axioms on athlete's heart. *Hosp Med* 13:70, 1977.

15. Sokolow M, McIlray MB: *Clinical Cardiology*. Los Altos, Calif, Lange Medical Publications, 1977, p 428.

16. Chung EK: *Principles of Cardiac Arrhythmias,* ed 2. Baltimore, Williams & Wilkins Co, 1977, p 617.

17. Taylor NB, McPhedran MC: *Basic Physiology and Anatomy*. New York, GP Putnam's Sons, 1965, p 250.

18. Anthony CP, Thibodeau G: *Textbook of Anatomy and Physiology,* ed 10. St. Louis, CV Mosby Co, 1979, p 418.

19. Corday E, Irving DW: *Disturbances of Heart Rate, Rhythm and Conduction*. Philadelphia, WB Saunders Co, 1962, p 26.

20. Cooksey JD, Dunn M, Massie E: *Clinical Vectorcardiography and Electrocardiography,* ed 2. Chicago, Year Book Medical Pub Inc, 1977, p 496.

21. Iruchijima J: *Cardiovascular Physiology*. Tokyo, Igaku Shoin Ltd, 1972, p 16.

22. Ferrer MI: Axioms on heart block. *Hosp Med* 13:25, 1977.

23. Goldberger AL, Goldberger E: *Clinical Electrocardiography*. St. Louis, CV Mosby Co, 1977, p 139.

24. Hatle L, Bathen J, Rokseth R: Sinoatrial disease in acute myocardial infarction. *Br Heart J* 38:410, 1976.

25. Dhingra RC, Amta-y-Leon F, Wyndham C, Deedwanla PC, Wu D, Denes P, Rosen KM: Clinical significance of prolonged sino atrial conduction time. *Circulation* 55:11, 1977.

26. Riseman JE, Segall E: *Cardiac Arrhythmia: Electrocardiogram, Diagnosis, Treatment*. New York, Macmillan Inc, 1963, p 228.

27. Bergersen BS, Goth A: *Pharmacology in Nursing*. St. Louis, CV Mosby Co, 1976, p 120, 139.

28. Ferrer MI: *Sick Sinus Syndrome*. Mt. Kisco, NY, Futura Pub Co Inc, 1974, p 31.

29. Fruehan CT: Sick Sinus Syndrome. *Cardiology Today* 6:14, 1978.

30. Jordan J, Yamoguchi I, Mandel WJ: Characteristics of sinoatrial conduction in patients with coronary artery disease. *Circulation* 55:572, 1977.

31. Winslow EH, Powell AH: Sick Sinus Syndrome. *Am J Nursing* 76:1262, 1976.

32. Kleinfeld MJ, Boal BH: Junctional escape rhythm in the sick sinus syndrome. *Cardiol* 63:198, 1978.

33. Walter PF: The sick sinus syndrome. *Med Times* 107:84, 1979.

6
Atrial Arrhythmias

An atrial arrhythmia, regardless of whether it is an isolated premature atrial contraction (PAC) or a sustained arrhythmia, may originate at any point in the atria except the SA node. Arrhythmias originating from the atria are usually categorized into four groups: premature atrial contraction (PAC), atrial tachycardia, atrial flutter, and atrial fibrillation.

PREMATURE ATRIAL CONTRACTIONS (PACs)

Pathogenesis

A PAC originates from an ectopic focus in any portion of the atria and activates the atria in an abnormal fashion. The P wave is usually distorted (P′), the proximity of the extopic focus to the SA node dictating the degree of distortion. If the extopic focus is located near the AV node, atrial activation occurs in a retrograde fashion, producing an inverted P wave in leads II, III, and aV_F and an upright P wave in lead aV_R. When the ectopic impulse is located near the SA node, the impulse travels in the usual antegrade fashion, producing a P wave that looks like a normal sinus P wave.

Electrocardiographic Features

1. The P wave (P′) appears earlier than the P waves of the basic rhythm.
2. The P wave (P′) has a different configuration from the sinus P wave, being upright, biphasic or inverted. If the P wave is inverted, its differentiation from a premature junctional contraction (PJC) is difficult or even impossible.
3. The P′R interval is usually 0.12 second or longer (1, 2, 3) and may be prolonged if the AV conduction of the basic rhythm is impaired.
4. The QRS complex is usually normal since conduction below the AV node is like the sinus beats. If aberrant conduction (see p. 109) is present, the QRS complex will be wide and bizarre, resembling a premature ventricular contraction (PVC).
5. The pause after the PAC is usually not a compensatory pause, meaning the P′P interval (measured from the ectopic P wave to the following sinus P wave) is less than two PP intervals of sinus beats (Fig. 6-1). The noncompensatory pause occurs because the ectopic focus which activated the atria also activates the SA node prematurely and temporarily suppresses it. PACs, however, may be associated with a complete compensatory pause if the ectopic focus appears late in the cycle.
6. The coupling interval (measured from the ectopic P wave to the P wave of the preceding cycle) is usually constant when the PACs originate from the same focus (Fig. 6-2). This interval will vary when the PACs are multifocal and when the atrial parasystole is

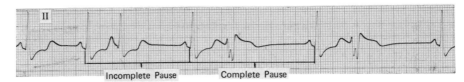

Figure 6-1. The third beat is a PAC and beats five and seven are PVCs. The PAC has a less than compensatory pause (incomplete pause) since it is less than two PP intervals of the patient's sinus beats. The PVCs have a complete pause. Note the increased PR interval with the PAC.

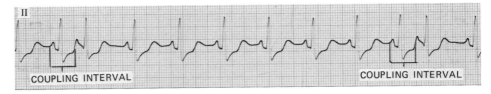

Figure 6-2. Coupling intervals for PACs are measured from the sinus P wave to the ectopic P wave (PP′) interval. The QRS configuration of PACs resembles the sinus beats.

present. The coupling interval is also more likely to vary with PACs as opposed to PVCs (2, 3). The coupling mechanism is thought to be the result of reentry (4) (See "Reentry Phenomenon," at the end of this chapter.)

If the ectopic focus discharges very early in the cycle, the impulse may find the AV node and the ventricles still refractory. The P′ wave will not be followed by a QRS complex and is termed a nonconducted PAC. Nonconducted PACs are the "commonest causes of pauses" (5, 3) that interrupt regular sinus rhythm (Fig. 6-3). Premature atrial contractions may appear alternately with the basic rhythm (bigeminy), as every third

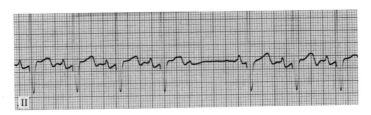

Figure 6-3. Nonconducted PAC produces an obvious pause.

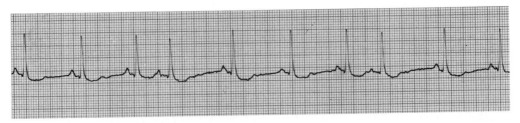

Figure 6-4. Atrial quadrigeminy (every fourth beat a PAC).

beat (trigeminy), or as every fourth beat (quadrigeminy) (Fig. 6-4). When five to six or more PACs occur in succession, a run of atrial tachycardia is present (3, 2). Frequent PACs may lead to atrial tachycardia, flutter, or fibrillation if the premature impulse fires during the vulnerable period of the atria. Killip (6) has developed a formula for determining whether the PAC falls in this vulnerable period. If the PP$'$ interval is greater than 60% of the previous PP interval, atrial arrhythmias are not likely to develop. If the interval is less than 50%, it may fire in the atrial vulnerable period and result in a tachyarrhythmia.

Differential Diagnosis

If a PAC has an invisible P wave, a wide, bizarre QRS complex (aberrant conduction), and a complete compensatory pause, it is almost identical with a PVC. Fortunately all three of these abnormalities usually do not occur at the same time (5).

When a PAC originates near the AV node it mimics a premature junctional contraction (PJC). PJCs usually have a PR interval less than 0.12 second, whereas the PR interval in PACs is usually greater than 0.12 second (6).

PACs may be interpreted as sinus bradycardia, sinus arrhythmia, sinus arrest, SA block, and second-degree AV block when the P$'$ wave is lost or buried in the preceding T wave (2).

Clinical Spectrum

Premature atrial contractions may occur in healthy persons as well as those with organic heart disease. Hinkle (7) found PACs and PJCs to be present in 76% of the people without organic heart disease. Secondary causes of PACs include emotional stress, tobacco, alcohol, coffee, tea, cola beverages, and fatigue. A higher incidence of coronary artery disease has not been found in people with PACs (8, 7).

Therapy

Therapy is usually directed toward the modification or removal of the secondary causes of PACs. If the premature atrial contractions are the result of congestive heart failure, digitalis is the drug of choice (2).

ATRIAL TACHYCARDIA

Pathogenesis

Atrial tachyarrhythmias, including atrial tachycardia, flutter, and fibrillation originate because of increased automaticity of the ectopic pacemaker (9, 10), reentry (11, 9), or the combined effects of both abnormalities. Atrial tachycardia usually begins and ends abruptly and is referred to as *paroxysmal atrial tachycardia* (PAT), the paroxysm lasting for seconds, hours, or days (Fig. 6-5).

Electrocardiographic Features

1. The atrial rate is usually between 160 to 250 beats per minute. Commonly the ventricular rate in untreated PAT ranges from 130 to 200 beats per minute owing to the refractoriness of the AV node (2). If the rate is relatively slow, 100 to 120 beats per minute, the term *nonparoxysmal tachycardia* has been used (5).

2. The presence of an abnormal P wave (P$'$) preceding each QRS complex is a key feature of PAT. Depending on the proximity of the ectopic focus, the P$'$ wave may be upright, biphasic, or inverted. Frequently the paroxysmal tachycardia has a ventricular rate of

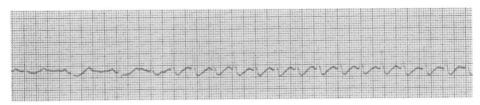

Figure 6-5. Atrial tachycardia suddenly develops in this patient at a rate of 187 beats per minute.

from 150 to 250 beats per minute, without a visible P wave, making it impossible to differentiate between PAT and paroxysmal junctional tachycardia (PJT). This is called *supraventricular tachycardia* (Fig. 6-6). The significance, treatment, and prognosis for both PAT and PJT is the same (3).

3. The P'P' and RR intervals are generally regular; however, the PP' intervals may vary during the first few beats of the paroxysm (12).
4. The QRS complex normally resembles the sinus beat unless aberration is present.
5. The P'R interval may be normal or prolonged.
6. Secondary ST and T wave changes may develop as a result of ischemia from decreased diastolic filling time in the coronary arteries. This abnormality has been called the *post-tachycardia syndrome* and may be present for hours or days after the tachycardia has stopped (5).

Differential Diagnosis

Sinus tachycardia at a rate of 140 to 160 beats per minute is similar to PAT if the ectopic focus is near the SA node. The RR interval may vary with sinus tachycardia but is usually constant with PAT. A carotid sinus message will either terminate paroxysmal atrial tachycardia or have no effect on it, whereas this vagal maneuver may produce a gradual slowing

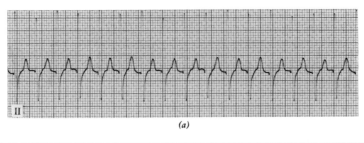

(a)

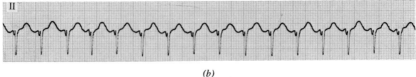

(b)

Figure 6-6. Both tracings show a rapid heart rate with no discernible P waves and a narrow QRS complex. (*a*) Ventricular rate is 180 beats per minute. (*b*) Ventricular rate is 136 beats per minute.

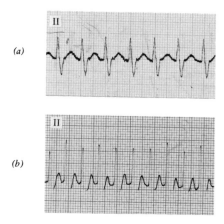

Figure 6-7. (*a*) Rapid supraventricular tachycardia with a ventricular rate of 150 per minute. The rhythm most likely is atrial flutter with 2:1 conduction. (*b*) The ventricular rate with this tachycardia is 230 per minute. The rhythm most probably is atrial tachycardia.

of the heart rate temporarily in sinus tachycardia. The clinical setting in which the tachycardia occurs often will provide information for distinguishing between these two tachycardias.

Atrial flutter with 2:1 conduction frequently has a regular ventricular rate of 150 beats per minute and flutter waves that are difficult to see because they are buried in the QRS-T complexes. This particular supraventricular tachycardia is usually atrial flutter with 2:1 conduction and is not paroxysmal atrial tachycardia. If the ventricular rate is greater than 200 beats per minute, atrial or junctional tachycardia is most likely, and if the ventricular rate is greater than 250 beats per minute, it is usually atrial flutter (2) (Fig. 6-7). Again, a carotid sinus message will help by revealing the flutter waves as the AV block is enhanced or if PAT is present; the vagal maneuver will either terminate the tachycardia or have no effect.

If the PAT is associated with wide, bizarre QRS complexes due to aberrant conduction, it mimics ventricular tachycardia.

Clinical Spectrum

PAT is commonly found in normal healthy people without heart disease. This tachyarrhythmia is associated with rheumatic heart disease, coronary heart disease, thyrotoxicosis, mitral valve prolapse, cardiomyopathy, hypertensive heart disease, chronic or acute cor-pulmonale, acute pericarditis, and the Wolff-Parkinson-White syndrome. The PAT may be provoked by emotional stress, physical fatigue, or excessive quantities of tobacco, coffee, or alcohol in some persons (1). The paroxysm may precipitate congestive heart failure (CHF) or aggravate preexisting CHF when the myocardium is already diseased. Coronary artery blood flow is reduced approximately 35% during PAT (13), and this may precipitate or aggravate coronary insufficiency (angina pectoris) in those persons with preexisting coronary artery disease. It must be emphasized that ventricular rates as slow as 120 to 140 beats per minute in the presence of myocardial disease may produce clinical signs and symptoms of CHF and/or coronary insufficiency, while ventricular rates much faster in a young otherwise healthy individual may produce little if any changes. Symptoms vary among palpitations, weakness, dizziness, anxiety, shortness of breath, chest pain, and syncope (Table 6-1).

Table 6-1. Hemodynamic Effects of Supraventricular Tachyarrhythmias

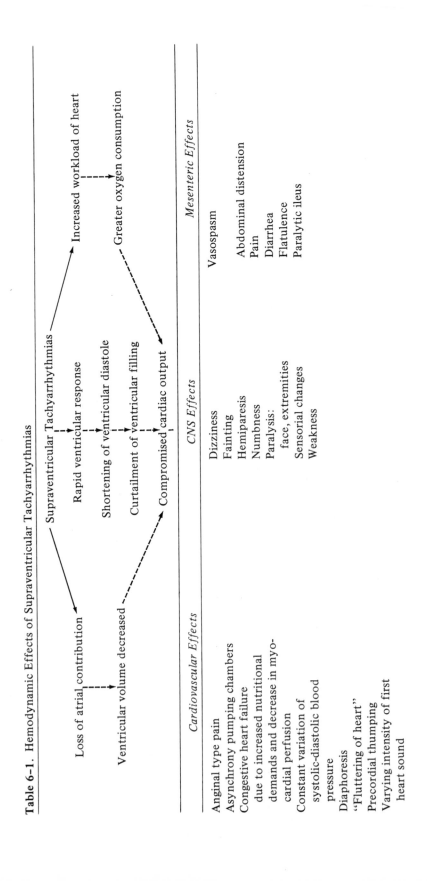

Supraventricular Tachyarrhythmias

Rapid ventricular response

Shortening of ventricular diastole

Curtailment of ventricular filling

Compromised cardiac output

Increased workload of heart

Greater oxygen consumption

Loss of atrial contribution

Ventricular volume decreased

Cardiovascular Effects

Anginal type pain
Asynchrony pumping chambers
Congestive heart failure
    due to increased nutritional
    demands and decrease in myo-
    cardial perfusion
Constant variation of
    systolic-diastolic blood
    pressure
Diaphoresis
"Fluttering of heart"
Precordial thumping
Varying intensity of first
    heart sound

CNS Effects

Dizziness
Fainting
Hemiparesis
Numbness
Paralysis:
    face, extremities
Sensorial changes
Weakness

Mesenteric Effects

Vasospasm

Abdominal distension
Pain
Diarrhea
Flatulence
Paralytic ileus

Peripheral Effects	Pulmonary Effects	Renal Effects
Cold, clammy skin	Dyspnea	Increased renal vascular resistance (homeostatic effort to divert blood to brain and heart)
Cyanotic hue to extremities	Pulmonary congestion	
Diaphoresis	Pulmonary edema	
Irregular pulse		↓ Urine volume (Ischemic tubular impairment of reabsorptive process)
Jugular venous engrogement		↑ Urine frequency
Pulse deficit		
"Thumping in head"		
Vascular collapse		Oliguria

Therapy

Persons without organic heart disease must be reassured that they have an excellent prognosis and usually are taught simple maneuvers such as carotid sinus message or the valsalva maneuver to terminate the PAT. Digitalis and/or quinidine may be used to help control and prevent PAT. If the PAT is associated with CHF, digitalis is the drug of choice (see Chap. 11).

PAROXYSMAL ATRIAL TACHYCARDIA WITH BLOCK

Pathogenesis

The majority of individuals with this rhythm disturbance have digitalis toxicity. Lown and Levine (14) in 1958 reported digitalis excess as the cause in 73% in their series.

Electrocardiographic Features

1. Presence of P′ waves in a regular rhythm.
2. Atrial rate usually from 150 to 250 beats per minute.
3. The P′ waves are separated by isoelectric intervals.
4. Second-degree AV block is present, 2:1 conduction being the most common (Fig. 6-8).

Differential Diagnosis

This arrhythmia is frequently confused with paroxysmal atrial tachycardia without block, junctional tachycardia, atrial flutter, or sinus tachycardia because the P waves are often difficult to see. Digitalis toxicity is rarely the cause of atrial flutter, whereas PAT with block is commonly caused by excessive digitalis (1).

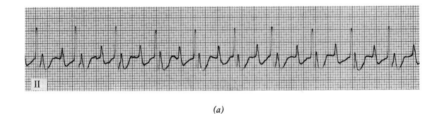

(a)

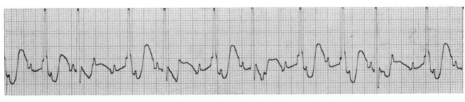

(b)

Figure 6-8. (a) Paroxysmal atrial tachycardia with 2:1 conduction. The atrial rate is 176 beats per minute and the ventricular rate is 88 beats per minute. (b) PAT with varying degree of block. The atrial rate is 166 beats per minute.

Clinical Spectrum

Digitalis toxicity is frequently associated with hypokalemia and the use of diuretics. Patients with advanced heart disease and impaired renal function frequently require the use of digitalis and diuretics and are at a higher risk of developing arrhythmias, owing to digitalis toxicity, even though they are given the usual maintenance doses. (See Chap. 11 for treatment of digitalis-induced arrhythmias.)

MULTIFOCAL ATRIAL TACHYCARDIA

Pathogenesis

This arrhythmia is also known as chaotic atrial rhythm or tachycardia and wandering pacemaker in the atria. The mechanism is the same as atrial tachycardia except that there is more than one ectopic focus located in the atria.

Electrocardiographic Features

1. P′ waves of varying configurations.
2. Variable PP, RR, and PR intervals.

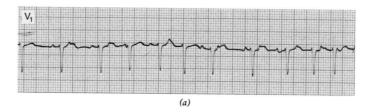

(a)

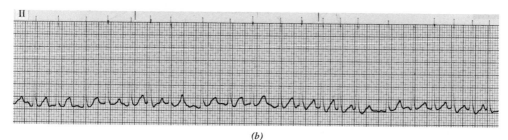

(b)

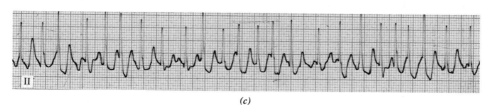

(c)

Figure 6-9. (*a*) Multifocal atrial tachycardia recorded from a woman with chronic cor pulmonale. The P waves appear different from each other, signifying many different foci. (*b*) Rapid multifocal atrial tachycardia with the ventricular rate as rapid as 214 beats per minute at times. (*c*) This rhythm was recorded from a patient with long-standing chronic obstructive lung disease. The patient was treated with digitalis IV in an attempt to convert the multifocal atrial tachycardia back to sinus rhythm. (See text on next page.)

3. Atrial rate of from 100 to 250 beats per minute.

4. Secondary ST and T wave changes.

Differential Diagnosis
A multifocal atrial tachycardia resembles atrial fibrillation or flutter owing to its irregularity (Fig. 6-9). The presence of ectopic P waves rather than flutter waves or a fibrillatory line helps separate multifocal atrial tachycardia from other arrhythmias.

Clinical Spectrum
This arrhythmia is frequently found in seriously ill patients and in older individuals. Patients with chronic obstructive lung disease have a high incidence of multifocal atrial tachycardia (Fig. 6-9). Digitalis toxicity is usually not a direct cause of this arrhythmia. It is interesting that a large number of patients have diabetes mellitus (15).

Therapy
Multifocal atrial tachycardia is usually associated with a high mortality rate since it is usually found in severely ill and elderly patients. This arrhythmia is fequently resistant to various antiarrhythmic agents.

ATRIAL FLUTTER

Pathogenesis
The controversy over the mechanism responsible for the production of atrial flutter has persisted for several years. The mechanisms responsible for atrial flutter and fibrillation may be identical. Currently, four phenomena are proposed as possible mechanisms, and they include: (*1*) circus movement, (*2*) unifocal atrial impulse formation, (*3*) multiple reentry, and (*4*) multifocal atrial impulse formation. One or a combination of these may be responsible for the initiation of such tachyarrhythmias (2, 1). Lewis et al (16) did extensive studies based on the circus movement theory, which proposes the presence of a primary impulse that activates the atria and is called a mother circus ring. This ring is a circular path around the ostia of the superior and inferior vena cavae in which the impulse travels in a unidirectional fashion. Other atrial waves called daughter waves leave the path of the mother circus ring and pass through both atria (Fig. 6-10). The head and tail of the mother circus ring are separated by an area of muscle that is in a nonrefractory state. This allows the impulse to immediately reenter the same path and produce a new cycle to perpetuate the circus movement. Obliteration of the area of muscle in a nonrefractory state that precedes the front of the mother circus ring would terminate the circus movement. Recent studies by Leier et al (197) have shown that atrial conduction disease may be major factor in the development of atrial flutter or fibrillation regardless of the underlying mechanism.

Electrocardiographic Features

1. The rapid atrial deflections, which resemble a sawtooth or a picket fence, are called F waves (Fig. 6-11).

2. The atrial rate is usually from 250 to 350 beats per minute, a rate of 300 being the most common.

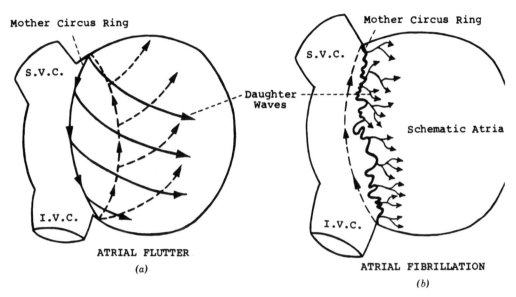

Figure 6-10. The diagrammatic representation of the circus movement of atrial flutter (*a*) and fibrillation (*b*). (SVC: superior vena cava; IVC: inferior vena cava.) The circus movement theory of atrial flutter (*a*) and fibrillation (*b*) includes the presence of a mother circus ring and daughter waves. The path traveled by the mother circus ring in atrial flutter is longer than in atrial fibrillation, producing a slower atrial rate in flutter. The mother circus waves and daughter waves are thought to travel a constant path in atrial flutter producing a regular flutter cycle. This is not true in atrial fibrillation, where both mother circus waves and daughter waves travel an irregular path with a varying speed producing the fibrillatory f waves. (Reproduced with permission from Chung EK: *Principles of Cardiac Arrhythmias.* Copyright © 1977, The Williams and Wilkins Co., Baltimore.)

3. The rate and regularity of the QRS complex is variable and depends upon conduction through the AV node. The conduction ratio ranges from 2:1 to 8:1, 2:1 being the most common ratio and the odd-numbered ratios (3:1 and 5:1) being rare (Fig. 6-12). Usually the ventricular rate in untreated atrial flutter is half of the atrial rate (2).

4. The QRS complex is usually normal unless aberration or preexisting conduction disease is present.

Prinzmetal (18) has described two components of the saw-toothed waves of atrial flutter. The first part of the F wave is the P′ wave, which signifies atrial depolarization and has a downward deflection (Fig. 6-13). This is followed by an upward deflection, the

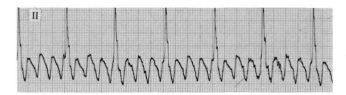

Figure 6-11. Tracing of standard lead II shows the characteristic sawtooth appearance of F (flutter) waves.

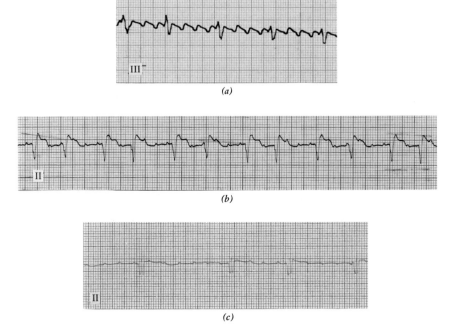

(a)

(b)

(c)

Figure 6-12. (*a*) Conduction ratio is 4:1 in this tracing. (*b*) Odd-numbered conduction ratios (3:1, 5:1) are rare, the even-numbered ratios being the most common. This tracing shows a varying degree of conduction between a 3:1 and 2:1 ratio. (*c*) Six flutter waves are present in the first RR interval.

Ta wave, which signifies atrial repolarization. The flutter waves are usually easily identified in leads II, III aV_F, V_{1-2}, and MCl_1 (Fig. 6-14).

When the flutter cycle is faster than 350 beats per minute, the term atrial impure flutter has been used. The F waves tend to vary slightly in their configuration also.

Differential Diagnosis

Atrial flutter with 2:1 AV conduction is very similar to atrial tachycardia and junctional tachycardia (Fig. 6-15). Careful inspection of several ECG leads is often necessary to discern the presence of flutter waves. Vagal stimulation may help increase the AV block and make it easier to see flutter waves or to convert the atrial tachycardia to sinus rhythm. Atrial flutter may resemble atrial fibrillation or PAT with variable block if the ventricular rate is not constant. When the QRS complex is wide and bizarre in the presence of atrial flutter, the arrhythmia mimics ventricular tachycardia. Again, vagal stimulation is helpful because it may uncover the flutter waves if the rhythm is atrial flutter, but will have no effect if the rhythm is ventricular tachycardia. Usually a ventricular rate greater than 250 beats per minute favors the presence of atrial flutter (2).

Clinical Spectrum

Usually atrial flutter is seen in patients with organic heart disease. The arrhythmia may be paroxysmal or chronic, lasting from minutes to years. Diseases most commonly seen with this tachyarrhythmia include coronary artery disease and rheumatic heart disease

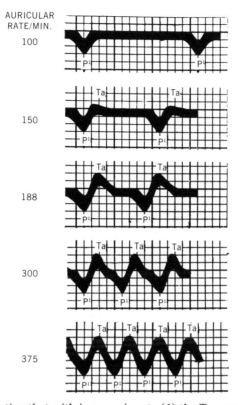

Figure 6-13. Illustrating that with increase in rate (*1*) the Ta wave assumes greater prominence and (*2*) the isoelectric shelf becomes shorter. (Reproduced with permission from Prinzmetal M: *The Auricular Arrhythmias,* 1951. Courtesy of Charles C Thomas, Springfield, Ill.)

(especially mitral valve disease) (Fig. 6-14). Atrial flutter is also seen with the Wolff-Parkinson-White syndrome, thyrotoxicosis, pericarditis, hypertensive heart disease, pulmonary embolism, and congenital heart disease (2, 1). Patients with preexisting significant coronary artery disease may develop or aggravate myocardial ischemia, which manifests itself as angina pectoris, myocardial infarction, or congestive heart failure when atrial flutter occurs. Atrial tachycardia, flutter, and fibrillation may reduce cerebral circulation, producing symptoms of blurred vision, confusion, weakness, dizziness, syncope, and psychosis.

Therapy
Atrial flutter rarely has 1:1 AV conduction; however, when it does, it is considered to be a medical emergency owing to the rapid ventricular response. The treatment of the patient with atrial flutter as well as any arrhythmia depends upon the total clinical picture, which includes underlying etiologic factors (metabolic and psychologic), the nature of heart disease (especially the presence or absence of CHF), and drug toxicity. Digitalis is the drug of choice in the conversion of atrial flutter, especially if congestive heart failure is present. Also frequently used as therapy is DC shock. Additional drugs include quinidine, propranolol (Inderal), procainamide (Pronestyl), and diphenylhydantoin (Dilantin) (see Chap. 11).

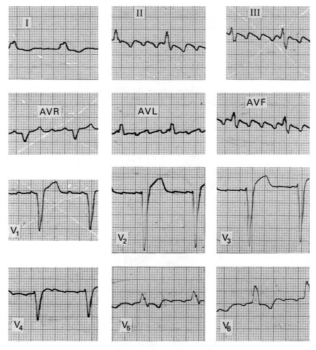

Figure 6-14. Atrial flutter developed in this patient with coronary artery disease. The F waves are poorly seen in the precordial leads but seen well in the limb leads. A LBBB pattern was present before the atrial flutter developed.

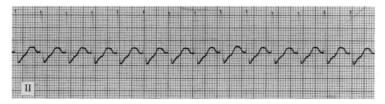

Figure 6-15. Typical atrial flutter with 2:1 conduction ratio. This produces a ventricular rate of 150 per minute with poorly visible flutter waves.

ATRIAL FIBRILLATION

Pathogenesis
The mechanisms involved in the production of atrial fibrillation are the same as those found in atrial flutter.

Electrocardiographic Features

1. The P waves are absent and replaced by an uneven, irregular wave, called an f wave. This fibrillatory line may be difficult to see and appears as a straight line between the QRS complexes. The f waves are best seen in leads II, V_1, and MCl_1 (Fig. 6-16).

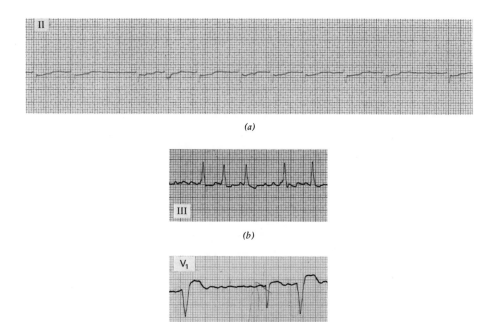

(a)

(b)

(c)

Figure 6-16. Fibrillatory line (f waves) of atrial fibrillation. (*a*) Often the f waves are difficult to see and the key finding is then the irregular RR intervals without visible P waves. (*b*) and (*c*) f waves are seen well in these two tracings.

2. The QRS complexes appear irregularly irregular. Unless aberration is present, the QRS complexes will be normal.

The atrial rate is usually impossible to determine since the rate is rapid—greater than 350 beats per minute. The f waves may be termed fine or coarse fibrillatory waves, depending on their size. An f wave greater than 0.5 mm is considered a coarse wave by some (19), whereas others use 1.0 mm (20) as the separation point between coarse and fine fibrillation. Atrial fibrillation with fine f waves are usually more difficult to convert to sinus rhythm (21).

Differential Diagnosis

Atrial fibrillation may resemble multifocal atrial tachycardia because of the rapid and irregular ventricular response. The presence of P' waves before each QRS complex is not present in atrial fibrillation as opposed to multifocal atrial tachycardia. Paroxysmal atrial tachycardia with variable degrees of block as well as atrial flutter with a varying ventricular response may appear like atrial fibrillation. A careful search for flutter waves or P' waves on the 12-lead ECG is essential.

Clinical Spectrum

Atrial fibrillation occurs 10 to 20 times more frequently than atrial flutter (2) and is one of the most common arrhythmias. Patients with atrial fibrillation usually have organic heart disease, the arrhythmia appearing in a paroxysmal form or typically the chronic

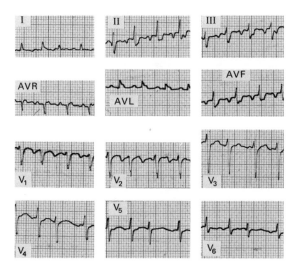

Figure 6-17. This 12-lead ECG was recorded from a man with coronary artery disease. He sought medical attention for shortness of breath and weakness. Rapid atrial fibrillation with a ventricular rate of 166 beats per minute is seen. The patient's chest x-ray revealed a left pneumothorax.

form. Diseases it is found with include coronary artery disease, rheumatic and hypertensive heart disease, congenital heart disease (atrial septal defect, Ebstein's anomaly, transposition of the great vessels), pericarditis, hyperthyroidism, cor pulmonale and Wolfe-Parkinson-White syndrome (Fig. 6-17). Digitalis toxicity rarely causes atrial fibrillation, whereas as many as 70% of patients with congestive heart failure have this tachyarrhythmia (2). Approximately 5% of patients with atrial fibrillation have no evidence of organic heart disease, the arrhythmia usually appearing in its paroxysmal form (22). These individuals may give a history of excessive ingestion of tobacco, alcohol, or coffee or emotional excitement, severe pain, or physical exhaustion as the precipitating factor.

Blood flow in the coronary arteries may be reduced by as much as 40% in untreated atrial fibrillation (13), which can account for the signs and symptoms of coronary insufficiency, that is, angina pectoris and congestive heart failure. Symptoms of cerebral ischemia, including dizziness, confusion, convulsions, and blurred vision, may develop owing to the average decrease of 23% in cerebral circulation with rapid atrial fibrillation (2). The atrial kick (atrial contraction) is absent in atrial fibrillation, which may be a critical problem in the decompensated heart. Patients with mitral stenosis and rapid atrial fibrillation may develop pulmonary edema because of a significant rise in left atrial pressure (2). The cardiac output increases by as much as 34% in patients in whom atrial fibrillation is converted to sinus rhythm by DC shock (24). A rapid ventricular response in atrial fibrillation may be associated with a 20% reduction in renal blood flow (25), producing symptoms of renal insufficiency, that is, oliguria and azotemia.

One of the most significant problems that develops because of atrial fibrillation is the formation of atrial thrombi. An ineffective squirming of the atria leads to stasis of blood flow in the atrial chambers and the formation of thrombi, which may travel in the circulatory system and produce a pulmonary and/or systemic arterial embolism.

Therapy

The decision to convert atrial fibrillation back to sinus rhythm is made on the basis of preventing pulmonary and/or systemic arterial emboli as well as reversing an embarrassed hemodynamic state. The drug of choice is digitalis for the termination of atrial fibrillation. Cardioversion, quinidine, propranolol, and procainamide may be used in addition to digitalis (see Chap. 11).

ABERRANT VENTRICULAR CONDUCTION
OF SUPRAVENTRICULAR ARRHYTHMIAS

Aberrant ventricular conduction refers to the temporary abnormal intraventricular conduction of a single beat or the constant aberrant conduction found with bundle branch blocks. Ventricular aberration produces a wide, bizarre QRS complex, which resembles a ventricular ectopic beat or ventricular tachycardia if a supraventricular tachycardia and aberration occur together. The differentiation between ventricular ectopy and aberration is very important because the therapy and clinical significance are different.

The mechanism responsible for the production of ventricular aberration is a change in the refractory state of the intraventricular specialized conducting fibers. If a supraventricular impulse arrives very early to find the specialized conducting fibers (right bundle branch, main left bundle branch, and the anterior and posterior fascicles of the left bundle) totally refractory, the impulse is not conducted. This situation typically occurs

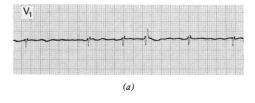

(a)

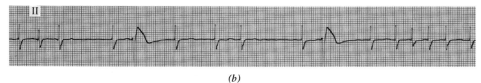

(b)

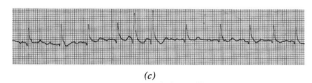

(c)

Figure 6-18. (*a*) Aberration usually produces a RBBB pattern in lead V_1, as seen by this rSR′ pattern of the fourth beat during atrial fibrillation. (*b*) Aberration is produced as a result of Ashman's phenomenon. The two aberrantly conducted beats are present in this tracing of atrial fibrillation. (*c*) When the ventricular rate increases in this patient with atrial fibrillation, aberration becomes evident. The initial deflection of the QRS complex of the aberrantly conducted beat is the same as the patient's other beats. (See text on next page.)

in blocked premature atrial contractions. If an impulse arrives at the ventricle before the entire conducting system has fully recovered, the ventricle will be activated abnormally. This alteration in intraventricular conduction produces the aberration. Commonly the right bundle branch system is found in a refractory state since this branch is longer and thinner, producing a longer action potential and thus a longer refractory period than the left bundle branch (26). The refractory period of the specialized conducting fibers is proportional to the length of the preceding ventricular cycle (RR interval) as originally described by Ashman. A slow heart rate produces a long RR interval and a long refractory period, and a fast heart rate shortens both the RR interval and the refractory period. Ventricular aberration may develop because (1) the immediate cycle (RR interval) is shortened, (2) the preceding cycle (RR interval) is lengthened, or (3) a combination of both occurs (5). Ashman's phenomenon commonly occurs in atrial fibrillation with marked irregularity in the ventricular cycles (RR intervals) and with atrial or junctional bigeminy (2) (Fig. 6-18). As the heart rate increases, the RR cycle as well as the refractory period shorten. Eventually the rate reaches a point in which intraventricular conduction is altered, producing intermittent bundle branch block. The heart rate at which ventricular

Table 6-2. The ECG Differentiation Between Ventricular Aberration and Ectopy

Ventricular Aberration Favored	*Ventricular Ectopy Favored*
1. Initial r wave in V_1.[a]	1. Initial q wave in V_1.
2. A triphasic QRS (rsR' or rSR') complex in V_1 with a triphasic QRS (qRs) complex in V_6 as well.	2. A biphasic QRS complex (qR, RS, or QR) in V_1, or QS complex in V_6.
3. Fixed coupling is absent.	3. Fixed coupling interval with similar QRS complexes.
4. P' wave precedes the wide, bizarre QRS complex.	4. A ventricular fusion beat may also have a P' wave preceeding the QRS complex.
5. The second beat is bizarre in a goup of beats (Ashman's phenomenon). The RR cycle, which contains the bizarre QRS complex is shorter than the previous RR cycle.	5. The RR cycle with the bizarre QRS complex is longer than the previous RR cycle.
6. The initial QRS vector is identical with that of the normally conducted beats.	6. Initial QRS vector is not identical.
7. No ventricular fusion beats are present.	7. Tachycardia with wide, bizarre QRS complexes which have some ventricular fusion beats (Dressler's beats).
8. Axis may vary.	8. Indeterminate frontal plane axis ($+180°$ to $-90°$).
9. WPW syndrome with tachyarrhythmias may produce this QRS configuration in the precordial leads also.	9. All QRS complexes in the precordial leads (V_1-V_6) are positive or all are negative.
10. A less than compensatory pause usually follows a PAC or PJC with aberration.	10. Full compensatory pause usually follows a PVC.

Source: Limpan BS: Aberrancy, ectopy, and reentry in the electrocardiogram (*Practical Cardiol* 4:107, 1978)

[a] *MCL$_1$ and MCL$_6$ may be used instead of V_1 and V_6.

conduction changes is called the critical rate. Rate-dependent–bundle branch block usually appears if the heart rate increases; however, it may appear as the heart rate slows.

The right bundle is usually found in a refractory state in aberration, which accounts for approximately 80% of all aberrant conduction presenting a right bundle branch block appearance (5). Since the initial vector in right bundle branch block (see Chap. 8) is unchanged, the initial part of the QRS complex in aberration should be the same as the QRS complex seen with normal intraventricular conduction. It usually is necessary to record the bizarre-looking beats or rhythm from several different leads. Leads V_1 and V_6 or MCl_1 and MC_6 provide the most useful information.

It also is usually helpful to compare the tracing with previous ECG tracings and rhythm strips. The ECG differentiation between aberration and ectopy is listed in Table 6-2.

Additional clinical examinations to make include inspection of the neck veins and auscultation of the heart. The presence of irregular cannon waves in the neck and/or a varying intensity of the first heart sound favors ventricular tachycardia. These features are produced by a dissociation between the atria and ventricles that occurs in ventricular tachycardia. His bundle electrograms may provide the only definitive diagnosis in the differentiation of ventricular aberration from ectopy.

Tachycardias with a wide, bizarre QRS complex that cause a loss of consciousness as well as a loss of pulse are usually terminated immediately with DC shock. Any tachycardia, regardless of its origin, that produces this type of altered clinical state demands prompt treatment. A delay in this treatment because of attempts at interpretation of the ECG is unwarranted and may prove fatal to the patient.

REENTRY PHENOMENON

Reentry, as a mechanism implicated in the genesis of ectopic beats and/or rhythm, may be of the circus movement type or of focal reentry activity. Circus reentry requires the presence of a unidirectional block as well as an alternate route of excitable tissue. As the propagated impulse traverses cardiac tissue such as the Purkinje system of the ventricles, it may encounter fibers with varying degrees of conduction velocity. The wave front may proceed normally down one fiber segment but can be impeded in its passage through the other, which may still be refractory to the passage of the impulse. As the fibers recover, the impulse which originally had been conducted in an antegrade manner along the uninvolved fiber segment, may then travel retrograde through the initially nonresponsive fiber (27) (Fig. 6-19). Reentry frequently occurs at the level of the atrioventricular node, which, according to Watanabe and Dreifus (28), can have differing conduction velocity within its fibers (longitudinal dissociation). This then can precipitate a reciprocal junctional tachycardia. Other types of reentry tachycardias frequently seen are sinoatrial reentry, intra-atrial reentry, and intraventricular reentry (29). Alternate factors that may predispose cardiac tissue to the reentrant phenomena are depressed conduction velocity and/or shortened refractory periods. Thus with vagal stimulation and nonuniform shortening of the refractory period in atrial muscle fibers, reentry of atrial fibers will occur.

The presence of paroxysmal atrial tachycardia associated with the Wolff-Parkinson-White syndrome (Chap. 7) is likewise the result of the passage of an impulse over two pathways with varying refractory periods—the normal conducting pathway and the accessory bundle pathway. Electrocardiographically, as outlined by Lipman and associates

A–BLOCK

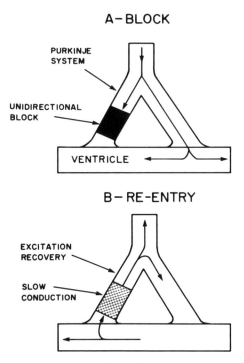

B–RE-ENTRY

Figure 6-19. Diagrammatic representation of circus type of reentry. The diagram shows a peripheral segment of the Purkinje system and the adjoining ventricular cell. In panel (*a*) there is impaired conduction in one branch of the Purkinje system owing to unidirectional block. The same impulse, however, is conducted through an alternate normal branch to the ventricle. In panel (*b*) the impulse travels from the ventricle through the area of unidirectional block in a retrograde course, arrives in the Purkinje system after recovery of excitation, and reenters the circuit. (Reproduced with permission from Naimi S: Electrophysiologic basis for arrhythmias, in Levine H [ed] : *Clinical Cardiovascular Physiology*. New York, Grune & Stratton Inc, 1976.)

(30), a reentrant or reciprocal beat of junctional origin may be recognized by the following features:

1. The presence of a junctional rhythm with prolonged retrograde conduction as evidenced by an RP interval greater than 0.20 second.

2. An identifiable retrograde P wave or fusion P wave preceding the reentrant beat.

3. Prolongation of the PR interval of the reentrant beat but not beyond that of the RP interval.

4. The occurrence of a reciprocal (reentrant beat) 0.50 second or less after the preceding QRS complex.

Focal reexcitation, according to Fowler (31), occurs secondary to differences in membrane potential of contiguous tissue. Therefore, an ischemic myocardium, an infarction, and/or a myocardial fibrosis tends to alter membrane responsiveness, thus precipitating focal reexcitation. This is most likely the mechanism involved in the lowering of the ventricular fibrillation threshold. In the presence of ventricular slowing, which accompanies ischemia of the myocardium, dispersion refractoriness can likewise occur (27).

REVIEW QUESTIONS

1. List the ECG features of a PAC. What is Killip's formula for determining the vulnerable period of the atria?
2. Describe the differences between atrial flutter and atrial fibrillation.
3. Explain the mechanisms responsible for the production of a cerebral infarction in a patient after atrial fibrillation has occurred.
4. List the ECG differences between ventricular aberration and ectopy.
5. How does atrial fibrillation affect the cardiac cycle?

REFERENCES

1. Chou TC: *Electrocardiography in Clinical Practice.* New York, Grune & Stratton Inc, 1979, p 350.
2. Chung, EK: *Principles of Cardiac Arrhythmias,* ed 2. Baltimore, Williams & Wilkins Co, 1977, p 99.
3. Lipman BS, Massie E, Kleiger RE: *Clinical Scalar Electrocardiography*, ed 6. Chicago, Year Book Medical Pub Inc, 1972, p 400.
4. Beckwith JR: *Grant's Clinical Electrocardiography: The Spatial Vector Approach,* New York, McGraw-Hill Book Co, 1970, p 196.
5. Marriott HJL: *Practical Electrocardiography,* ed 6. Baltimore, Williams & Wilkins Co, 1977, p 133.
6. Killip T, Gault JH: Mode of onset of atrial fibrillation in man. *Am Heart J* 70:172, 1965.
7. Hinkle LE, Carver ST, Stevens M: The frequency of asymptomatic disturbance of cardiac rhythm and conduction in middle-aged men. *Am J Cardiol* 24:629, 1969.
8. Chiang BN, Perlman LV, et al: Relationship of premature systoles to coronary heart disease and sudden death in the Tecumseh epidemiologic study. *Ann Intern Med* 70:1159, 1969.
9. Josephson ME, Kastor JA: Supraventricular tachycardia. Mechanisms and management. *Ann Intern Med* 87:346, 1977.
10. Goldreyer BN, Gallagher JJ, Damato AN: The electrophysiologic demonstration of atrial ectopic tachycardia in man. *Am Heart J* 85:205, 1973.
11. Han J: The mechanism of paroxysmal atrial tachycardia. Sustained reciprociation. *Am J Cardiol* 26:329, 1970.
12. Gilette PC, Garson A: Electrophysiologic and pharmacologic characteristics of automatic ectopic atrial tachycardia. *Circulation* 56:571, 1977.
13. Corday E, Gold H, et al: Effect of the cardiac arrhythmias on the coronary circulation. *Ann Intern Med* 50:535, 1959.
14. Lown B, Levine HD: *Atrial Arrhythmias, Digitalis and Potassium,* New York, Landsberger Medical Books, 1958, p 39.
15. Kones RJ, Phillips JH, Hersh J: Mechanism and management of chaotic atrial mechanism. *Cardiol* 59:92, 1974.
16. Lewis T, Feil HS, Stroud WD: Observations upon flutter and fibrillation. *Heart* 7:191, 1918-20.
17. Leier CV, Meachom JA, Schaal SF: Prolonged atrial conduction. A major predisposing factor for the development of atrial flutter. *Circulation* 57:213, 1978.
18. Prinzmetal M, Corday E, et al: *The Auricular Arrhythmias,* Springfield, Ill, Charles C Thomas Pub, 1952, p 145.
19. Thurmann M, Janney JR Jr: The diagnostic importance of fibrillatory wave size. *Circulation* 25:991, 1962.
20. Peter RH, Morris JJ Jr, McIntosh HD: Relationship of fibrillatory waves and P waves in the electrocardiogram. *Circulation* 33:599, 1966.
21. Hall JI, Wood DR: Factors affecting cardioversion of atrial arrhythmias with special reference to quinidine. *Br Heart J* 30:84, 1968.

22. Orgain ES, Wolff L, White PD: Uncomplicated auricular fibrillation and auricular flutter. *Arch Intern Med* 57:493, 1936.

23. Singh S: Hemodynamic evaluation of the patient with supraventricular tachycardia. *Practical Cardiol.* 5:131, 1979.

24. Morris JJ Jr, Entman ML, et al: The changes in cardiac output with reversion of atrial fibrillation to sinus rhythm. *Circulation* 31:670, 1964.

25. Irving DW, Corday E: Effect of the cardiac arrhythmias on the renal and mesenteric circulation. *Am J Cardiol* 8:32, 1961.

26. Limpan BS: Aberrancy, ectopy, and reentry in the electrocardiogram. *Practical Cardiol.* 4:107, 1978.

27. Naimi S: Electrophysiological basis for arrhythmias and their therapy, in Levine, H. (ed): *Clinical Cardiovascular.* New York, Grune & Stratton Inc, 1976, p 318.

28. Wantanabe Y, Dreifus L: *Cardiac Arrhythmias: Electrophysiologic Basis for Clinical Interpretation.* New York, Grune & Stratton Inc, 1977, p 20.

29. Berne RM, Levy MN: *Cardiovascular Physiology,* ed 3. St. Louis, CV Mosby Co, 1977, p 30.

30. Lipman BS, Massie E, Kleiger RE: *Clinical Scalar Electrocardiography,* ed 6. Chicago, Year Book Medical Pub Inc, 1972, p 405.

31. Fowler NO: *Cardiac Diagnosis and Treatment,* ed 2. Hagerstown, Md, Harper & Row Pub Inc, 1976, p 1028.

7
Disturbances of Atrioventricular Conduction

Automaticity and spontaneous depolarization are characteristics identifiable not only with the sinus node but also with the junctional tissue. As such, each can assume a pacemaking function either by usurpation or through default. This may be in the form of an individual beat or an established rhythm.

The process of usurpation is recognized electrocardiographically by the early appearance of the ectopic beat and is related to an increase in automaticity. The escape beat, however, would occur later than the expected sinus beat (Fig. 7-1). Both can be a result of the depression of impulse formation or conduction secondary to pronounced vagal stimulation, ischemia, infarction (atrial), overdigitalization, hyperkalemia, and excessive tobacco or coffee consumption. Depression of sinoatrial activity, however, can occur in healthy, young individuals.

JUNCTIONAL ESCAPE BEATS; RHYTHM

When the sinus node is unduly suppressed or impulse formation and/or conduction are affected by pathological processes, the junctional tissue, although having a slower inherent rate (30–60 beats per minute) can pace the heart. If the sinus node fails to function for one beat, the atrioventricular junctional escape beat will follow the prolonged pause for that one beat and allow for the sinoatrial node to regain its function. However, if the sinus beat is ineffective, atrioventricular junctional rhythm supervenes. Electrocardiographically, one would note the presence of an established rhythm initiated by an escape AV junctional beat, that is, a junctional beat that occurred somewhat later than the expected sinus beat.

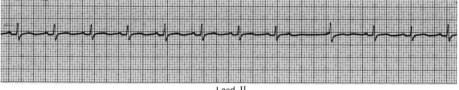

Lead II

Figure 7-1. Junctional escape beat.

115

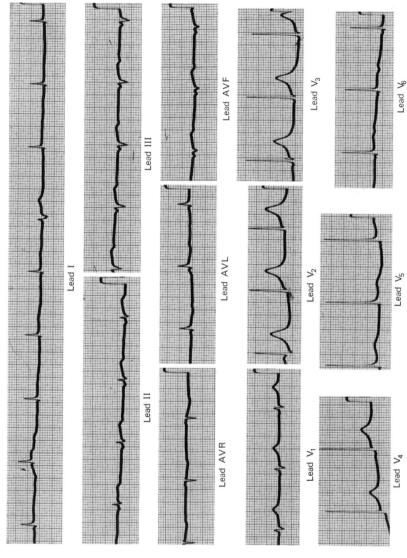

Figure 7-2. Junctional rhythm with retrograde activation of the atria. The PR interval is 0.10 second.

Lead I

Lead II

Lead III

Lead AVR

Lead AVL

Lead AVF

Lead V_1

Lead V_2

Lead V_3

Lead V_4

Lead V_5

Lead V_6

Controversy still exists about whether there are pacemaking cells within the atrioventricular node itself or whether these cells are found primarily in the surrounding junctional tissue. In this text, the term *junctional* will be used. The junctional ectopic beats are usually classified as occurring from the upper, mid, or lower junctional areas.

Electrocardiographic Features

If the escape focus is located in the uppermost part of the junctional tissue, antegrade conduction (to the ventricles) will proceed normally and the atria will be activated in a retrograde manner (Fig. 7-2). The P wave therefore will be inverted in leads II, III, and aV_F and upright in aV_R, but will appear before the QRS-T complexes. The axis of the P wave, instead of being around +60 will be located in the superior axis around –90. The PR interval will be less than 0.12 second (1). If the escape focus is located in the central area of the atrioventricular junction, both antegrade and retrograde activation will occur simultaneously and the P wave will be overshadowed by the QRS complex; thus only an R wave will be identifiable (Fig. 7-3). Location of the escape focus in the lower end of the junctional tissue would reveal that antegrade conduction of the impulse to the ventricles precedes retrograde activation of the atria, hence an inverted P wave will follow the R wave in leads II, III, and aV_F (Fig. 7-4). In this situation the RP interval rarely exceeds 0.11 second. As depicted on an electrocardiogram the presence and configuration of the P wave depnds upon the site of the escape focus. Chung (2) emphasizes the fact that not only must the proximity of the ectopic pacemaker to the atria and

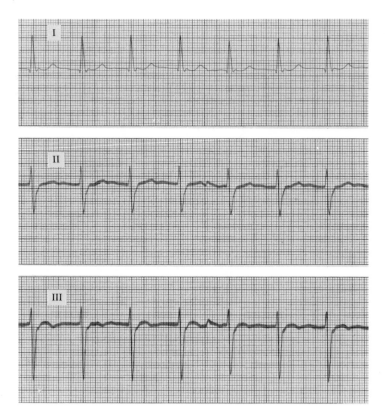

Figure 7-3. Midjunctional mechanism.

AGE 63

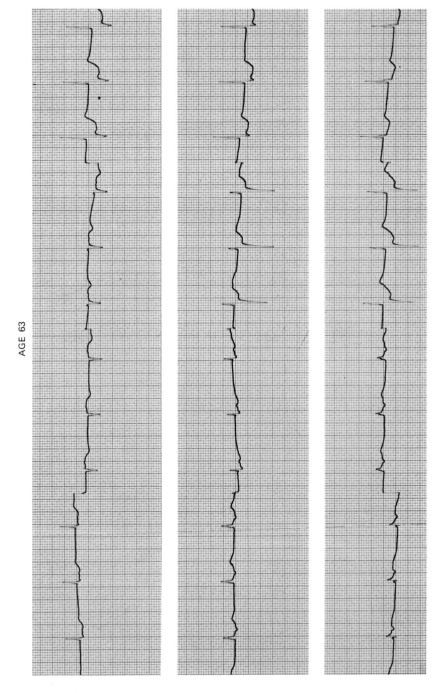

Figure 7–4. Low junctional mechanism with retrograde activation of the atria. Ventricular activation precedes retrograde activation of the atria.

ventricles be taken into consideration, but other factors such as the speed of impulse conduction must be weighed.

Junctional escape beats are usually associated with sinoatrial block or arrest. They serve as a safety factor when the normal pacemaker of the heart is functionally inefficient.

PREMATURE JUNCTIONAL CONTRACTION (PJC)

As previously mentioned, the atrioventricular junction can also be the site of premature impulse contraction (PJC). The premature junctional contraction, like the escape beat, may occur as a result of sinus node depression, ischemia of tissue, and overdigitalization.

A series of three consecutive premature junctional beats constitutes junctional tachycardia which can arbitrarily be categorized as slow junctional tachycardia and rapid junctional tachycardia. In slow junctional tachycardia the rate is greater than 60 beats per minute. Rapid junctional tachycardia indicates that the ventricular rate is in excess of 100 beats per minute. The usual range is 100 to 220.

Other terms associated with junctional rhythm are paroxysmal and nonparoxysmal (accelerated) junctional tachycardis. The former is related to a sudden onset of junctional tachycardia, which may occur with a rate of 130 to 220 beats per minute, whereas the latter is usually gradual in onset and associated with a ventricular rate of 70 to 130 beats per minute (3).

The premature junctional beat, like premature atrial contraction, may be associated with congestive heart failure, myocardial infarction, rheumatic heart disease, and increased sympahtetic tone.

Electrocardiographic Features

The QRS morphology associated with a premature junctional beat is similar to that of the sinus complex unless it is associated with ventricular aberration (4) (see p. 109). Differentiation between a low atrial premature contraction and a junctional premature beat is usually made on the basis of the P′R interval, which in the PJC is less than 0.11 second.

One can likewise measure the interval between the end of the P′ wave and the onset of the R wave. In premature atrial contractions the interval may be shortened or normal; however, it is usually greater than 0.05 second, which is the normal delay time in the atrioventricular junction.

In the event that a premature junctional beat is accompanied by a bizarre QRS complex, consideration must be given to whether the impulse is conducted aberrantly or whether a premature ventricular contraction exists. An RP interval of 0.11 second or less suggests the presence of a premature junctional beat with aberration, whereas an RP of 0.12 second or greater is more frequently associated with a ventricular beat with retrograde conduction to the atria (5).

ATRIOVENTRICULAR (AV) BLOCKS

Delay in transmission or complete blocking of an impulse indicates a derangement in the functional property of the N fibers within the atrioventricular node (see Chap. 1). In normal hearts, conduction from the atria to the His bundle is from 50 to 120 msec (6).

Since the junctional tissue is abundantly supplied with vagal and sympathetic nerve fibers, prolonged vagal stimulation and/or the blocking of B-adrenergic fibers will result in the slowing of impulse transmission to the ventricles.

Although the delay in transmission of an impulse can occur at any site of the conduction system (Fig. 7-5), prolongation of the passage of an impulse from the sinus node through the junctional region and His bundle reflects first-degree AV block and is identified electrocardiographically by a PR interval beyond the normal range for a designated age group (Fig. 7-6). The His bundle recording will depict prolongation of the AH interval (7). According to Corday (8), the normal PR interval differs with age groups and heart rate. The maximal PR interval for a person within the age group of 17 years and older, is 0.20 second, while 0.18 second is maximal for the 14 to 17-year-old group. The fourteen years and younger age groups manifest a maximal PR interval of 0.16 second. Thus the PR interval tends to lengthen with age and shorten with rapid heart rates.

Another variable influencing the PR interval is that of body position and maneuvers. Shortening of the PR interval occurs with an upright position, which is associated with an increase in sympathetic activity and vagal depression (9); and lengthening of the PR interval usually occurs with carotid sinus pressure (8).

Atrioventricular blocks are generally classified as first-degree, second-degree, and third-degree, or complete, according to severity and location of lesion (Table 7-1). They may be further categorized as incomplete, complete, transient, and/or permanent.

First-degree AV Block

Since the PR interval represents the total time of impulse transmission from the atria to the ventricles, the exact site of delay in impulse transmission is not reflected on the surface electrocardiogram. Yet, according to Goldschlager and Scheinman (10), the

---

Figure 7-5. (a) Simultaneous recording of unipolar and bipolar electrograms from the area of the AV junction and lead II electrocardiogram. The components of the PR interval are (1) PA time, (2) AH time, and (3) HV time. PA time: the time interval from the onset of the P wave to the A wave. AH time: the time interval from the A wave to the bundle of His (BH) deflection. HV time: the time interval from BH to the onset of ventricular activation (V). A: bipolar atrial electrogram from the area of the AV junction. BH: bipolar electrogram of the bundle of His. V: bipolar ventricular electrogram from the area of the AV junction. UE: unipolar electrogram from the area of the AV junction. BE: bipolar electrogram from the area of the AV junction. L2: lead II of the standard lead electrocardiogram. (b) Diagrammatic representation of the AV conduction system illustrating that the different varieties of the AV block can occur as a result of lesions in different segments of the conducting system. At the bottom left-hand corner are the simultaneous recordings of a standard electrocardiograph lead II (L-2) and a typical bipolar electrogram (BE) from the area of the AV junction. SAN: sinoatrial node. AVN: atrioventricular node. BH: bundle of His. RB and LB: right and left bundle branches, respectively. AH: conduction time through the AVN. HV: conduction time through the His-Purkinje system. A: bipolar atrial electrogram. V: the ventricular electrogram recorded from the area of the AV junction. (Reproduced with permission from Narula OS et al: Atrioventricular block-localization and classification by His bundle recordings. *Am J Med* 50:147, 1971.)

site of atrioventricular block has greater significance than the degree of block. For this reason, there is wider use of the His bundle recording in delineating the exact site of delay or block. (See Chap. 6 for further discussion of His bundle recordings.)

Goldschlager and Scheinman (10) further suggest that a prolonged PR interval in association with a normal QRS complex may indicate a delay in conduction within the AV node or His bundle, whereas a prolonged PR interval and widened QRS complex greater than 0.12 second is highly suggestive of a transmission delay beyond the His bundle.

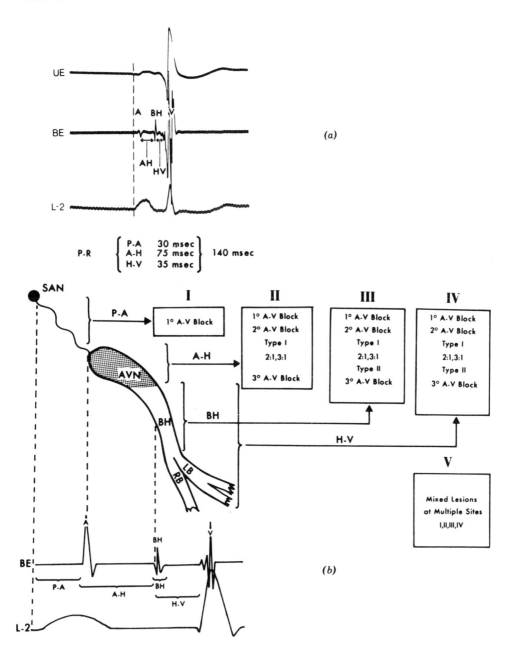

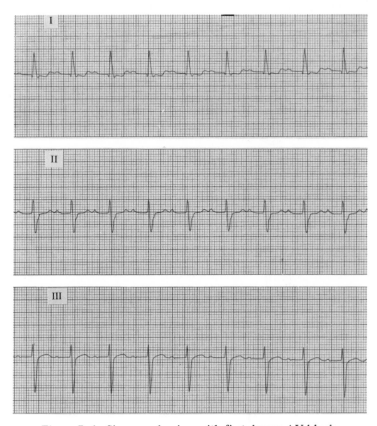

Figure 7-6. Sinus mechanism with first-degree AV block.

Table 7-1. Types of Conduction Disturbances

Atrioventricular
  First degree
  Second degree
  Third degree
  AV dissociation

Intraventricular
  Monofascicular
    RBB
    LBB
    LAFB
  Bifascicular
    RBB + LAFB
    LPFB
    RBB + LBBB
  Trifascicular
    RBBB + LAH +
      1st degree AV block

Electrocardiographic Features

P Wave   Precedes every QRS deflection.
PR interval   Prolonged beyond range for age and heart rate.
                    Adult 0.20 second with heart rate 60 to 100 beats per minute.
                    Child 0.16.
QRS complex   Normal in configuration and duration.
                    Follows every P wave.
RR Interval   Regular.

Second–degree AV Block

Two forms of second-degree atrioventricular block generally are identifiable: Mobitz type I and Mobitz type II block. Mobitz type I block (11) may be recognized by a progressive prolongation of the PR interval until there is failure of an atrial beat to be conducted to the ventricles (Fig. 7-7). According to Guntheroth (12), the mechanism attributed to the periodic failure of the transmission of an impulse through the atrioventricular node (junction) in Wenckebach's phenomenon is the fatiguing of the atrioventricular node in a cumulative manner. Although this type of conduction disturbance is usually associated with transient ischemia of the atrioventricular node, it may be a naturally occurring phenomenon in some athletes. The block is usually confined to the area preceding the bifurcation of the His bundle. His bundle recordings of the Wenckebach phenomenon (Mobitz type I block) would reveal progressive lengthening of the AH interval until the dropping of the beat. The P wave therefore would not be followed by a His bundle spike (13).

A criterion for the diagnosis of Mobitz type II AV block according to Phibbs (14) is the presence of two or more normally conducted sinus beats associated with a PR interval that is constant and that occurs before a P wave not followed by a QRS complex.

Goldman (15) categorized Mobitz II AV block into two subsets: second–degree periodic block, in which there is failure of the ventricles to respond periodically (after every fifth or sixth beat), and second–degree constant block, in which the ventricular response to atrial stimulation is after every second impulse, thus giving a ratio of 2:1.

The advanced form of second-degree heart block characterized by a fixed 2:1 ratio is associated with a distinctive pattern of the PP interval. The PP interval, which includes a QRS complex, is shorter in duration than the PP interval not containing a QRS complex. Stock and Williams (16), offer several explanations for this particular pattern. The first is related to coronary blood flow changes where in the shorter PP cycle is most likely associated with improved corony perfusion subsequent to ventricular systole, and the second is related to a baroreceptor response. The latter is associated with a reduction of vagal tone in response to ventricular systole, and the former is identified as a form of sinus arrhythmia (ventriculophasic) (see Chap. 5).

As mentioned previously, unlike the Wenckebach phenomenon (Mobitz type I AV Block), the PR interval in Mobitz II is constant (Fig. 7-8). The His bundle recording usually identifies the block to be distal to the His bundle or intermediate between the His bundle and Purkinje system (see Fig. 7-5). The AH interval remains normal. However, there is periodic absence of a QRS complex following a His bundle spike. Mobitz II AV block, when associated with extensive anterior myocardial infarction, is of greater significance than in the absence of a myocardial infarction. Digitalis as well as sclerodegenerative disease cause this type of second-degree AV block. The disorder is usually

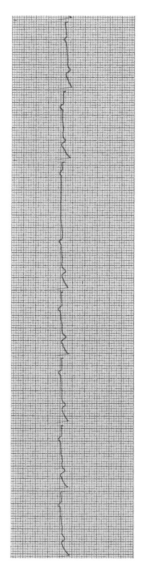

Figure 7-7. Mobitz type I (Wenckebach) AV block.

124

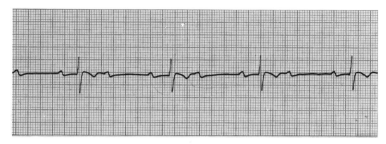

Figure 7-8. Mobitz type II second-degree AV block with 2:1 response.

chronic and frequently is an indication for electrical pacing, since it is considered to be a precursor of complete heart block (17). Prognostically, Mobitz II is thought to be of graver significance than Mobitz I, for Adams-Stokes attacks occur more frequently and the block is frequently associated with a right bundle branch block (18).

Electrocardiographic Features
Mobitz type I block

P wave   Precedes the majority of QRS complexes.

PR interval   Progressively prolonged; greatest increment between the first and second conducted beats; shortest increment between the second and third conducted beats.

Pause   Duration of pause is shorter than twice the preceding sinus intervals. According to Goldschlager and Scheinman, is equal to two sinus beats minus the PR interval.

QRS complex   Usually normal in configuration; an indication that the block is within the AV node.
                Occasionally, the block may occur within the His–Purkinje system; thus the QRS complex will be widened.

RR interval   Slightly irregular. As PR interval increases, the RR decreases.

Mobitz Type II Block

P wave   Every 2nd, 3rd, or 4th atrial complex is followed by a QRS complex.

PR interval   Constant; may be normal or prolonged.

QRS complex   Periodic and/or regular failure of QRS to follow sinus conducted impulse. Block may occur as 2:1, 3:1 conduction ratio. The conduction ratio may be fixed or varying. Since the block is infrajunctional, the QRS complex may be widened 0.12 second.

RR interval   Usually regular.

Third-degree AV Block (Complete Heart Block)

In complete heart block, the heart is paced from two independent pacemaking sites. The atria respond to a stimulus orginating usually in the sinus node, and the ventricles respond to the impulse originating either in the AV node, His bundle, bundle branches, or Purkinje network. The location of the pacemaking site to which the ventricles respond will have an effect upon heart rate and ultimately cardiac output. If the ventricles are paced by the impulse from the AV node (junction), the heart rate will be in the range of 50 to 60, which is the inherent rate of the AV node, and the QRS complex will resemble that responding to a sinus pacemaker. However, if the pacemaking site is located in the lower sections of the ventricles, the heart rate usually is in the range of 20 to 30 beats per minute, a rate not well tolerated by an active individual. Consequently, Adams-Stokes attacks can occur.

According to Cosby and associates (19), in addition to the syncopal episodes associated with Adams-Stokes attacks, several accompanying signs may be present. The individual may become very pale and lose consciousness and may have an absence of peripheral pulses. Prolongation of the syncopal attack is associated with a color change—from paleness to ashen gray. Stertorous breathing may become evident, and absence of sphincter control and seizures are additional features associated with the Adams-Stokes episodes. Occasionally, flushing of the face may occur as a response to vasodilation associated with hypoxia. The mechanism most commonly involved in producing Adams-Stokes attacks is that of ventricular standstill or fibrillation in the presence or absence of sino-atrial activity.

The electrocardiographic features peculiar to complete heart block and which distinguish this conduction disturbance from that of other forms of AV dissociation are an atrial rate that is faster than the ventricular rate and the presence of a latent pacemaker that is not necessarily accelerated. That is to say, if the ventricles respond to a junctional pacemaker, the rate will usually be less than 60 beats per minute rather than the rate expected of tachycardia. If the escape pacemaker is within the ventricles, the rate will most likely be less than 40 beats per minute (20) (Fig. 7–9).

Electrocardiographic Features

Corday and Irving (8) consider five features essential in the diagnosis of complete heart block:

1. The absence of an existent relationship between atrial and ventricular complexes.
2. The presence of more frequent atrial complexes than ventricular deflections.
3. A varying PR interval.
4. Regularity of both atrial and ventricular rhythms, each related to the inherent rate of the driving pacemaker.
5. Normally appearing P waves and QRS deflections. The QRS complex is influenced by the site of the subsidiary pacemaker to which the ventricles respond. If the latent pacemaker is the AV node, the QRS complex will be normal in configuration and

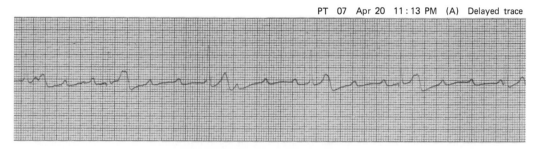

PT 07 Apr 20 11 : 13 PM (A) Delayed trace

Figure 7–9. Complete heart block.

duration. However, if the ventricles respond to an infranodal, infra-His bundle pacemaker, the QRS complex may be bizarre in configuration and abnormal in duration.

Despite the fact that complete heart block is characterized by complete dissociation between atrial and ventricular rhythms, occasionally, the atrial rhythm may be influenced by ventricular activity. A PP interval encompassing a ventricular complex in complete heart block is usually shorter than the PP interval without a QRS complex. In the former, it is thought that the ventricular activity precipitates and/or accelerates the presence of the ensuing P wave, which results in a shortened PP interval. The presence of a shortened PP interval (one encompassing a QRS complex) accompanied by a longer PP interval (without an intervening QRS complex) denotes the presence of ventricular sinus arrhythmia. Schamroth (4) identifies certain factors that contribute to the initiation of ventriculophasic sinus arrhythmia in the presence of complete heart block:

1. A rise in intra-atrial pressure after ventricular contraction. The sequence initiates the Bainbridge reflex, resulting in vagal inhibition and sinoatrial acceleration.
2. Following ventricular contraction, the sinoatrial node may discharge more rapidly as a result of receiving a greater blood supply.
3. The mechanical effect of ventricular contraction causes traction to be placed upon the atria. Consequently, the traction stimulates the sinoatrial node to a more rapid discharge.

Etiology

The pathogenesis of atrioventricular block may be considered multifactorial. Vagal stimulation, blocking of the B-adrenergic fibers, total absence of the atrioventricular node, and/or degenerative lesions can affect the conduction system. In addition, drug toxicity, electrolyte imbalances, and/or inflammatory lesions can produce prolongation or complete cessation of impulse conductance (Table 7-2).

Clinical Manifestations

First-degree AV Block. Usually there are no symptoms associated with first-degree atrioventricular block. A direct relationship exists between the length of the PR interval and the intensity of the first heart sound. Generally when the PR interval is short (0.12), the first heart sound is sharp and loud; at a PR interval of 0.14 second, the first heart sound is moderately sharp; and as the PR interval lengthens beyond 0.20 second, the first heart sound is faint (21). Therefore in first-degree AV block, the first heart sound would be very faint. The physiological basis associated with the varying intensity of the first heart sound is related to the position of the atrioventricular valves during a cardiac cycle. When a long interval occurs between atrial and ventricular contraction, the atrioventricular valves have floated back to their normal position and initial closure has begun (11). The significance of first-degree AV block lies in the fact that there may be progression to a more severe degree of heart block. This is particularly true when first-degree AV block accompanies myocardial infarction.

Second-degree AV Block (Mobitz type 1: Wenckbach). A pause of the dropped beat followed by a slight acceleration of heart rate might be suggestive of the Wenckebach phenomenon. Palpitations are commonly experienced by the individual. This may be attributed to a greater ventricular filling subsequent to the dropped beat, resulting in greater myocardial fiber stretch and more vigorous chamber contraction. Auscultation

Table 7-2. Etiologic Factors Implicated in Conduction Impairment

Vagotonia	*Drug-Related*	*Electrolyte Imbalance*	*Inflammatory Disease*
Vagal maneuvers eyeball pressure carotid massage	Quinindine Procaine amide Norpace	K^+	Rheumatic Viral Myocarditis

Iatrogenic	*Congenital*	*Degenerative Conditions*	
Surgical trauma	Absence of AV node	Coronary artery disease Myocardial infarction (see Chap. 10) Sclerotic changes Lev's disease Lenegre's disease	

of the chest would reveal a rhythmically varying intensity of the first heart sound. As the PR progressively lengthens, the intensity of the first heart sound decreases.

Second-degree AV Block (Mobitz type II). This type of conduction disturbance may be accompanied by Adams-Stokes attacks, which are minifested by facial pallor, absence of pulse, and loss of consciousness with or without seizures. There is a greater tendency for Adams-Stokes attacks to occur during the transition of Mobitz type II AV block to complete heart block (10). The individual may complain of "chest or head thumping" or palpitations secondary to greater filling of the ventricles following the dropped beat. Since the PR interval is constant, varrying intensity of the first heart sound will not be evident.

Third-degree AV block (Complete Heart Block). The clinical manifestations associated with complete heart block are related, according to Haft (7), to the two effects of the block. They may be related to the inability of the heart to increase its rate when needed and secondly to the unreliability of the low ventricular pacemaker. The bradycardia-related symptoms associated with complete heart block are activity-related fatigue, precordial discomfort, palpitations, Stokes-Adams syncope, and/or shortness of breath. Alterations in blood pressure may also become evident in the presence of complete heart block. The systolic pressure occasionally may be elevated, whereas the diastolic pressure is lowered, resulting in a wide pulse pressure.

A variation in the intensity of the first heart sound is evident upon auscultation of the anterior chest wall (21). Auscultation of the anterior chest in the presence of right bundle branch block reveals distinct splitting of the first heart sound, heard best at the left sternal border and the apicosternal sternal region. Abnormal splitting of the second heart sound is evident both during expiration and to a greater degree on inspiration. Paradoxical splitting of the second heart sound occurs in the presence of left bundle branch block.

Therapy

In the presence of first- and second-degree (Mobitz I type) atrioventricular blocks that are not associated with alterations in hemodynamics, no treatment is indicated. Mobitz type II atrioventricular blocks may be associated with significant slowing of ventricular rate; thus temporary transvenous pacing may be indicated. This is especially true when this type of block is associated with an anterior myocardial infarction (see Chap. 10). Treatment for complete heart block is dependent upon the ventricular rate.

Atropine and isoproterenol are drugs capable of suppressing the vagal effect upon the AV node and thus are indications of whether the ectopic pacemaker "driving" the ventricles in complete heart block is located in the atrioventricular node (14). These drugs, however, have little or no effect upon an ectopic site within the ventricles, and an electrical pacemaker must be inserted. Thus the width of the QRS reflects site of the ectopic pacemaker. If atrioventricular block is a response to toxic effects of drugs and/or to electrolyte imbalance (potassium excess), efforts to correct the toxicity and/or imbalance must be undertaken (22).

ATRIOVENTRICULAR DISSOCIATION

Atrioventricular dissociation as described by Lipman and associates (23) is always a secondary rhythm in which there are two independent pacemakers. The atria respond to one pacemaker and the ventricles are governed by another. Although the atrial and ventri-

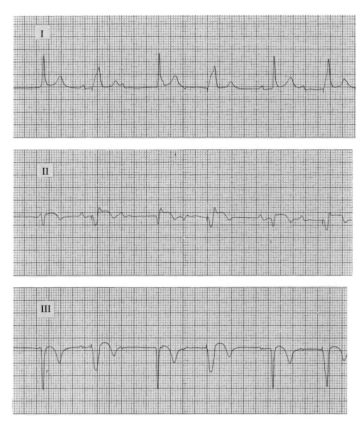

Figure 7-10. Junctional tachycardia with AV dissociation. Sinus pauses of brief duration are noted with escape junctional rhythm.

cular rhythms are regular, the ventricular rate usually is faster than the atrial rate (Fig. 7-10).

According to Schamroth (24), two basic arrhythmic disturbances lead to AV dissociation, namely, an impulse-formation disturbance and/or an impulse-conduction disturbance. The discharge sequence of the sinus node occasionally may be delayed or impaired secondary to vagal stimulation and/or drug therapy. When this occurs, a subsidiary pacemaker with an inherent rate slower than the normal sinus pacing rate but somewhat faster at the time of depression and/or sinoatrial blocking gains control of ventricular activation. In this situation, the subsidiary pacemaker, usually the AV node (junction), assumes the pacemaking function by default (25). The pacemaker role can likewise be unsurped by irritable foci in the atria, AV junction, and/or ventricles.

A functional rather than organic block distinguishes AV dissociation from third-degree heart block. Impulses of sinus or atrial origin are usually not conducted to the ventricles nor can retrograde activation of the atria occur. The reason for the antegrade and retrograde blocking is related to the refractoriness of depolarized tissue. Impulse transmission from both pacemaking sites is impeded (26). Occasionally, a sinoatrial impulse may occur at a time when the junctional tissue is nonrefractory and therefore is transmitted to activate the ventricle. This sequence results in a ventricular capture beat (24). According to Marriott (27), the capture beat interferes with the ventricular rhythm and hence the event is termed *interference dissociation*. Recognition of a capture beat is possible if the following features are evident (24):

1. An association of the capture beat with the preceding P wave.
2. The morphology of the capture beat differs from that of the configuration of the subsidiary pacemaker (if ventricular in origin).
3. In the presence of a subsidiary pacemaker within the AV junction, the QRS complex may be normal in configuration, reflecting antegrade conduction or the morphology of the capture beat may be altered owing to aberrant ventricular conduction (see Chap. 6).

At times, the rate of the independent pacemakers may be similar. The term *isorhythmic dissociation* is used to identify this feature (24). Other descriptive terms related to the above features are synchronization and accrochage. The former term as used by Schamroth (24) implies the presence of a relatively long sequence of identical rates by the independent pacemakers, whereas the latter denotes the presence of the phenomenon for a shorter period of time.

Since AV dissociation is a secondary dysrhythmia, intervention is directed toward the identification of the cause. The dysrhythmia can be distinguished from third-degree AV block by the atrial and ventricular rates. Atrial rate is more rapid than the ventricular rate in third-degree AV block, whereas in AV dissociation, the ventricular rate is more rapid.

HIS BUNDLE ELECTROCARDIOGRAPHY

A diagnostic tool available to the cardiologist in delineating more precisely the location of atrioventricular conduction blocks is the His bundle electrocardiogram (28). In addition, it is commonly utilized in the following situations: (*1*) differentiating complex rhythm disturbances such as paroxysmal supraventricular tachycardia with aberrancy from that of ventricular tachycardia, (*2*) in the identification of preexcitation of the ventricles, and (*3*) the determination of site of reentry associated with paroxysmal supraventricular tachycardia (29).

According to Aranda and associates (30) the His bundle electrocardiogram may be valuable in the determination of prognosis in the patient who has sustained a myocardial infarction and whose basic problem is complicated by the presence of an incomplete bundle branch block. A more current use of the His bundle recording is its application in evaluating the effects of pharmacokinetic agents.

The surface electrocardiogram identifies depolarization of the atria (P wave), depolarization of the ventricles (QRS complex), conduction from the SA node through the ventricular muscle (PR interval), and repolarization of the ventricles (T wave). Thus a prolonged PR interval merely indicates that there is a delay in transmission of the impulse somewhere from the sinus node to the ventricular muscle. The His bundle recording, on the other hand, as depicted in Figure 7-5 identifies more precisely the timing of of impulse conduction through the PR subintervals:

1. Sinus node through the atrial conduction: PA segment.
2. Impulse transmission from the low atrium to the His bundle: AH interval.

3. His bundle to the beginning of ventricular activation: HV interval. The latter is a direct measurement of conduction time through the His bundle just beyond the site of the recording electrode, the left and right bundle branches, and the Purkinje fibers of the ventricular myocardium (29).

The technique involved in obtaining a His bundle recording is the insertion of a bipolar or tripolar electrode catheter percutaneously through a femoral or arm vein to the level of the septal leaflet of the tricuspid valve (31). The advancement of the electrode catheter to the site of the tricuspid valve is possible through the use of fluoroscopy, although when a balloon-tip catheter is utilized, fluoroscopy is not always necessary (28). As can be seen in Figure 7–5 there is a direct correlation between the events of a cardiac conduction of an impulse, a surface electrocardiogram, and a His bundle recording.

The accepted normal range for the PA interval is 25 to 46 msec (28). An AH interval prolonged beyond the upper limits of normal, 140 msec, reflects a delay in transmission of the impulse through the artioventricular junctional tissue (32). Prolongation of transmission impulse through the bundle of His and initial ventricular activation is reflected by an HV interval in excess of 55 msec. Information-reflecting activity within the His bundle is identified by the H spike. Impaired conduction at this site is reflected by a time interval in excess of the normal His bundle duration of 15 to 20 msec (28).

In conjunction with the His bundle recording, atrial pacing is frequently employed as a means of stress testing the conduction system. Frequently, abnormalities are identified during the stress testing with rapid atrial rates which are perhaps not evident during a resting state. During rapid atrial pacing, the AH interval usually increases, but the HV interval remains unchanged (33). Further discussion of His bundle recordings will be in association with specific rhythm/conduction disturbances.

WOLF-PARKINSON-WHITE (WPW) SYNDROME

The ECG findings of a short PR interval with an abnormal QRS complex were initially described by Wilson (34) in 1915. In 1930 Wolff, Parkinson, and White (34) jointly collected eleven patients whose ECGs showed the abnormal PR interval and QRS complex. Their patients were relatively young and healthy, but prone to bouts of paroxysmal tachycardias, and this clinical entity became known as the Wolff-Parkinson-White syndrome. Öhnell (35) in 1944 incorporated the word preexcitation (PES or preexcitation syndrome) to explain the premature activation of a portion of the ventricle before the impulse could have arrived by the normal conduction pathway to activate the ventricle.

The incidence of the WPW syndrome is difficult to assess because it alone does not produce symptoms unless rapid tachycardias develop. Additionally, the conduction abnormality in the WPW syndrome is often intermittent. The WPW syndrome has been estimated to occur in 0.15% to 0.20% of the general population (36). It occurs more frequently in males than in females (37), and the incidence of tachycardia is related to the population sampled. Tachyarrhythmias were found in only 13% (34) of patients when the WPW syndrome was diagnosed from a routine ECG as opposed to a 40% to 80% incidence in hospitalized or cardiac clinic patients (38). The preexcitation syndrome is not associated with organic heart disease about two-thirds of the time (38,36).

Patients with hyperthyroidism have been shown to have a higher incidence (39). The WPW syndrome is found frequently in patients with idopathic hypertrophic subaortic stenosis, Ebstein's anomaly, mitral valve prolapse, rheumatic heart disease, atrial septal defect, familial cardiomyopathy, tricuspid atresia, and transposition of the great vessels (40, 41, 42, 43, 36).

Pathogenesis

Premature stimulation of the ventricles through accessory pathways from the atria to the ventricles is the mechanism responsible for ventricular preexcitation. Various pathways have been identified, and they include Kent's bundle, Mahaim fibers, and James fibers (Fig. 7-11). The bundle of Kent is located between the free wall of the left or right atrium and the corresponding ventricle, which accounts for the bypassing of the AV node and subsequent short PR interval on the ECG. The abnormal premature activation of a portion of the ventricle changes the initial part of the QRS complex and is called the delta wave. Ventricular depolarization is abnormal and produces a wide QRS, which resembles a bundle branch block pattern. Repolarization is affected secondarily, producing the ST and T wave changes (45). The James fibers insert themselves into the distal part of the AV node or the proximal part of the His bundle bypassing the upper or central AV node, where the impulse is normally delayed. Ventricular depolarization is not altered, which leaves a normal QRS complex, and only the PR interval is affected (shortened) (37) (Fig. 7-12). The James fibers are thought to be responsible for the Lown-Ganong-Levine syndrome (46). The Mahaim fibers are short fibers connecting the lower AV node region and the bundle of His with the ventricular septum (45). When conduction occurs along these fibers a normal PR interval is recorded since the impulse may travel normally through the AV node, but an abnormal QRS (delta wave with wide QRS) is produced since the ventricles are preexcited (47) (Fig. 7-12). Combinations of abnormal conduction through the Mahaim fibers as well as the James fibers could produce a short PR interval, delta wave, and wide QRS stimulating conduction through either bundle of Kent (37).

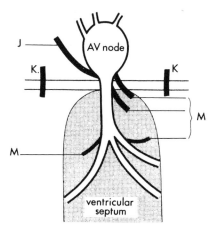

Figure 7-11. Schematic representation of the location of the anomalous AV pathways playing a possible role in the preexcitation syndrome. J: James fibers; K: Kent fibers; M: Mahaim fibers. (Reproduced with permission from Durrer D, Schuilenburg RM and Wellens HJJ: Pre-excitation revisited. *Am. J. Cardiol* 25:690, 1970.)

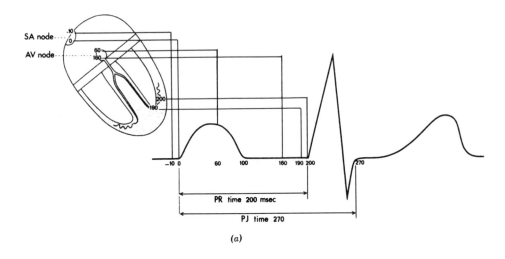

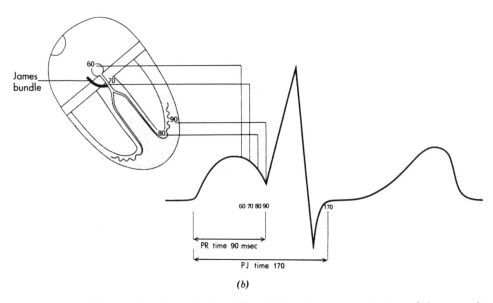

Figure 7-12. (*a*) Normal AV conduction. The relation between excitation of the normal human heart and its electrocardiogram as recorded from a standard lead (values in milliseconds). (*b*) James fibers. Schematic representation of the relation between excitation of the heart with James fibers and its electrocardiogram as recorded from a standard lead. (*c*) Mahaim bundle. Relation between excitation of the heart with a Mahaim bundle and its electrocardiogram as recorded from a standard lead. (Reproduced with permission from Durrer D, Schuilenburg RM, Wellens HJJ: Pre-excitation revisited. *Am J Cardiol* 25:690, 1970.)

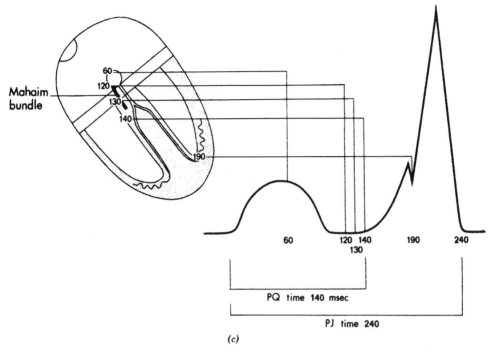

(c)

Figure 7-12. (Continued)

Electrocardiographic Features

The diagnosis of the WPW syndrome rests entirely on the ECG findings since there are no hemodynamic alterations or symptoms produced. The classic findings on the ECG include (*1*) a PR interval less than 0.12 second, (*2*) a delta wave on the initial part of the QRS complex, and (*3*) a QRS wider than 0.12 second (34) (Fig. 7-13). There are variants of this syndrome that do not meet all these criteria (36). The Lown-Ganong-Levine syndrome is included as a preexcitation syndrome, and it is characterized by a PR interval less than 0.12 second, a normal QRS complex, and paroxysmal tachycardias (44) (Fig. 7-14).

Classification

The WPW syndrome was classified into type A and type B by Rosenbaum and associates in 1945 (48). These two classes are based on the QRS morphology and the direction of the delta wave in the precordial leads. In type A, the delta wave and the remainder of the QRS are upright in leads V_{1-2} owing to early activation of the left ventricle (37) (Fig. 7-15). In type B, the delta wave is negative as is the remainder of the QRS complex in V_{1-2} (Fig. 7-15). Type A WPW syndrome produces a premature activation of the left ventricle, which may be misdiagnosed on the ECG as right bundle branch block, right ventricular hypertrophy, or true posterior myocardial infarction because of the tall R waves in the right precordial leads (Fig. 7-16). The delta wave tends to be more prominent and the QRS complex wider in type A as opposed to type B (50). The T waves are usually inverted in V_{1-3} in type A. The WPW syndrome of the type A classi-

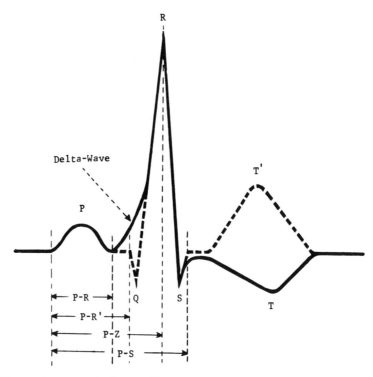

Figure 7-13. The uninterrupted line indicates an anomalous conduction in Wolff-Parkinson-White syndrome, whereas the dotted line indicates a normal conduction. PR and PR′ intervals are AV conduction times in Wolff-Parkinson-White syndrome and normal conduction, respectively. The PR interval is shorter than the PR′ interval because of a delta wave. Note that the PZ and PS intervals are constant during anomalous and normal conduction. The T wave in Wolff-Parkinson-White syndrome is inverted because of secondary T wave change. (Reproduced with permission from Chung EK: *Principles of Cardiac Arrhythmias.* Copyright © 1977, Williams and Wilkins Co., Baltimore.)

fication is found less frequently than type B (49). Premature activation of the right ventricle occurs in type B and accounts for the Q or QS deflection seen in the right precordial leads and the secondary ST and T wave changes in the left precordial leads (Fig. 7-17). This ECG pattern may be misinterpreted as anterior or anteroseptal myocardial infarction. Tall R waves in leads I, aV_L and V_{4-6} along with the ST and T wave changes, can mimic left ventricular hypertrophy (50) or left bundle branch block (wide QRS) (45). Abnormal Q waves may be seen in both type A and type B in leads II, III, and aV_F, which may be misdiagnosed as an inferior myocardial infarction (45) (Fig. 7-18). When the WPW syndrome occurs intermittently it mimics junctional or ventricular premature contractions as well as short runs of ventricular tachycardia. Patients with type B preexcitation syndrome commonly have false-positive exercise ECGs (51). His bundle electrocardiography has played a tremendous role in the accurate diagnosis of the preexcitation syndrome as well as differentiating the mechanism of the tachycardia.

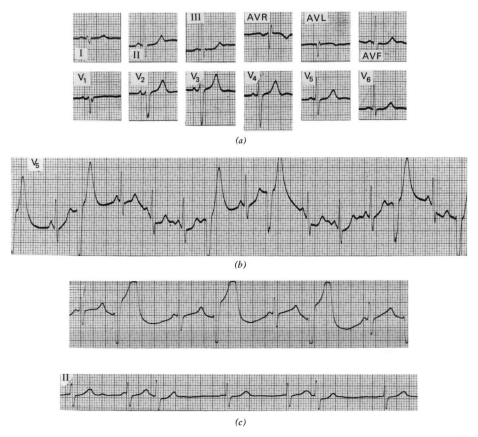

(a)

(b)

(c)

Figure 7-14. (a) 12-lead ECG recorded from a patient with the Lown-Ganong-Levine syndrome. (b) Postexercise rhythm strip reveals PVCs. (c) Two rhythm strips taken from a 24-hour continuous monitoring of the same patient. PVCs (first tracing) as well as PACs (second tracing) are present in a bigeminal pattern. The PR interval of the sinus beats is short.

Clinical Spectrum

The WPW syndrome alone does not compromise circulatory dynamics and therefore is void of symptoms; however, it may be associated with tachyarrhythmias that do produce symptoms, congestive heart failure, and (rarely) death. Paroxysmal supraventricular arrhythmias are commonly encountered and are the result of reentry (52, 53) (Fig. 7-19). (see Chap. 6 for a review of reentry mechanisms.) The impulse may be conducted in an antegrade fashion to the ventricles by the normal pathway and then retrogradely to the atria by the anomalous pathway, which produces a normal QRS configuration (Fig. 7-20). The majority of tachycardias in the WPW syndrome have a normal QRS complex (50) (Fig. 7-21). A wide, bizarre QRS is recorded if the reentry impulse is conducted antegradely to the ventricles by the anomalous pathway and regrogradely to the atria by the normal pathway and mimics ventricular tachycardia (54) (Fig. 7-21). The frequency of tachyarrhythmias varies from 13% to 80% (36, 55). Paroxysmal atrial tachycardia is the most common form of tachyarrhythmia (70 to 80%) seen in patients with WPW syndrome (36, 39). This type of tachycardia is usually regular, with a rate of 140 to 250 beats per minute and a normal QRS configuration (45). Reports from European countries use the term circus movement tachycardia instead of reentry tachycardia (56, 57). Atrial fibrillation or flutter is uncommon in the WPW syndrome and constitutes 10% to 25% of all the tachyarrhythmias (36, 51). Type A WPW syndrome has a higher incidence of atrial fibrillation or flutter than type B and is associated with a wide QRS and rapid ventricular rates (250 to 300 beats per minute) (36, 51). The reentry mechanism alone may not be responsible for the atrial fibrillation or flutter;

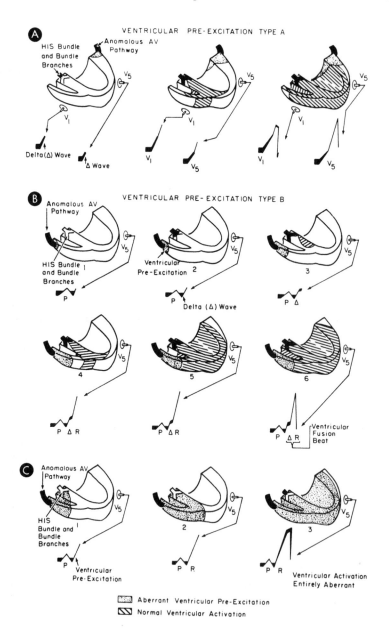

instead a supraventricular premature impulse occurring during the vulnerable period of the atria may initiate the arrhythmia (37). These two types of tachyarrhythmias may produce death, and therefore prompt treatment is necessary (50). Ventricular tachycardia and fibrillation are rare in the WPW syndrome and are often diagnosed incorrectly; however they can be present (58, 59).

Therapy

The management of the patient with Wolff-Parkinson-White syndrome depends upon the presence or absence of tachyarrhythmias. No treatment is indicated in patients free of

---

Figure 7-15. Ventricular preexcitation type A. (*a*) Manner in which the interventricular septum and ventricular muscle are activated in cases of type A ventricular preexcitation. The characteristic features of ventricular preexcitation in the ECG are a short PR interval [the P wave is not shown in (*a*)], an initial slurred component of the first limb of the QRS deflection, the delta wave Δ, and widening of the QRS. In the type A pattern, upright QRS deflections are written in all precordial leads. Since this is the case, it is generally conceded that the anomalous AV pathway must insert posteriorly on the left or right ventricular wall. In the first figure in (*a*), it can be seen that excitation has arrived in the posterobasal region of the left ventricle and is spreading anteriorly, while at the same time the excitation impulse traveling over normal pathways has just reached the bifurcation of the bundle of His. The aberrant spread of the preexcitation wave produces delta waves in leads V_1 and V_5. In the middle figure, the preexcitation wave front continues to spread in an anterior and somewhat rightward direction; but in the meantime, excitation has been distributed over normal pathways to the septum and apicoanterior regions of the ventricles, so that at this point the delta waves inscribed in leads V_1 and V_5 merge with the more steeply rising upstrokes of R waves. In the figure on the right, ventricular activation is nearing completion, the greater portion of the ventricles having been depolarized in normal fashion. Late activation of posterolateral and lateral walls of the left ventricle projects a terminal small S wave on lead V_1 and diminishing positive voltage on lead V_5. (*b*) The sequence of ventricular activation in preexcitation type B. In this pattern, the right precordial leads register essentially downward QRS deflections, while the left precordial leads record upright QRS deflections. This precordial lead pattern may be determined by the fact that the anomalous AV pathway is inserted either on the anterior wall of the right ventricle or somewhere anteriorly in the left ventricle. In type B ventricular preexcitation, the delta wave is produced by spread of the preexcitation wave front in a leftward and posterior direction before the arrival of excitation in the bundle branches. In part 3 of (*b*) septal activation via the normal conducting pathways has begun and produces forces, directed to the right and anteriorly, which tend to nullify the forces produced by the preexcitation process. Consequently, a short plateau appears at the peak of the delta wave. In part 4, as activation of apicoanterior walls of the ventricles occurs, the rapid, steep upstroke of a R wave begins to be written in lead V_5. In parts 5 and 6, ventricular activation continues primarily via the normal conducting pathways and in a normal fashion, so that the remainder of the QRS deflection is essentially like that present during totally normal intraventricular conduction. Consequently, the QRS deflection written in lead V_5 is a ventricular fusion beat, since it represents a fusion of early electrical forces produced by the preexcitation impulse and later electric forces generated by normal ventricular activation. (Reproduced with permission from Cooksey JD, Dunn M, Massie E: *Clinical Vectorcardiography and Electrocardiography,* 2nd edition. Copyright ©1977, Year Book Medical Publishers, Inc., Chicago.)

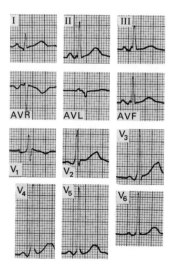

Figure 7-16. Type A WPW was recorded on the ECG of a 45-year-old man. The tall R waves in the right precordial leads mimic RVH or a true posterior MI.

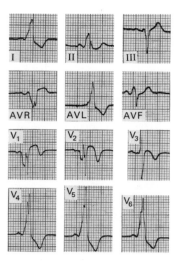

Figure 7-17. Type A WPW produces a LBBB pattern and mimics an anteroseptal MI. Prominent delta waves are present.

arrhythmias and therapy for those with the tachycardias is directed toward interruption of the reentry circuit. This goal can be attained in the following ways: (1) producing equal conduction times in both pathways by slowing conduction in the anomalous pathway or enhancing conduction through the normal pathway, or (2) producing a block (organic or functional) in one or both pathways (50). Lidocaine has been found

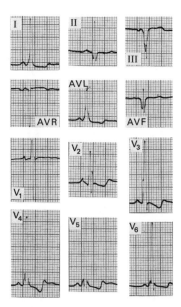

Figure 7-18. Prominent Q waves are seen in leads II, III, and aV$_F$ in this tracing of WPW recorded from a 15-year-old boy.

very useful in terminating supraventricular tacharrhythmias, especially atrial fibrillation and flutter. Conduction through the anomalous pathway is depressed by lidocaine and interrupts the reentry circuit (60, 61). Propranolol (Inderal) is considered to be the drug of first choice in the treatment of supraventricular tachycardias with a normal QRS complex because this drug depresses the normal pathway for conduction (62, 63, 51).

Procainamide (Pronestyl) and quinidine slow conduction (lengthen) effective refractory period) in the accessory pathway and promote conduction through the normal pathway (39). Quinidine also has the beneficial effect of suppressing atrial premature beats which may initiate the tachycardia. Digitalis depresses the normal AV conduction but may accelerate conduction through the anomalous pathway to further promote the reentry circuit (64). It is therefore dangerous to use digitalis alone in patients with atrial fibrillation or flutter and a wide QRS complex (62, 58). Digitalis may be used in the treatment and prevention of tachycardias with a normal QRS complex; however, propranolol is usually the drug of choice (50, 62) (Table 7-3).

Direct current (DC) shock may be used in the treatment of tachyarrhythmias in the WPW syndrome (51, 50, 62), and artificial pacemakers may be used to interrupt the reentry circuit when the arrhythmia is resistant to drug therapy (51, 65). The surgical interruption of the reentry circuit may also be employed but is usually reserved for those arrhythmias that are not controlled by drug therapy and produce significant problems for the patient (58) (Fig. 7-22).

The appearance of the WPW syndrome on the ECG may mimic ischemic heart disease and be associated with paroxysmal tachycardias. Life insurance companies rate the patient with the WPW syndrome at a risk even though the syndrome is considered to be benign for the most part (37, 62).

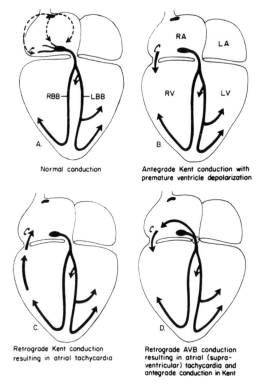

Normal conduction	Antegrade Kent conduction with premature ventricle depolarization
Retrograde Kent conduction resulting in atrial tachycardia	Retrograde AVB conduction resulting in atrial (supra-ventricular) tachycardia and antegrade conduction in Kent

Figure 7-19. (*a*) Normal conduction pathways of atria and ventricles (*b*) The excitation impulse is conducted antegrade through the normal AV conduction system and returns to the atrium via retrograde conduction through the accessory bundle. A circus movement is therefore established, resulting in atrial tachycardia. (*d*) Retrograde AV bundle (AVB) conduction resulting in atrial (supraventricular) tachycardia and antegrade conduction in Kent. QRS may be wide and bizarre and suggests ventricular tachycardia. (Reproduced by permission of the American Heart Association, Inc., from Dreifus LS et al: Control of recurrent tachycardia of Wolff-Parkinson-White syndrome by surgical ligature of the A–V bundle. *Circulation* 38:1030, 1968.)

Figure 7-20. Diagram illustrating the mechanism of a reciprocating tachycardia with normal QRS complex in the WPW syndrome. In diagram (*a*), an atrial premature impulse (marked A) is conducted to the AV node (marked N), but the atrial premature impulse is blocked in the anomalous pathway. The atrial premature impulse is then conducted to both ventricles via the bundle branch system (diagram *a*). In diagram (*b*), the atrial impulse is conducted to the atria in retrograde fashion to produce an inverted P wave. In diagram (*c*), the impulse is conducted in a clockwise fashion, producing reciprocating (reentry) cycle, and the same cycle may repeat indefinitely. Note that the QRS complex during the tachycardia is normal. (S: sinus node; d: delta wave; P: inverted P wave.) In diagrams (*d*), (*e*), and (*f*), a reciprocating tachycardia with anomalous conduction in the WPW syndrome is illustrated. The rentry cycle is counterclockwise, which is exactly the reverse direction to that shown with a narrow QRS tachycardia. (Reproduced with permission from Chung EK: *Principles of Cardiac Arrhythmias.* Copyright © 1977, Williams and Wilkins Co., Baltimore.)

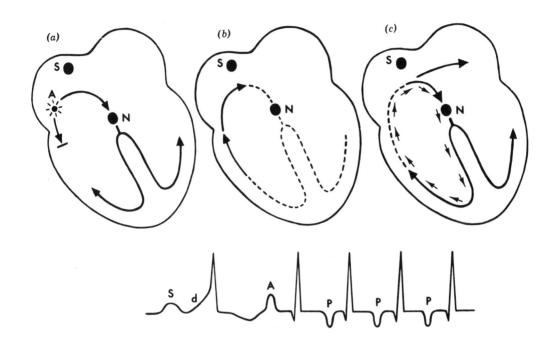

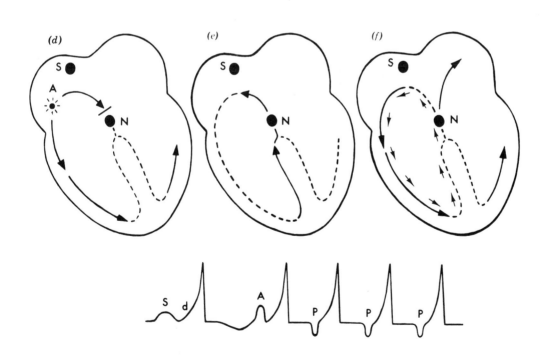

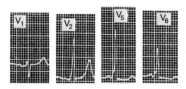
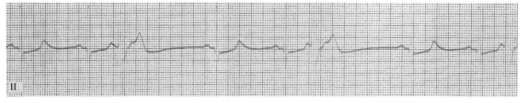
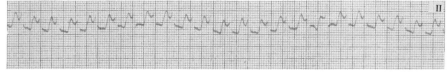

Figure 7-21. Typical WPW complexes are seen in the precordial leads of a patient prone to bouts of paroxysmal tachycardias. The middle tracing is a rhythm strip of the same patient in atrial bigeminy, which ultimately leads to an episode of the rapid supraventricular tachycardia (bottom tracing).

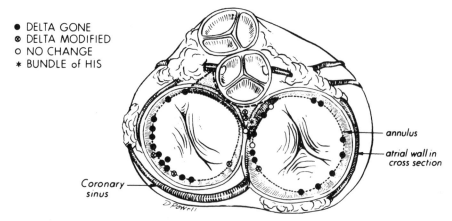

Figure 7-22. Composite of presumptive sites of preexcitation in 29 WPW patients who had surgery. The heart is viewed from above with the atria removed. The stippled triangles represent the fibrous trigones. Pathways are located on the mitral and tricuspid annuli, as well as in the true septum between atrium and ventricle. Thirty-two pathways are depicted because of the presence of two separate pathways in three patients. When the annulus was incised at the area of the solid circle, the delta wave and preexcitation were abolished. When the areas with an encircled X were incised, the delta wave and preexcitation were diminished but not abolished. The areas chosen for incision were identified by epicardial mapping and ventricular stimulation to localize the anomalous pathway. (Reproduced by permission of The American Heart Association, Inc., from Gallagher JJ, Gilbert M, Svenson RH, Sealy WC, Kasell J, Wallace AG: Wolff-Parkinson-White syndrome: the problem, evaluation, and surgical correction, *Circulation* 51:767, 1975.)

144

Table 7–3. Wolff-Parkinson-White Syndrome (Effect of Various Maneuvers and Drugs on the Impulse Conduction in the Accessory Pathway and Normal AV Conduction System.)

Agent	Accessory Pathway	AV Conduction	Result
Vagal stimulation	0	Depress	Favor WPW
Propranolol	0	Depress	Favor WPW
Digitalis	Enhance	Depress	Favor WPW
Parasympathomimetic drugs	0	Depress	Favor WPW
Quinindine	Depress	a	Favor normal AV conduction
Pronestyl	Depress	0	Favor normal AV conduction
Lidocaine	Depress	0	Favor normal AV conduction
Sympathomimetic drugs	0	Enhance	Favor normal AV conduction
Exercise	0	Enhance	Favor normal AV conduction
Atropine	0	Enhance	Favor normal AV conduction
Amyl nitrite	0	Enhance	Favor normal AV conduction
Diphenylhydantoin	0 or depress	Enhance or 0	

Source: Reproduced with permission from Chou, TC: *Electrocardiography in Clinical Practice* (New York, Grune & Stratton, Inc, 1979).
[a] May depress or enhance normal AV conduction.

REVIEW QUESTIONS

1. What is the inherent rate of the junctional tissue?
2. How can the junction assume control of the heart?
3. How do the following pharmacologic agents affect cardiac activity?
   a. Digoxin
   b. Quinidine
   c. Inderal
   d. Pronestyl
4. How can a premature junctional contraction (PJC) be differentiated from a premature atrial contraction (PAC)?
5. What are the criteria for the differentiating paroxysmal junctional tachycardia from the nonparoxysmal type?
6. Second degree AV block is subdivided into two forms, Mobitz I and Mobitz II. Electrocardiographically, how do they differ?
7. How is third-degree AV block differentiated from AV dissociation?

8. The AH interval of the His bundle recording reflects the transmission of impulse from one area of the heart to another. Identify the area of conduction system that is represented by this interval?

9. What are the indications for His bundle recordings?

10. The diagnosis of the Wolff-Parkinson-White syndrome is made strictly on the basis of the electrocardiogram. List the ECG criteria that can be present with this abnormality.

11. Why are these patients predisposed to the development of tachyarrhythmias?

REFERENCES

1. Mariott HJL: *Practical Electrocardiography*, ed 5. Baltimore, Williams & Wilkins Co, 1972, p 158.

2. Chung EK: *Principles of Cardiac Arrhythmias,* ed 2. Baltimore, Williams & Wilkins Co, 1977, p 192.

3. Fowler NO: *Cardiac Diagnosis and Treatment*, ed 2. Hagerstown, Md, Harper & Row Pub Inc, 1976, p 924.

4. Schamroth L: *The Disorders of Cardiac Rhythm*. Oxford, Blackwell Scientific Publications, 1971, p 74.

5. Bilitch M: *A Manual of Cardiac Arrhythmias*. Boston, Little Brown & Co, 1971, p 167.

6. Helfant RH: Current clinical status of His bundle electrocardiography. *Practical Cardiol.* 5:88, 1979.

7. Haft JI: Clinical implications of atrioventricular and intraventricular conduction abnormalities, in Brest and Rios (eds): *Cardiovascular Clinics*. Philadelphia, FA Davis Co, 1977, p 2.

8. Corday E. Irving DW: *Disturbances of Heart Rate, Rhythm and Conduction*. Philadelphia, WB Saunders Co, 1962, p 78.

9. Cosby RS, Bilitch M: *Heart Block*. New York, McGraw-Hill Book Co, 1972, p 116.

10. Goldschlager N, Scheinman MM: Diagnosis and clinical significance of atrioventricular (AV) conduction disturbances. *Practical Cardiol* 4:43, 1978.

11. Lipman BS, Massie E. Kleiger RE: *Clinical Scalar Electrocardiography*, ed 6. Chicago, Year Book Medical Pub Inc, 1972, p 433.

12. Guntheroth WG: Disorder of heart rate and rhythm. *Pediatr Clin North Am* 25:881, 1978.

13. Cantwell JD: *Modern Cardiology*. Boston Butterworth & Co, 1977, p 358.

14. Phibbs B: *The Cardiac Arrhythmias,* ed 3. St. Louis, CV Mosby Co, 1978, p 74.

15. Goldman MJ: *Principles of Clinical Electrocardiography*. Los Altos, Calif, Lange Medical Publications, 1979, p 230.

16. Stock JP, Williams MB: *Diagnosis and Treatment of Cardiac Arrhythmias*, ed 3. Boston, Butterworth & Co, 1974, p 239.

17. Wantanabe Y, Dreifus LS: *Cardiac Arrhythmias: Electrophysiologic Basis for Clinical Interpretation*. New York, Grune & Stratton Inc, 1977, p 164.

18. Bilitch M: *A Manual of Cardiac Arrhythmias*. Boston Little Brown & Co, 1971, p 193.

19. Cosby RS, Bilitch M: *Heart Block*. New York, McGraw-Hill Book Co, 1972, p 116.

20. Bellet S: *Essentials of Cardiac Arrhythmias: Diagnosis and Management*. Philadelphia, WB Saunders Co, 1972, p 127.

21. Ravin A: *Auscultation of the Heart*, ed 2. Chicago, Year Book Medical Pub Inc, 1979, p 149.

22. Ferrer, MI: Axioms on heart block. *Hosp Med* 13:37, 1977.

23. Lipman BS, Massie E, Kleiger RE: *Clinical Scalar Electrocardiography,* ed 6. Chicago, Year Book Medical Pub Inc, 1972, p 445.

24. Schamroth L: *The Disorders of Cardiac Rhythm*. Oxford, Blackwell Scientific Publications, 1971, p 253.

25. Chung EK: *Principles of Cardiac Arrhythmias,* ed 2. Baltimore, Williams & Wilkins Co, 1977, p 240.

26. Naimi S: Electrophysiological basis for arrhythmias, in Levine E (ed): *Clinical Cardiovascular Physiology*. New York, Grune & Stratton Inc, 1976, p 31.

27. Marriott HJL: *Practical Electrocardiography*, ed 5. Baltimore, Williams & Wilkins Co, 1976, p 215.

28. Cantwell JD: *Modern Cardiology*. Boston, Butterworth & Co, 1977, p 356.

29. Lipman BS, Massie E, Kleiger RE: *Clinical Scalar Electrocardiography*, ed 6. Chicago, Year Book Medical Pub Inc, 1972, p 251.

30. Aranda JM, Befelar B, Castellanos A, El-Sherif N: His bundle recordings: their contribution to understanding of human electrophysiology. *Heart Lung* 5:907, 1976.

31. Gallagher JJ, Damato AN, Lau SH: Antecubital vein approach for recording His bundle activity in man. *Am Heart J* 85:199, 1973.

32. Fowler NO: *Cardiac Diagnosis and Treatment*, ed 2. Hagerstown, Md, Harper & Row Pub Inc, 1976, p 980.

33. Helfant RH: Current clinicial status of His bundle electrocardiography. *Practical Cardiol* 5:88, 1979.

34. Wolff L, Parkinson J, White PD: Bundle branch block with short RP interval in healthy young people prone to paroxysmal tachycardia. *Am Heart J* 5:685, 1930.

35. Öhnell RF: Pre-excitation, a cardiac abnormality. *Acta Med Scand* [suppl] 152, 1944.

36. Chung KY, Walsh TJ, Massie E: Wolff-Parkinson-White syndrome. *Am Heart J* 69:116, 1965.

37. Cooksey JD, Dunn M, Massie E: *Clinical Vectorcardiography and Electrocardiography*, Chicago, Year Book Medical Pub Inc, 1977, p 642.

38. Hejtmancik MT, Herrmann GR: The electrocardiographic syndrome of short PR interval and broad QRS complexes. A clinical study of 80 cases. *Am Heart J* 54:708, 1957.

39. Chung EK: Tachyarrhythmias in Wolff-Parkinson-White sysdrome. *JAMA* 237:376, 1977.

40. Schiebler GL, Adams P, Jr. Anderson RC: Familial cardiomegaly in association with the Wolff-Parkinson-White syndrome. *Am Heart J* 58:113, 1959.

41. Frank S. Braunwald E: Idiopathic hypertrophic subaortic stenosis. Clinical analysis of 126 patients with emphasis on the natural history. *Circulation* 37:759, 1968.

42. Swiderski J, Lees MH, Nadas AS: The Wolff-Parkinson-White syndrome in infancy and childhood. *Br Heart J* 24:561, 1962.

43. Schiebler GL, Adams P, Jr, Anderson RC: The Wolff-Parkinson-White syndrome in infancy and childhood. *Pediatrics* 24:585, 1959.

44. Lown B, Ganong WF, Levine SA: The syndrome of short PR interval, normal QRS complex and paroxysmal rapid heart action. *Circulation* 5:693, 1952.

45. Chou TC: *Electrocardiography in Clinical Practice*, New York, Grune & Stratton Inc, 1979, p 476.

46. Hecht HH, Kennamer R, et al: Anomalous atrioventricular excitation. Panel discussion. *Ann NY Acad Sci* 65:826, 1956.

47. Lipman BS, Massie E, Kleiger RE: *Clinical Scalar Electrocardiography*, ed 6. Chicago, Year Book Medical Pub Inc, 1972, p 244.

48. Rosenbaum FF, Hecht HH, et al: Potential variations of the thorax and the esophagus in anomalous atrioventricular excitation (Wolff-Parkinson-White syndrome). *Am Heart J* 29: 281, 1945.

49. Spurrell RAJ, Krikler DM, Sowton E: Problems in the assessment of the location of the accessory pathway in the Woff-Parkinson-White syndrome. *Br Heart J* 37:127, 1975.

50. Chung EK: *Principles of Cardiac Arrhythmias,* ed 2. Baltimore, Williams & Wilkins Co, 1977, p 423.

51. Chung EK: Wolff-Parkinson-White syndrome. Current views. *Am J Med* 62:252, 1977.

52. Durrer D, Schuilenburg RM, Wellens HJJ: Pre-excitation revisited. *Am J Cardiol* 25:690, 1970.

53. Castillo CA, Castellanos A: His bundle recordings in patients with reciprocating tachycardias and Wolff-Parkinson-White syndrome. *Circulation* 42:271, 1970.

54. Goldman MJ: *Principles of Clinical Electrocardiography*, ed 10. Los Altos, Calif, Lange Medical Publications, 1979, p 265.

55. Berkman NL, Lamb LE: The Wolff-Parkinson-White electrocardiogram. Follow-up study of five to twenty-eight years. *N Engl J Med* 278:492, 1968.

56. Smithen CS, Krikler DM: Aspects of pre-excitation and its elucidation by His bundle electrograms. *Br Heart J* 34:735, 1973.

57. Wellens HJ, Durrer D: Wolff-Parkinson-White syndrome and atrial fibrillation. Relation between refractory period of accessory pathway and ventricular rate during atrial fibrillation. *Am J Cardiol* 34:777, 1974.

58. Dreifus LS, Haiat R, et al: Ventricular fibrillation. A possible mechanism of sudden death in patients with Wolff-Parkinson-White syndrome. *Circulation* 43:520, 1971.

59. Gallagher JJ, Gilbert M et al: Wolff-Parkinson-White syndrome. The problem, evaluation, and surgical correction. *Circulation* 51:767, 1975.

60. Kaplan MA, Cohen KL: Ventricular fibrillation in the Wolf-Parkinson-White syndrome, *Am J Cardiol* 24:259, 1969.

61. Rosen KM, Barwolf C: Effects of lidocaine and propranolol on the normal and anomalous pathways in patients with pre-excitation. *Am J Cardiol* 30:801, 1972.

62. Dye CL: Atrial tachycardias in Wolff-Parkinson-White syndrome. Conversion to normal sinus rhythm with lidocaine. *Am J Cardiol* 24:265, 1969.

63. Burchell HB: Management of tachycardias associated with Wolff-Parkinson-White syndrome, in Dreifus LS, Likoff W (ed): *Cardiac Arrhythmias*. New York, Grune & Stratton Inc, 1973, p 476.

64. Reynolds EW: Beta-blocking agents in the management of cardiac arrhythmias. Arrhythmia Symposium. Part 3. *Geriatrics* 16:150, 1971.

65. Wellens HJ, Durrer D: Effect of digitalis on atrioventricular conduction and circus-movement tachycardias in patients with Wolff-Parkinson-White syndrome. *Circulation* 47:1229, 1973.

66. Barold SS, Linhart JS: Recent advances in the treatment of ectopic tachycardias by electrical pacing. *Am J Cardiol* 25:698, 1970.

8
Impaired
Intraventricular
Conduction

Common conduction disturbances occurring infranodally are usually perceived as mono-fascicular (right bundle branch or left main stem bundle branch); bifascicular (right bundle branch and left anterior fascicle); and/or trifascicular (right bundle branch, left anterior fascicle and posterior fascicle and/or first-degree AV block).

As was mentioned in Chapter 1, the terminal His bundle bifurcates into a right and left bundle branch. The latter further subdivides to form two main fascicles, the anterior superior and the posterior inferior. The degree of vulnerability differs in each of the fascicles. The right bundle branch, because of its length and thinness, is more frequently involved in conduction delays or block. Next in order of vulnerability is the left anterior fascicle, which is located in a significantly high-pressure and turbulent area of the outflow tract of the left ventricle. The left anterior fascicle also has a single source of blood, the left anterior descending coronary artery. The left posterior fascicle is the least frequently involved. It has a dual blood supply, is located in a low-pressure area at the inflow tract of the left ventricle, and is a short and wide divisional branch. When it is involved, prog-nostically it is of graver significance than the delay or blocking in the other fascicles.

To understand the electrocardiographic changes inherent in the various forms of intra-ventricular conduction disturbances, it is important to be able to visualize the course of events associated with normal ventricular activation. As depicted in Figure 8-1, septal and right ventricular activation proceed in a rightward direction. Lead V_1 views this activity as coming toward it; consequently a positive wave is inscribed (r) on the electro-cardiogram. This same activity is viewed as receding from V_6, and thus a negative q wave is seen. The third vector denotes left ventricular depolarization and a leftward-directed vector. This accounts for the R wave in V_6 and S wave in V_1.

The degree of block in the bundle branch system may vary from a simple delay of im-pulse transmission in one or more branches to an intermittent failure of conductance and/or complete interruption of sinus impulses infranodally. If there is a delay in con-duction of the impulse in both main bundle branches (first-degree AV block), the PR interval will be prolonged; and since antegrade conduction is normal through the ven-tricles, a normal QRS complex will be seen. However, the complete blocking of one bundle and simple delay in passage of the impulse in the other bundle, the prolonged PR interval will be associated with QRS complex which is bizarre in configuration.

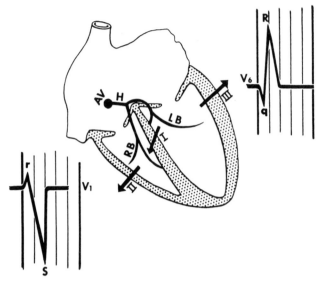

Figure 8-1. Normal ventricular activation. Depolarization of interventricular septum from left to right plus depolarization of the right ventricle (arrow I plus arrow II) travel in the general direction of V_1 and therefore produce a positive deflection (r wave) in that lead. These same forces face away from V_6 and therefore produce a negative deflection (q wave) in this lead. This is called a septal q. The final and most powerful force representing left ventricular depolarization (arrow III) is directed to the left, in the general direction of V_6 and away from V_1. Therefore, it produces a strong positive deflection (R wave) in V_6 and a deep negative deflection (S wave) in V_1. The intrinsicoid deflection in V_1 (peak of r) represents the arrival of the depolarization wave in the epicardial surface of the right ventricle. In occurs 0.02 second after the beginning of the QRS complex. The intrinsicoid deflection in V_6 (peak of R) represents the arrival of the depolarization wave in the epicardial surface of the left ventricle. It occurs 0.04 second after the beginning of the QRS complex. The QRS interval in both leads is 0.08 second. (Reproduced with permission from Bernreiter, M.: *Electrocardiography*, ed 2. Philadelphia, JB Lippincott Co, 1963.)

Second-degree AV block occurring within the infranodal tissue could indicate that one bundle may be blocked and there is a delay in transmission of the impulse in the remaining bundle branch. Second-degree infranodal conduction delays or interruption can take the form of the Wenckebach phenomenon (progressive prolongation of the PR interval) in association with a widened QRS complex, indicating that one bundle is completely blocked and in the other there is a progressive delay until one ventricular complex is dropped. (Widened QRS complex; PR interval which progressively becomes longer until there is failure of the impulse to be conducted to the ventricles.) In the event that conduction through one bundle branch is completely blocked and periodic blocking occurs in the other, Mobitz Type II block becomes evident. (Widened QRS as well as intermittent absence of the QRS complex.) Third-degree block denotes complete absence of impulse transmission through the bundle branches, and therefore two pacemakers must be present.

RIGHT BUNDLE BRANCH BLOCK (RBBB)

Involvement of the right bundle branch may occur with conditions associated with increased pressure of the right ventricular chamber, congenital absence of intraventricular tissue, and/or anteroseptal myocardial infarction. Occasionally it is found in normal individuals as a congenital aberrancy without clinical significance.

Interruption of impulse transmission through the right bundle branch may result in the electrocardiographic features as depicted in Figure 8-2. Septal activation occurs in a normal sequence, that is, from left to right. The right precordial leads view the activity as coming toward their placement, and hence a positive wave (r) is inscribed on the electrocardiographic tracing. Activation of the intact bundle (left) occurs in a leftward direction, with the resultant deflection appearing as a negative wave (S); since from this vantage point, the vector recedes from leads V_1 and V_2. Subsequent excitation of the affected ventricle beyond the area of the block is provided by the transmission of the impulse

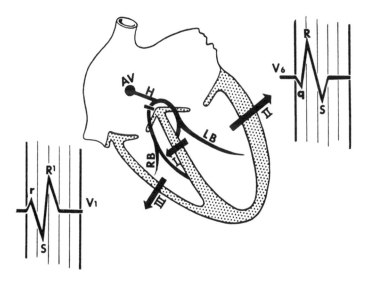

Figure 8-2. Right bundle branch block. The septum depolarizes from left to right as it normally does. This force (arrow I) produces a small negative deflection (septal q wave) in V_6 and a small positive deflection (r wave) in V_1. The left ventricle is next to be activated (arrow II). This is a strong force, traveling in the general direction of V_6. Therefore it will produce a strong positive deflection (R wave) in V_6 and a deep negative deflection (S wave) in V_1. Depolarization of the right ventricle (arrow III) is delayed because the right bundle is blocked, and the impulse reaches the right ventricle slowly through the muscle mass instead of the rapid specialized bundle tissue. This force (arrow III), traveling in the general direction of V_1, will produce a positive deflection (R^1 wave) in lead V_1 and a negative deflection (S wave) in V_6. As a result of the right bundle branch block the QRS interval is prolonged to 0.12 second or more in V_1 as well as V_6, but the intrinsicoid deflection arrives normally in V_6 within 0.04 second, as represented by the peak of the R wave in that lead. The intrinsicoid deflection is much delayed in V_1. It is represented by the peak of R' which occurs 0.08 second after the beginning of the QRS complex (normally 0.02 second). (Reproduced with permission from Bernreiter, M.: *Electrocardiography*, ed 2. Philadelphia, JB Lippincott Co, 1963.)

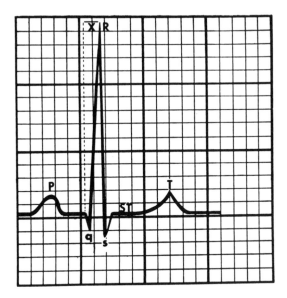

Figure 8-3. Ventricular activation time. The tip of the R wave occurs about 0.05 second after the beginning of a q wave. This is the intrinsicoid deflection (X). The intrinsicoid deflection occurs over the right ventricle within 0.02 second or less and over the left ventricle within 0.05 second or less. The ST segment is the state of electrical systole. No electric potential is apparent during this period, and thereafter the ST segment is on the isoelectric line. The T wave represents the forces active during repolarization. (Reproduced with permission from Bernreiter, M.: *Electrocardiography*, ed 2. Philadelphia, JB Lippincott Co, 1963.)

through septal muscle in a left to rightward direction. Thus, the aberrant activation of the right bundle branch produces the second positive wave (R). As a result, an rSR[1] complex is identified in the precordial lead V_1. Another feature of right bundle branch block is the prolongation of ventricular activation time (VAT) over leads overlying the right ventricle. Ventricular activation time, or the intrinsicoid deflection, represents the time it takes the impulse to travel from endocardium to epicardium under a specific exploring electrode. Normally, right ventricular activation time is within 0.02 second or less in a right epicardial lead and that of the left ventricle, according to Bernreiter (1), is 0.04 second or less as viewed in a left epicardial lead. It can be measured by determining the time in seconds from the beginning of the QRS complex to the tip of the R wave (Fig. 8-3).

The activity associated with right bundle branch block as viewed from a left precordial lead (V_5) is as follows:

1. Septal activation occurring in a normal sequence from left to right produces a q wave.
2. Impulse transmission down the intact left bundle and free left ventricular wall is manifest by an R wave.
3. The late activation of the right bundle beyond block is indicated by a broad S wave.
4. The intrinsicoid deflection time or ventricular activation time (VAT) of the left ventricle is within the normal range, that is 0.04 second or less.

Lead I is likewise helpful in identifying the presence of RBBB on the electrocardiogram. In this lead the S wave, which reflects a rightward direction of the vector, is widened and

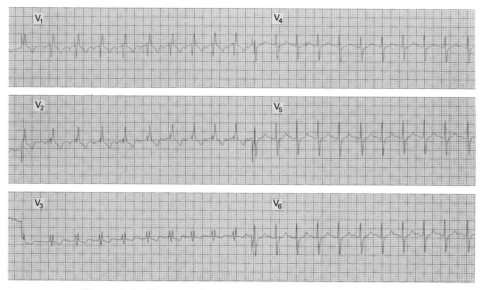

Figure 8-4. Sinus mechanism with right bundle branch block.

slurred. The duration of the QRS complex is prolonged in excess of 0.12 second, indicating complete right bundle branch block; whereas if the bundle is partially blocked the duration of the QRS complex would be in the range of 0.10 to 0.12 second. The T wave is asymmetrical and appears in the opposite direction to the wave form, reflecting delayed activation of the right ventricle (2) (Fig. 8-4).

LEFT MAIN BUNDLE BRANCH BLOCK (LMBBB)

Left bundle branch block is almost always associated with some form of acquired cardiac disease. Among the most common lesions affecting the left main bundle are aortic stenosis, left ventricular hypertrophy, coronary artery disease, and an associated anterior myocardial infarction. Since the affected ventricle must be activated in an aberrant manner, the QRS complex is both widened and distorted. In complete left main bundle branch block the QRS duration time is usually 0.12 second or longer. Incomplete left main bundle branch block produces a QRS complex that is within the range of 0.10 to 0.11 second in duration. The ventricular activation time (VAT) is greater than 0.05 second over the left ventricular precordial leads (V_5, V_6) (Fig. 8-5).

The factors responsible for the specific electrocardiographic wave form alterations are depicted in Figure 8-6.

In addition to the presence of a widened QRS complex and increased VAT, other electrocardiographic findings are the absence of a q wave in V_5 and V_6 secondary to the abnormal initial septal activation. Owing to the block of the left bundle branch, septal activation according to Lipman and associates (3) occurs initially in the region of the right mid and lower septal muscle. The vector thus travels in a right to leftward direction, resulting usually in a QS deflection in V_1. If, however, an r wave is seen as in Figure 8-6, it is representative of the activation of the free right ventricular wall. The late activation of the left ventricular wall in left bundle branch block produces changes in the process of

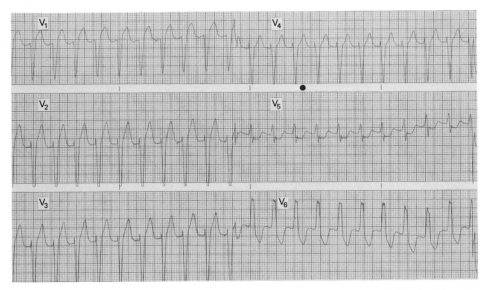

Figure 8-5. This 72-year-old patient has developed a left bundle branch block. There is sinus tachycardia.

repolarization. Therefore the T wave will be asymmetrical and opposite in direction to the widened ventricular complex.

As was mentioned on the first page of this chapter, bundle branch involvement may vary from simple to more complex degrees of blocking. In first-degree block of the left bundle branch, according to Bellet (4), the following characteristics are usually identifiable:

1. The voltage of the q wave is decreased or it is entirely absent in the leads overlying the left ventricle.
2. Initial slurring of the R wave is identifiable.
3. The QRS complex may range from 0.07 to 0.12 second.
4. The intrinsicoid deflection in lead V_6 is prolonged beyond the expected 0.04 second.
5. The right precordial leads reflect a small QRS rather than the rS complex.

Second-degree LBB is commonly associated with the following characteristics:

1. A greater degree of slurring of the R wave.
2. Absence of the q wave in the left-sided chest leads (V_5 and V_6).
3. Inversion and asymmetry of the T wave in the leads overlying the left ventricle.
4. Further prolongation of the QRS complex ranging from 0.11 to 0.15 second.
5. Absence of rightward vector, which is responsible for the r wave in the right-sided chest leads (V_1, V_2), indicating that the intitial septal depolarization occurs abnormally from right to left.
6. Presence of a leftward axis.

In third-degree LBBB Lipman and associates (1) describe several factors that are responsible for the configuration of the wave forms:

1. There is greater slurring and duration of the QRS complex than is evident in a lesser degree of block.

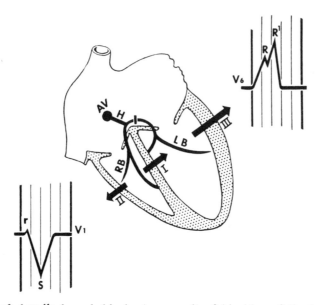

Figure 8-6. Left bundle branch block. As a result of blocking of the left bundle, the interventricular septum is activated by the right bundle in the direction from right to left (arrow I). This force produces an upright deflection in V_6 (R wave). This same force may produce a small negative deflection (q wave) in V_1. But frequently the stronger depolarization force of the right ventricle (arrow II) traveling in the opposite direction will outbalance the septal forces (arrow I) and produce a small positive deflection (r wave) in V_1. The forces representing right ventricular activation (arrow II) traveling away from the V_6 position usually are adequate to produce a small negative deflection (notching) on the upstroke of the R wave. Activation of the left ventricle is delayed because it receives the impulse slowly through the musculature of the interventricular septum rather than through the rapid left bundle. It is a final and powerful force (arrow III) that produces a strong, upright deflection (R^1) in V_6 and a deep, wide negative deflection (S wave) in V_1. As a result of the aberrant depolarization wave, the QRS complex is prolonged to 0.12 second in V_1 and V_6, but the intrinsicoid deflection (r wave) in V_1 arrives 0.02 second after the beginning of the QRS complex. In V_6 the intrinsicoid deflection (R') is delayed and arrives approximately 0.10 second after the beginning of the QRS complex. The intrinsicoid deflection is the last positive deflection (R') in V_6. Septum depolarization from right to left produces an initial positivity in the left ventricular cavity, doing away with the septal q waves usually seen in leads facing the left ventricle. (Reproduced with permission from Bernreiter M.: *Electrocardiography*, ed 2. Philadelphia, JB Lippincott Co, 1963.)

2. The intrinsicoid deflection time (VAT) exceeds the expected 0.04 second.

3. A more leftward axis deviation than in the second-degree type of LBBB is noted.

4. The T wave in the right precordial leads is upright, whereas it is inverted in the left precordial leads. This characteristic differs from the previous degrees of block since the T wave usually appears to be inverted in both right and left precordial leads.

Infranodal conduction disturbances may be related to isolated lesions involving primarily the divisions of the left main bundle branch or in combination with the right bundle branch. Thus the features of the electrocardiogram will vary accordingly.

LEFT ANTERIOR HEMIBLOCK (LAH)

Delay or blocking of an impulse within the anterior fascicle of the left bundle branch produces a shift of the axis to the position of $-45°$ to $-90°$ on the hexaxial sphere. The mechanism implicated in the vector shift toward the abnormal leftward axis deviation may be explained in terms of the vector traveling initially toward the uninvolved inferior (posterior) division and then toward the affected fascicle (Fig. 8-7). This accounts for the various configurations of the QRS in the lead system (Fig. 8-8). Albion and associates (5), have found in a series of patients, the presence of a q wave in the right precordial leads associated with left anteiror hemiblock. They attribute the presence of the q wave to modification of septal activation caused by the anterior hemiblock.

LEFT POSTERIOR HEMIBLOCK (LPH)

Involvement of the posterior division of the left bundle produces a right axis deviation in the area of $+120°$ or greater. The impulse is conducted through the uninvolved anterior fascicle, resulting in an initial positive deflection in lead I and a small negative deflection in the leads aV_F, II, and III (Fig. 8-9). The terminal deflection in these leads is reflective of the vector activating the obstructed fascicle. Thus lead I views this activity as receding from it and in leads aV_F, II, and III the vector is seen as approaching the positive pole of each lead (Fig. 8-10).

In addition to the factors mentioned earlier relative to the predisposition of the left

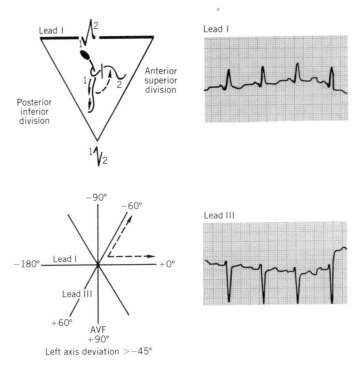

Figure 8-7. Left anterior hemiblock. The mechanism involved in the configuration of the electrocardiographic tracing.

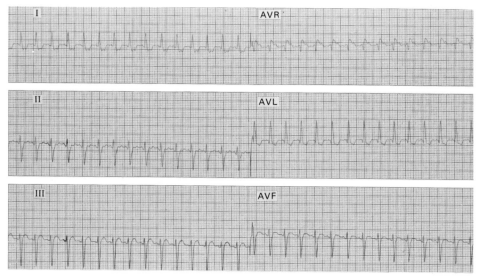

Figure 8-8. Left axis deviation of the QRS, left anterior hemiblock. The conduction defect has masked the changes of an inferolateral infarction present 4 days before this tracing.

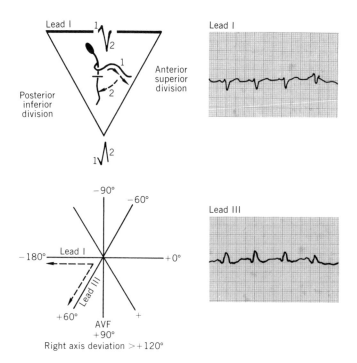

Figure 8-9. Left posterior hemiblock. The pathway of the vector in producing the electrocardiographic wave form.

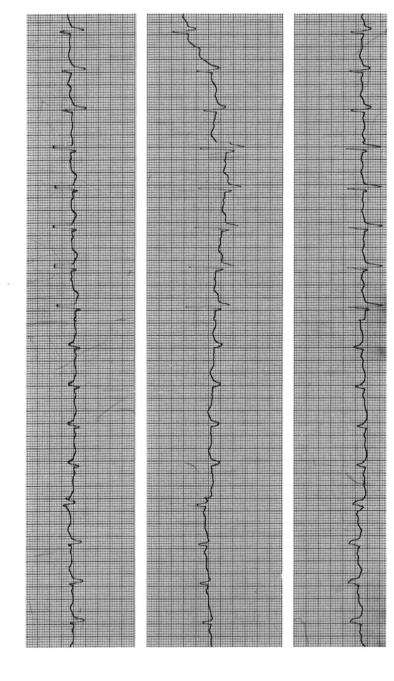

Figure 8-10. A rightward axis of the QRS is present as well as evidence of right bundle branch block. The tracing is suggestive of the presence of posterior hemiblock.

anterior and posterior divisions of the let bundle branch to interruption or delay in conduction of the impulse, certain degenerative disease processes can likewise be confined to the area of the cardiac skeleton. Fibrotic changes may invade the conduction tissue directly (Lenegre's disease), while sclerotic lesions produce changes in areas adjacent to the conduction (Lev's disease). The latter condition is seen more frequently in old people. The presence of posterior hemiblock is highly suggestive of diffuse coronary artery disease since the fascicle is served normally by both the right coronary artery and the anterior descending branch of the left coronary artery.

According to a study cited by Levy and associates (6), transient left anterior hemiblock may be related to attacks of angina pectoris. The results of the study indicate that under these conditions, left anterior hemiblock is thought to indicate severe obstructive lesions of the left anterior descending coronary artery and may suggest impending myocardial infarction.

Therapy

The therapeutic approach to conduction disturbances associated with the various degrees of block involving the atrioventricular and intraventricular conducting tissue usually is determined on the basis of whether or not cardiac function has become compromised.

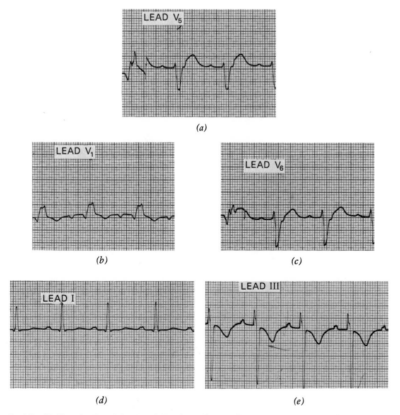

Figure 8-11. Trifascicular block. Criterion for trifascicular block. (*a*) First degree A-V block. (*b–c*) Right bundle branch block. (*d–e*) Left anterior hemiblock. (See text on page 161.)

Drug therapy may be indicated in certain conditions to increase the ventricular rate. This is especially true when the conduction disturbances are a result of vagal effects (7). Pacemaker insertion (Chap. 14) may be indicated in the presence of an anterior myocardial infarction with associated forms of intraventricular conduction disturbances.

Nursing Intervention

The patient with conduction disturbances presents a challenge for the nurse, for it is by her evaluation of the state of vital measurements that decisions relative to therapy are made. The detection of a progression of the block and the subsequent intervention may significantly reduce morbidity and mortality.

According to Costellanos and associates (8), the coronary care nurse in particular can play a vital role in the detection of fascicular blocks which so often are harbingers of symptomatic atrioventricular blocks. The group further identifies guides as part of nursing care of the acutely ill patient.

1. One must know the type of myocardial infarction (by location) the patient may have sustained.
2. Specific placement of the chest electrodes should be maintained on a daily basis. Any change in site should be noted on the plan of care.
3. Changes in wave form gain should be noted.
4. If feasible, hourly strips of the heart's electrical activity should be available.
5. The utilization of lead II in the absence of known fascicular blocks enables one to

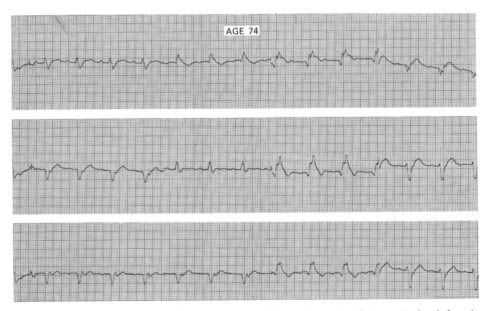

Figure 8-12. The PR interval is prolonged (first-degree AV block) there is also left axis deviation of the QRS complex; right bundle branch block; left anterior hemiblock as well as evidence of an anterior myocardial infarction. This would represent a trifascicular block.

detect the emergence or presence of left-axis deviation and left anterior hemiblock. This is particularly important in the presence of documented right bundle branch block.

6. The ability to recognize the onset of first- or second-degree block in the presence of existing bifascicular block alerts one to the presence of more progressive and symptomatic degrees of block, namely, trifascicular block (Figs. 8-11, 8-12).

In addition to the above, utilization of the lead MCL$_1$ is often helpful in the detection of right bundle branch block.

REVIEW QUESTIONS

1. In assessing the patient's condition at the bedside, what is the clinical feature that is highly suggestive of right bundle branch block? Left bundle branch block?

2. What clinical finding is pathognomonic of third-degree heart block?

3. Draw the shape of the QRS complex that is associated with left anterior hemiblock.

4. The onset of first-degree AV block in the presence of a right bundle branch block and left anterior hemiblock is said to be of prognostic significance. Why is this true?

5. Does the anatomical location of the left posterior fascicle somewhat protect it from ischemia and/or injury?

6. Based on the presence of the following tracing, would you agree that left anterior hemiblock is present?

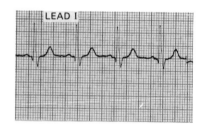 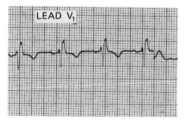

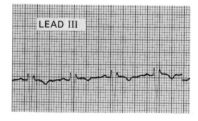

REFERENCES

1. Bernreiter M: *Electrocardiography*. Philadelphia, JB Lippincott Co, 1958, p 83.

2. McLachlan EM: *The Highways of Electrocardiography*. New Zealand, Logan Print Ltd, 1975, p 19.

3. Lipman BS, Massie E, Kleiger RE: *Clinical Scalar Electrocardiography*, ed 6. Chicago, Year Book Medical Pub Inc, 1972, p 162.

4. Bellet S: *Essentials of Cardiac Arrhythmias: Diagnosis and Management*. Philadelphia, WB Saunders Co, 1972, p 128.

5. Alboni P, Malacarne C, DeLorenzi E, Pirani R, Baldassari F, Masoni A: Right precordial Q waves due to anterior fascicular block. Clinical and vectorcardiographic study. *J Electrocardiog* 12:41, 1979.

6. Levy S, Gerard R. Castellanos A, Gharhamani A, Sommer L: Transient left anterior hemiblock during angina pectoris: coronarographic aspects and clinical significance. *Eur J Cardiol* 9:215, 1979.

7. Phibbs B: *The Cardiac Arrhythmias*, ed 3. St. Louis, CV Mosby Co, 1978, p 28.

8. Castellanos A, Spence MI, Chapell DE: Hemiblock and bundle branch block: a nursing approach. *Heart Lung* 1:43, 1972.

9
Ventricular Arrhythmias

Ventricular arryhthmias are characterized by the appearance of wide, bizarre QRS complexes. The bizarre QRS complex is a result of abnormal ventricular depolarization since the pacemaker has an ectopic focus located in the ventricles. The terms ectopic beat, extrasystole, and premature beat are used interchangeably today; however, all ectopic beats are not premature. A ventricular escape beat is late, but it is an ectopic beat nevertheless. An isolated beat or a rhythm that originates in the ventricles may then be divided into two categories: (*1*) active impulse formation (usurpation) and (*2*) passive impulse formation (default). Examples of active impulse formation include premature ventricular contractions (PVCs), ventricular tachycardia, flutter, and fibrillation. In contrast to active impulse formation, ventricular escape beats or rhythm (idioventricular rhythm) develop in response to the absence of conduction from the SA node, atria, or AV junction.

VENTRICULAR ESCAPE BEATS AND IDIOVENTRICULAR RHYTHM

Pathogenesis

This ventricular disturbance is produced by passive impulse formation as a result of supraventricular impulses arriving at a slower rate than the rate of the ectopic ventricular pacemaker. This most commonly is the result of AV block but is also seen with sinus bradycardia, sinus arrest, and SA block.

Electrocardiographic Features

1. The QRS complex occurs late in relation to the prevailing rhythm.
2. QRS complex is wide and bizarre.
3. When three or more ventricular escape beats occur consecutively, the phenomenon is called idioventricular rhythm.
4. The rate of the idioventricular rhythm is usually from 30 to 40 beats per minute (Fig. 9-1).

Clinical Significance

The ventricular rate in idioventricular rhythm is usually so slow that symptoms of cerebral ischemia are manifested. These include syncope, confusion, and blurred vision. All vital organs may develop ischemia and produce signs and symptoms. This arrhythmia is usually found in patients with advanced heart disease.

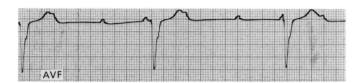

Figure 9-1. Idioventricular rhythm is seen in this patient with complete heart block. The QRS is wide and the ventricular rate is 27 beats per minute.

Therapy

Emphasis must be placed on the fact that ventricular escape beats as well idioventricular rhythms are passive. Abolishment of them through the use of a drug such as lidocaine may result in asystole. Therefore, therapeutic measures are directed at increasing the impulse formation in the SA node (atropine) or using an electrical pacemaker if AV block is the cause.

PREMATURE VENTRICULAR CONTRACTIONS (PVCs)

Pathogenesis

Two mechanisms have been postulated in the production of premature ventricular contractions: (*1*) theory of reentry (Chap. 6) and (*2*) increased automaticity. The ventricular arrhythmias which develop on the basis of usurpation or active impulse formation are also thought to be the result of one of these mechanisms.

Electrocardiographic Features

1. The QRS complex is early (premature) in relation to the prevailing rhythm.
2. The QRS complex is wide and bizarre.
3. Secondary ST and T wave changes develop. Usually the ST and T wave is opposite in direction to the QRS complex.
4. A full compensatory pause usually follows the premature ventricular contraction.
5. Unifocal PVCs (ectopic beats from the same focus) generally have a fixed or constant coupling interval. The coupling interval is the interval between the ectopic beat and the preceding beat of the prevailing rhythm (Fig. 9-2).

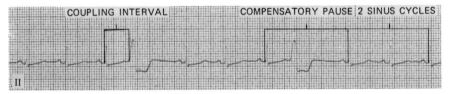

Figure 9-2. Characteristic features of PVCs are seen in this tracing. Both PVCs have the same coupling interval (fixed coupling) and both have a compensatory pause (same as two sinus cycles). The PVCs are early (occur before the next expected sinus beat), and both are wide and bizarre. The PVCs do not have P waves; the ST and T wave are opposite directions of the QRS complex and are unifocal (identical in appearance).

6. The P wave is usually lost (buried in the QRS complex) or may appear inverted after the QRS complex indicating retrograde activation of the atria.

The QRS complex is usually wide and bizarre owing to asynchronous activation of the two ventricles. When the ectopic focus is located in the left ventricle, a right bundle branch block pattern is produced; if the ectopic focus is located in the right ventricle, a left bundle branch block pattern is seen. The value in identifying the origin of the PVC from the right or left ventricle is unclear. Rosenbaum (1) reported that healthy individuals with no heart disease generally have PVCs that have a left bundle branch block configuration, indicating that the PVCs originated from the right ventricle. Lewis and Konakis (2) reported that 74% of persons with no organic heart disease had right ventricular PVCs and 17% had left ventricular PVCs. In contrast, Lewis found 46% of patients with organic heart disease had left ventricular PVCs and 45% had right ventricular PVCs. However, recent electrophysiologic studies by Josephson et al (3) have shown that the expected origin of the ectopic beats made on the basis of the QRS morphology is not always accurate.

When the QRS complex is wide and bizarre, the ectopic focus is usually located near the peripheral part of the Purkinje system (4). If the ectopic impulse originates high in the interventricular septum near the bundle of His, a near normal QRS configuration may result. These PVCs are called septal beats or *main stem beats* (5) (Fig. 9-3). The PVC may also show a near normal configuration if it occurs in the presence of a bundle branch block. For example, if a left bundle branch block exists and an ectopic focus located in the left ventricle fires, the impulse reaches the conduction system of both ventricles in a shorter time, producing normalization of the QRS complex (6).

The P wave is usually lost in the PVC because the QRS complex occurs early. However, the impulse from the PVC may activate the atria in a retrograde fashion, producing inverted P waves following the QRS complex. These will be seen in leads II, III, and aV_F with an upright P wave after the QRS complex in lead aV_R. Premature atrial contractions with retrograde conduction of the atria are likely to occur during sinus bradycardia (6). The P^1P interval (interval from the ectopic P wave to the following sinus P wave) is usually longer than the PP interval of the prevailing rhythm (7). Occasionally, retro-

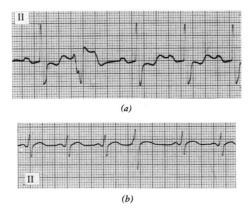

(a)

(b)

Figure 9-3. (*a*) PVCs that originate in the Purkinje system produce obviously bizarre QRS complexes as compared with (*b*), PVCs originating near the His bundle, producing a more normal looking complex.

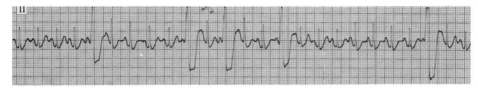

Figure 9-4. End-diastolic PVCs are present, producing fusion between the sinus P wave (P waves before the bizarre QRS complexes) and the bizarre QRS complex from the PVCs. The PR interval is very short in these PVCs.

grade conduction from the PVC reaches the AV junction and stops. The atria are not activated retrogradely in this circumstance, but the AV junction may be left refractory. When the next sinus impulse travels down toward the ventricles, the AV junction is still found refractory and a long PR interval is produced (8). This effect on the PR interval from the previous PVC is referred to as concealed retrograde conduction (9). A normal P wave preceding a PVC may appear if the premature beat occurs late in diastole. This PVC is called an *end-diastolic PVC* and is only slightly premature. The P wave is sinus in origin and will appear normal and at the expected time; but the QRS complex appears early, resulting in a shorter PR interval (Fig. 9-4). The P wave and the QRS complex are dissociated from each other in the end-diastolic PVC. The sinus impulse and the end-diastolic PVC may activate the ventricular myocardium together, resulting in a *ventricular fusion beat* (6).

The pause following most PVCs is generally fully compensatory in contrast to the pause that follows supraventricular impulses. A full compensatory pause follows a PVC because the premature beat does not depolarize the SA node, and therefore the rhythm of the sinus node is undisturbed (7). If the PVC depolarizes the SA node, its rhythm is disturbed and the PVC may be followed by less-than-compensatory pause.

Unifocal premature ventricular contractions usually have a constant coupling interval because the abnormal impulse in the ventricle is somehow related to the preceding beat of the prevailing rhythm (6). The variation of the coupling interval should not be greater than 0.08 second (10). Multifocal PVCs (occurring from different foci) do not exhibit fixed or constant coupling intervals and ventricular parasystole also characteristically produces varying coupling intervals.

The pattern PVCs present may vary from bigeminy (the PVC alternates with the basic beat) (Fig. 9-5), to trigeminy (PVC is every third beat) (Fig. 9-6), to quadrigeminy (PVC is every foruth beat) (Fig. 9-7). Two consecutive PVCs are termed a couplet, or pair. When PVCs occur at a rate of six or more per minute, they are considered to be

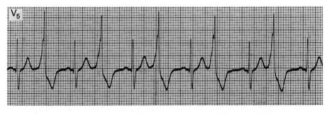

Figure 9-5. Ventricular bigeminy developed in a patient immediately after exercise during a stress test.

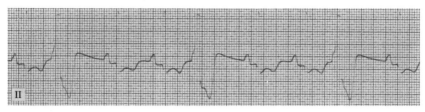

Figure 9-6. Ventricular trigeminy is present. Every third beat is a PVC.

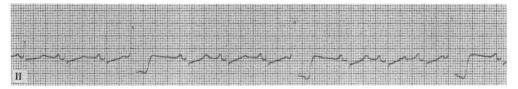

Figure 9-7. Ventricular quadrigeminy.

frequent. Ventricular tachycardia is present when three or more premature ventricular contractions occur in rapid succession (4, 6) (Fig. 9-8). Multi-form PVCs (not to be confused with multifocal PVCs, whose configuration obviously varies and fixed coupling is absent) are present when the QRS configuration varies but a constant coupling interval remains (5) (Fig. 9-9). The same lead must be used to diagnose multifocal as well as multiform PVCs. When a premature ventricular contraction is sandwiched between two sinus beats, the PVC is called an interpolated beat (Fig. 9-10).

Clinical Spectrum
The most common arrhythmia in normal, healthy individuals as well as those with organic heart disease is PVCs (4). Excessive use of alcohol, tea, coffee, or tobacco as well as fatigue and anxiety may produce PVCs in normal individuals. Premature ventricular contractions often decrease or disappear during exercise in healthy individuals (7, 11) (Fig. 9-11). Organic heart disease and/or digitalis toxicity are usually present when the PVCs are multiform or multifocal, or are also found in the presence of atrial or junctional premature contractions (7). Studies which have utilized continuous ECG recording have reported a 100% incidence of PVCs in acute myocardial infarction (13, 14). It is unclear from the literature whether the frequency of PVCs is related to coronary artery disease alone, ventricular asynergy, or a combination of these two variables. Califf et al (15) and Sharma et al (16) found that the frequency of PVCs was related

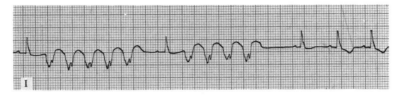

Figure 9-8. Lead I recording of two brief runs of ventricular tachycardia.

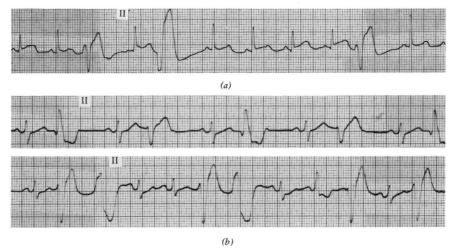

(a)

(b)

Figure 9-9. (*a*) Multiform PVCs are present in this tracing recorded from a patient with digitalis toxicity. (*b*) Multifocal PVCs produce varying coupling intervals and different QRS deflections as seen in these two tracings recorded from the same patient on the same lead approximately 2 minutes apart.

to the degree of coronary artery disease and not to ventricular asynergy; whereas Calvert et al (17) reported that the incidence of ventricular arrhythmias was directly related to both the extent of left ventricular dysfunction and the number of diseased coronary arteries. Ventricular arrhythmias are more likely to develop during exercise in those individuals with coronary artery disease (18). However, the mere presence of exercise-induced PVCs is not a good predictor of coronary disease (19, 20). Premature ventricular contractions are also seen in the following organic heart diseases: Cardiomyopathy, rheumatic heart disease, and hypertensive heart disease. Patients with mitral valve prolapse syndrome have PVCs as their most common arrhythmia (21). Additional causes of PVCs and other ventricular arrhythmias include digitalis toxicity, hypokalemia (with or without digitalis toxicity), and hypercalcemia and administration of quinidine, procainamide, and tricyclic antidepressants (4). Bigeminal PVCs appearing in a patient receiving digitalis has been taught as a classic indication of digitalis toxicity. Constant

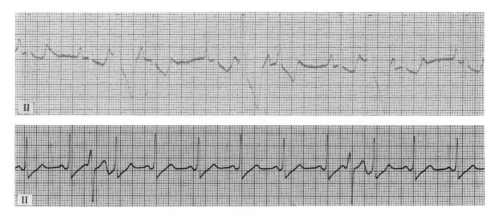

Figure 9-10. Interpolated PVCs from two different patients.

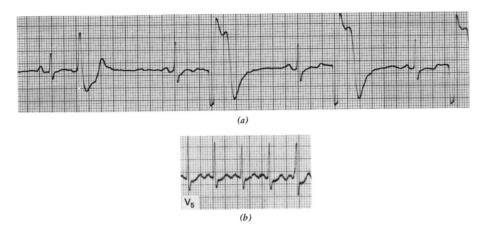

Figure 9-11. (a) Bigeminal PVCs were recorded in a patient at rest. (b) Exercise abolished the PVCs in this patient who had a positive stress test (ST depression in V_5).

(22), however, has found this classic teaching to be exaggerated in comparison with clincial occurrence.

Premature ventricular contractions which occur occasionally seldom produce symptoms. Sensitive individuals, nevertheless, may experience palpitations and a feeling of "skipped beats" or "flip-flops of the heart." Physical examination usually reveals a pulse deficit during a PVC, since the cardiac output is temporarily decreased. Coronary artery blood flow may be diminished by 12% with occasional PVCs but may be reduced as much as 25% when the PVCs appear frequently (23). This reduction takes on a greater significance when the patient has preexisting heart disease. Symptoms of cerebral and renal ischemia likewise may develop with frequent premature ventricular contractions.

Therapy

Treatment of individuals with PVCs depends on several points: (*1*) the frequency of the PVCs, (*2*) the configuration of the PVCs, and (*3*) presence or absence of organic heart disease. The removal of precipitating factors such as tobacoo, coffee, tea, cola beverages, and alcohol is warranted. Correction of acid-base imbalances, electrolyte imbalances, as well as the removel of digitalis, must be considered. Complex PVCs which include multifocal and multiform PVCs, couplets (pairs), and PVCs occurring more than six times per minute are generally thought of as precursors to ventricular tachycardia and fibrillation and therefore are treated.

The significance of the R-on-T phenomenon (PVC occurring on the upstroke or peak of the preceding T wave) has been stressed as a precursor to the development of ventricular tachycardia and fibrillation (24) (Fig. 9-12). Recent studies have questioned the importance of the R-on-T phenomenon. Bleifer and associates (25, 26) found the presence of the R-on-T phenomenon alone was not associated with the development of ventricular tachycardia. However, if this phenomenon was also associated with paired PVCs, the incidence of ventricular tachycardia was high. Chou (27) found the R-on-T phenomenon produced ventricular tachycardia in only 6 of 44 patients. In contrast, 16 of his 44 patients developed ventricular tachycardia from late cycled PVCs.

Patients with acute myocardial infarction who develop frequent or complex PVCs have a high incidence of ventricular tachycardia and fibrillation and require prompt therapy (28) (Fig. 9-13).

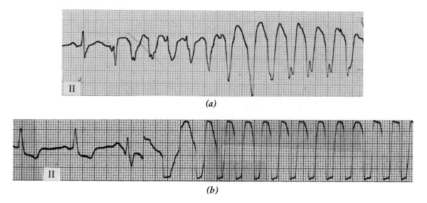

Figure 9-12. (*a*) Late cycled (away from T wave) PVC produces ventricular tachycardia. (*b*) PVC falls on the T wave and produced ventricular tachycardia in this patient who was wearing a 24-hour continuous ECG monitoring device.

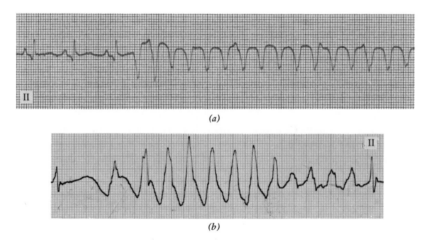

Figure 9-13. (*a*) Tracing was recorded from a 65-year-old woman with multivessel coronary artery disease and left ventricular dysfunction. This episode of ventricular tachycardia produced loss of consciousness. (*b*) Ventricular tachycardia developed in a man with an acute myocardial infarction.

Therapeutic regimens include lidocaine, procainamide, quinidine, propranolol, diphenyl-hydantoin, disopyramide, and bretylium tosylate (see Chap. 11).

VENTRICULAR TACHYCARDIA

Pathogenesis

The mechanisms responsible for the production of PVCs, namely, reentry and enhanced automaticity, also are thought to be responsible for the production of ventricular tachycardias. Recent studies by Wellens (29) and Josephson (3) indicate reentry as the most likely cause of recurrent sustained ventricular tachycardias.

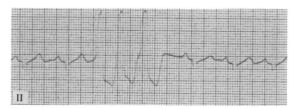

Figure 9-14. Three-beat run of ventricular tachycardia.

Electrocardiographic Features

1. Wide, bizarre QRS complexes.
2. Rapid succession of three or more PVCs (Fig. 9-14).
3. The ventricular rate is usually between 140 to 200 beats per minute with regular or slightly irregular rhythm.
4. Secondary ST and T wave changes are present (their direction is usually opposite to that of the QRS complex).
5. Absent P waves or, if they are present, P waves dissociated from the QRS complex.
6. Paroxysmal nature (abrupt onset and termination) (Fig. 9-15).
7. Presence of fusion beats.

The RR interval in ventricular tachycardia may be slightly irregular, but any gross irregularity should raise the possibility of atrial fibrillation with a ventricular conduction defect. The appearance of either all positive or all negative QRS complexes in leads V_1 to V_6 is a point usually in favor of ventricular ectopy as well as the appearance of an indeterminate axis (+180° to -90°) in the frontal plane (8). Bidirectional ventricular tachycardia is present when the wide QRS complexes alternate polarity.

Digitalis toxicity is usually the cause of bidirectional ventricular tachycardia (7, 8). Fusion beats which interrupt a suspected ventricular tachycardia are a very important finding. These fusion beats are called *Dressler beats* (30) and indicate that an ectopic impulse originates in the ventricles. Unfortunately, they are seldom found in paroxysmal

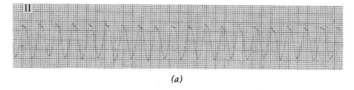

(a)

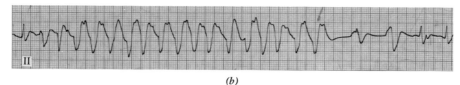

(b)

Figure 9-15. (*a*) Ventricular tachycardia (ventricular flutter) produced wide bizarre QRS complexes without P waves. The rate is 187 beats per minute and regular. (*b*) Ventricular tachycardia produces QRS complexes that merge with the ST and T wave segments, giving a zigzag appearance.

ventricular tachycardia (4). Some authorities differentiate ventricular tachycardia from flutter based on the fact that the QRS complex merges with the ST and T wave, producing a zigzag appearance (continuous sine wave) and/or a slightly faster rate (6, 7, 4). The significance of ventricular flutter is the same as that of ventricular tachycardia.

Clinical Spectrum

Ventricular tachycardia is nearly always found in persons with organic heart disease, especially acute myocardial infarction (31). Other organic heart diseases in which ventricular tachycardia may develop include rheumatic and hypertensive heart disease, mitral valve prolapse syndrome, and ventricular aneurysm. Digitalis toxicity, hyper and hypokalemia, WPW syndrome, and hereditary prolongation of the QT interval with or without congenital deafness are other additional causes of ventricular tachycardia. A mechanical irritation of the ventricles may develop during cardiac catheterization or the insertion of a transvenous pacemaker and may precipitate ventricular tachycardia. Digitalized patients who undergo DC shock for treatment of their arrhythmias can develop ventricular tachycardia. Coronary blood flow may be reduced as much as 60% during ventricular tachycardia (23), the cerebral blood flow decreasing as much as 40% to 75%. Quite frequently an altered state of consciousness develops during ventricular tachycardia.

Therapy

Since ventricular tachycardia is considered to be a life-threatening arrhythmia, prompt therapy is necessary. Various antiarrhythmic agents include lidocaine, procainamide, quinidine, diphenylhydantoin, propranolol, and bretylium tosylate (Chap. 11). Extremely effective in the treatment of ventricular tachycardia is DC shock, unless the tachycardia is a result of digitalis toxicity. The use of an artificial pacemaker may be necessary in the treatment of drug-resistant ventricular tachycardia (7).

ACCELERATED IDIOVENTRICULAR RHYTHM

This rhythm is also called nonparoxysmal ventricular tachycardia, idioventricular tachycardia, and slow ventricular tachycardia.

Electrocardiographic Features

1. Wide, bizarre QRS complexes.
2. QRS complexes appear in a regular fashion at a rate from 60 to 100 beats per minute.
3. Ventricular fusion beats are common.

This rhythm often has a heart rate similar to the prevailing sinus rate and therefore appears if the ectopic focus accelerates slightly or the sinus mechanism slows slightly (Fig. 9-16). Since these two mechanisms (the sinus and the ventricular ectopic mechanism) have similar rates, it is quite common for the accelerated rhythm to begin with and end with ventricular fusion beats (8).

Clinical Spectrum

Accelerated idioventricular rhythm usually is a benign rhythm and is generally not considered to be a precursor of paroxysmal ventricular tachycardia or fibrillation (8). Hemo-

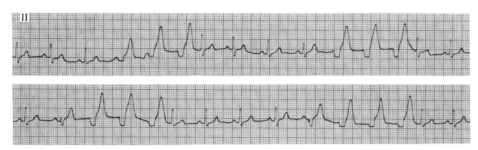

Figure 9-16. Continuous tracing of lead II was recorded from a man with an acute myocardial infarction. The rhythm is an accelerated idoventricular rhythm at a rate of 95 beats per minute. The patient was asymptomatic during these runs.

dynamic changes are not usually produced by this arrhythmia, which is frequently seen in patients with acute myocardial infarction. Therapy is usually not required.

VENTRICULAR FIBRILLATION

The mechanisms responsible for the development of ventricular fibrillation are the same as those for atrial flutter and fibrillation (see Chap. 6).

Electrocardiographic Features
Unevenly appearing deflections with no clear-cut P, QRS, or T waves (Fig. 9-17).

Clinical Spectrum
Ventricular fibrillation is a lethal arrhythmia leading to sudden death unless promptly treated. The pulse is not detectable and the person loses consciousness rapidly. The

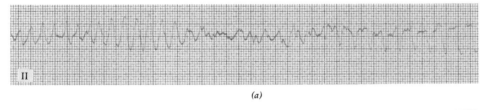

(a)

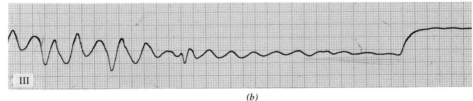

(b)

Figure 9-17. (*a*) Ventricular tachycardia leading to a period of ventricular fibrillation was recorded from a young woman with mitral valve prolapse. (*b*) Ventricular fibrillation deteriorating to asystole in a man with chronic cor pulmonale.

arrhythmia is nearly always associated with organic heart disease and frequently develops during the terminal stage of noncardiac disease (7).

Therapy
The treatment of choice in patients with ventricular fibrillation is DC shock.

VENTRICULAR PARASYSTOLE

Pathogenesis
In ventricular parasystole, two independent pacemakers compete with each other to gain control of the heart rate. An ectopic focus with its origin in the ventricles and the normal focus of the SA node are usually the location for these independent pacemakers. The parasystolic focus located in the ventricles is protected from the sinus node impulse by an entrance block. The parasystolic focus is protected by the entrance block and forms impulses at a set rate (usually slower than the sinus rate). However, its impulse is allowed conduction (PVC) only when the ventricles are in a nonrefractory state. These PVCs bear no fixed relationship with the normally conducted sinus beats (5).

Electrocardiographic Features

1. Variable coupling intervals since the PVCs bear no constant relationship with the previous sinus beat. The coupling interval usually varies more than 0.08 second.
2. The interectopic intervals (measured from one PVC to the next) will be equal to or multiples of the shortest interectopic interval. This is present because the parasystolic beats bear a relationship to each other.

Clinical Spectrum
Ventricular parasystole will not be recognized unless a long rhythm strip is used to calculate the interectopic intervals and absence of fixed coupling. Baxter and associates (32) found ventricular parasystole to be present in 4% of patients who had recently suffered a myocardial infarction. This arrhythmia was found to be relatively benign (32, 33).

REVIEW QUESTIONS

1. Accelerated idioventricular rhythm is usually considered a benign arrhythmia requiring no treatment. How does this rhythm differ from ventricular tachycardia? What clinical setting is this rhythm disturbance frequently seen with?
2. Why is ventricular tachycardia considered a life-threatening arrhythmia? What is the treatment of choice with this arrhythmia?
3. Describe the ECG appearance of an end-diastolic PVC.

REFERENCES

1. Rosenbaum MB: Classification of ventricular extrasystoles according to form. *J. Electrocardiol* 2:298, 1969.
2. Lewis S, Konakis C: Significance of site of origin of premature ventricular contractions. *Am Heart J* 97:159, 1979.

3. Josephson ME, Harowitz, et al: Recurrent sustained ventricular tachycardia. 2. Endocardial mapping. *Circulation* 57:431, 1978.

4. Chou TC: *Electrocardiography in Clinical Practice,* New York, Grune & Stratton Inc, 1979, p 419.

5. Lipman BS, Massie E, Kleiger RE: *Clinical Scalar Electrocardiography,* ed 6. Chicago, Year Book Medical Publishers Inc, 1972, p 403.

6. Schamroth L: *The Disorders of Cardiac Rhythm,* Oxford, Blackwell Scientific Publications, 1971, p. 89.

7. Chung EK: *Principles of Cardiac Arrhythmias,* ed 2. Baltimore, Williams & Wilkins Co, 1977, p 376.

8. Marriott HJL: Practical Electrocardiography, ed 6. Baltimore, Williams & Wilkins Co, 1977, p 103.

9. Langendorf R: Concealed A-V conduction. *Am Heart J* 35:542, 1948.

10. Langendorf R, Pick A, Winternitz M: Mechanisms of intermittent ventricular bigeminy. I. Appearance of ectopic beats dependent upon length of cycle, the "rule of bigeminy". *Circulation* 11:422, 1955.

11. Kennedy HL, Underhill SJ: Frequent or complex ventricular ectopy in apparently healthy subjects. A clinical study of 25 cases. *Am J Cardiol* 38:141, 1976.

12. McHenry PL, Fisch C, et al: Cardiac arrhythmias observed during maximal treadmill exercise testing in clinically normal men. *Am J Cardiol* 29:331, 1972.

13. Romhilt DW, Bloomfield SS, et al: Unreliability of conventional electrocardiographic monitoring for arrhythmia detection in coronary care units. *Am J Cardiol* 31:457, 1973.

14. Morgensen L: A controlled trial of lignocaine prophylaxis in the prevention of ventricular tachyarrhythmias in acute myocardial infarction. *Acta Med Scand* 513:1, 1971.

15. Califf RM, Burks JM, et al: Relationship among ventricular arrhythmias, coronary artery disease, and angiographic and electrocardiographic indicators of myocardial fibrosis. *Circulation* 57: 725, 1978.

16. Sharma SD, Ballantyne F, Goldstein S: The relationship of ventricular asynergy in coronary artery disease to ventricular premature beats. *Chest* 66:358, 1974.

17. Calvert A, Lown B, Gorlin R: Ventricular premature beats and anatomically defined coronary heart disease, *Am J Cardiol* 39:627, 1977.

18. McHenry PL, Morris SN, et al: Comparative study of exercise–induced ventricular arrhythmias in normal subjects and patients with documented coronary artery disease. *Am J Cardiol* 37: 609, 1976.

19. Froelicher VF, Thomas MM, et al: Epidemiologic study of asymptomatic men screened by maximal treadmill testing for latent coronary artery disease. *Am J Cardiol* 34:770, 1974.

20. Faris JV, McHenry PL, et al: Prevalence and reproducibility of exercise induced ventricular arrhythmias during maximal exercise testing in normal man. *Am J Cardiol* 37:617, 1976.

21. Winkel RA, Lopes MG, et al: Arrhythmias in patients with mitral valve prolapse. *Circulation* 52:73, 1975.

22. Constant J: Management of arrhythmias in patients with ischemic heart disease. Part II. PVC's in patients who have never had an infarct. *Practical Cardiol* 5:49, 1979.

23. Corday E, Gold H, et al: Effect of the cardiac arrhythmias on the coronary circulation. *Ann Intern Med* 50:535, 1959.

24. Smirk FH, Palmer DG: A myocardial syndrome. With particular reference to the occurrence of sudden death and premature systoles interrupting antecedent T waves. *Am J Cardiol* 6:620, 1960.

25. Bleifer SB, Sheppard JJ, et al: Relationship of the R-on-T phenomenon to the development of ventricular tachycardia (abstr). *Circulation* 43 and 44 (Suppl II):142, 1971.

26. Bleifer SB, Karpman HL, et al: Relation between premature ventricular complexes and development of ventricular tachycardia. *Am J Cardiol* 31:400, 1973.

27. Chou TC, Wenzke F: The importance of the R on T phenomenon. *Am Heart J* 96:191, 1978.

28. Lown B, Fakhro AM, et al: The coronary care unit. New perspective and directions. *JAMA* 199: 188, 1967.

29. Wellens HJ: Pathophysiology of ventricular tachycardia in man. *Arch Intern Med* 135:473, 1975.

30. Dressler W, Roesler H: The occurrence in paroxysmal ventricular tachycardia of ventricular complexes transitional in shape to sinoauricular beats. *Am Heart J* 44:485, 1952.

31. MacKenzie GJ, Pascual S: Paroxysmal ventricular tachycardia. *Br Heart J* 26:441, 1964.

32. Baxter RH, McGuinness JB: Comparison of ventricular parasystole with other dysrhythmias after acute myocardial infarction. *Am Heart J* 88:443, 1974.

33. Salazar J, McKendrick CS: Ventricular parasystole in acute myocardial infarction. *Br Heart J* 32:377, 1970.

10
Degenerative Myocardial Changes

MYOCARDIAL ISCHEMIA; INFARCTION

Disparity between supply and demand of myocardial nutrient flow may render the heart ineffective as the propelling force necessary for tissue and organ perfusion. Circulatory deficits can occur subendocardially, subepicardially, and/or transmurally, resulting in episodes of ischemia and injury or infarction of cardiac tissue. The pathogenesis of myocardial ischemia is multifactorial (1, 2, 3). The most common conditions implicated in the imbalance of myocardial oxygen supply and demand are identified in Table 10-1.

Blood flow through the coronary arteries can be curtailed by obstructive conditions such as atherosclerosis, thrombosis, embolization, spasm, and/or epicardial compression by means of myocardial bridges. These conditions contribute to myocardial ischemia by a reduction in the intraluminal space through which blood can flow (4).

Other conditions reducing the amount of blood flow to the myocardium do so either by encroaching upon diastolic filling time or by prolonging the systolic phase of the cardiac cycle (5).

A rapid heart rate can compromise myocardial blood flow, especially to the left ventricle, by limiting the diastolic filling time. Ordinarily most persons can tolerate rapid heart rates without experiencing adverse effects; however, episodes of tachycardia become more significant in the presence of coronary vessels narrowed by atherosclerotic lesions. According to Corday and Irving (6), a heart rate of 180 in a diseased heart can predispose the person to severe chest discomfort or to congestive heart failure.

Dysfunction of the aortic valve can interfere with coronary flow in several ways:

1. In the presence of aortic insufficiency, the diastolic pressure is lowered, owing to the reflux of blood from the aortic compartment to the left ventricular chamber. Hence the blood that normally fills the aortic cusps and distends the coronary ostia is refluxly returned to the ejecting chamber.

2. Aortic stenosis by impeding the free flow of blood that is ejected from the left ventricle prolongs the period of isometric contraction of the cardiac cycle. The net result is shortening of diastole. In addition, the high intracavitary pressure of the left ventricle associated with impedance (afterload) to ventricular ejection exerts increased pressure and compression of subendocardial coronary vessels, thus limiting flow. The effect of the increased afterload is what Eliot and Holsinger (7) identify as a "hemodynamic vise" (Fig. 10-1).

Table 10-1. Pathogenic Factors in Myocardial Ischemia—Infarction

Flow Reduction	Increase in Oxygen Requirements
Obstructive Lesions	Augmented cardiac output
Coronary artery stenosis	Increase in body activity
Thrombus, embolus	Metabolic effects of
Spasm	Thyroxin
Myocardial bridges	Catecholamines
Nonobstructive luminal factors	Hyperglycemia
Rapid heart rate	Increase in myocardial wall tension
Aortic Valvular dysfunction	Systemic Impedance (afterload)
	Hypertrophy of cardiac muscle

Conditions imposing a greater workload upon the heart in effect evoke the need for greater myocardial oxygen consumption. Exercise, fever, and thyrotoxicosis are accompanied by an increase in cardiac output; thus greater requirements are imposed upon cardiac muscle to provide the necessary cardiac flow.

Effects related to endocrine system activity have been found to occur in association with an acute myocardial infarction. Enhanced glycogenolysis as well as the supression of insulin activity by catecholamines released in the bloodstream during the stressful state may precipitate hyperglycemic episodes (8, 9, 10). A schematic representation of the mechanisms involving the endocrine system in relation to the onset of hyperglycemia as identified by Prakosh and Chhablani (8) are depicted in Figure 10-2.

Preload (diastolic stretch of myocardial fiber) as an adaptive mechanism of the heart in providing an adequate stroke volume is reliant upon the end-diastolic volume within the cardiac chamber. Factors influencing end-diastolic volume are wall compliance, filling

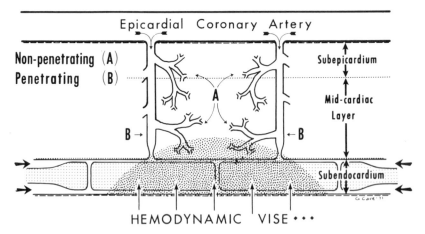

Figure 10-1. Subendocardial ischemia. Stippled area represents subendocardial ischemia resulting in obliteration of the microcirculation and producing an endarterial system. (a) Nonpenetrating coronary arteries; (b) penetrating coronary arteries; arrows demonstrate real and potential collateral flow. (Reproduced with permission from Holsinger JW Jr, Eliot RS: The potential role of the subendocardium in the pathogenesis of myocardial infarction. Heart Lung 1:356-361, 1972.)

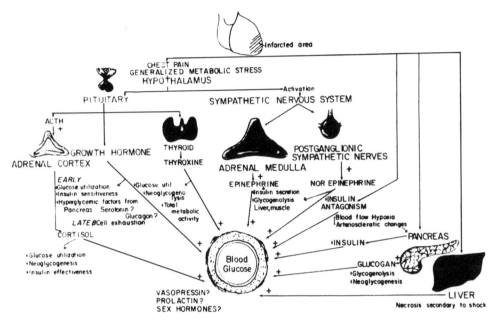

Figure 10-2. Possible factors contributing to hyperglycemia in patients with acute myocardial infarction are diagrammatically illustrated in this figure. Chest pain and generalized metabolic stress of acute myocardial infarction activates the pituitary, pancreas, and sympathetic nervous system, possibly via the hypothalamus. The growth hormone causes a decrease in glucose utilization and insulin sensitiveness and stimulates ? hyperglycemic factors from the pancreas (? serotonin, ? glucagon); may also cause late B cell exhaustion. Cortisol can decrease glucose utilization and insulin sensitiveness besides causing neoglucogenesis. The adrenal medulla releases epinephrine, and norepinephrine is released from postganglionic sympathetic nerves. These catecholamines cause glycogenolysis and insulin antagonism. Glucagon is released from the pancreas and has been shown to cause glycogenolysis and neoglycogenesis. The participation of other hormones such as thyroxin, vasopressin, prolactin, and sex hormones in causing hyperglycemia is not clear in acute myocardial infarction at present. Liver necrosis in patients with shock may also cause derangement of many metabolic pathways, thus leading to hyperglycemia. (Reproduced by permission from Prakosh R, Chhablani R: Immunoreactive serum insulin and growth hormone responses in patients with preinfarction angina and acute myocardial infarction. *Chest* 65:408–414, 1974.)

pressure, and filling time (11). Thus, the more compliant the chamber wall, the longer the filling time, and the lower the filling pressure, the greater is end-diastolic volume. This principle is in accordance with Starling's law of the heart, which states that the heart can deliver either a small amount of blood or a large amount, depending on the volume filling the chamber during diastole. Within physiologic limits, the greater the myocardial fiber stretch, the greater the stroke volume (12). The intramyocardial wall tension, as well as forceful contraction resulting from a maximal end-diastolic volume, requires greater oxygen consumption by cardiac muscle (13, 14).

Afterload, as defined by the clinical physiologist, refers to the level of pressure or force that the ventricle must utilize in ejecting its contents against impedance (resistance) in an effort to meet the circulatory needs of the body (11, 15). As vascular resistance increases, a greater amount of energy must be expended by the cardiac chambers in expelling their contents.

Hypertrophy of cardiac muscle alters the ratio of capillary proximity to myocardial fibers. As the muscle mass increases, the distance between the perfusing capillary and the fiber likewise increases (16). The net result usually is an underperfusion of the thickened cardiac muscle.

Regardless of whether myocardial ischemia occurs as a result of coronary artery occlusion or any other pathogenetic factor, the ischemic process evokes certain pathophysiologic events thought to lead to a further compromise of myocardial circulation. According to Pitt (17), the following can occur:

1. The left ventricular end-diastolic pressure may rise to a level of 30 to 40 mmHg in response to either left ventricular dysfunction and/or to a decrease in chamber compliance. Consequently the high pressure impedes blood flowing from the surface area of the heart to the subendocardium.

2. The distribution of blood flow to the endocardium may likewise be affected by what is thought to be a delayed phase of cardiac relaxation. Further compromise of blood flow to the subendocardial tissue occurs.

CLINICAL SYNDROME; ANGINA PECTORIS

Myocardial ischemia secondary to pathogenetic factors can be recognized clinically by the presence of chest discomfort (angina pectoris). According to Karlinger (18), the term angina as is commonly used refers to pain resulting from the inadequacy of myocardial perfusion in relationship to the demands placed upon it. The literature abounds in descriptive terms associated with angina pectoris. For purposes of this chapter, the most common terms, such as Heberden's (stable) angina, unstable angina, and Prinzmetal's angina, will be considered.

Classical angina (stable), as described by Heberden in 1786, is characterized by transient episodes of pain that are usually precipitated by effort and that are relieved by rest and nitroglycerin. It is associated with some coronary artery pathology and is said to be a "predictable" type of chest discomfort. Exercise, a heavy meal, and/or exposure to cold weather may precipitate the anginal pain (18), which generally is described as crushing, dull, aching, squeezing, or oppressive.

Unstable angina implies more progressive impairment of myocardial nutrient flow. Individuals who have experienced stable effort chest discomfort previously readily become aware of the fact that unpredictable variables progressively induce chest discomfort. The chest discomfort associated with unstable angina according to Falicev (19) differs from that of stable angina in that it is more progressive, unpredictable, more severe, and of longer duration.

Other terms included within the category of unstable angina are crescendo angina, decubitus angina, preinfarction angina, and impending infarction (19). Sodeman (16) associated the occurrence of nocturnal angina with the presence of diffuse cardiac disease.

Prinzmetal's (variant) angina, ascribed to spasm of the large coronary vessels, occurs at rest or during normal activity. The spasm has been found to occur in the absence of preexisting atherosclerotic lesions of the coronary vasculature as well as in the presence of

Table 10-2. Comparison of Clinical Features of Variant Angina and
Typical Exertional Angina

	Variant Angina	*"Usual" Angina*
ECG changes	Transient ST elevation	ST segment Depression or no change
Arrhythmias During pain	Ventricular Tachycardia, Heart block common	Uncommon Usually PVCs
Blood pressure, Heart rate at onset	Not increased	Almost always Increased

Source: Reproduced with permission from Johnson, A. Prinzmetal's Variant Angina:
Current Concepts and Management (*Practical Cardiology*, 1977).

such lesions (20, 21). Several explanations have been offered for the occurrence of
coronary artery spasm:

1. The spasm occurs secondary to hypersensitivity of the coronary artery to a localizing
   atheromatous plaque (21).
2. Alternations in sympathetic coronary innervation (22).
3. Humoral agents such as serotonin, histamine, and bradykinin within the circulating
   blood evoke contraction of smooth muscle within the vessel (21).
4. The withdrawal from prolonged exposure to the nitrite products of munitions
   factories (21).

In comparing the clinical features of Prinzmetal's angina with that of stable angina
(Heberden's), Johnson (21) has considered three variables (Table 10-2): the electrocardiographic manifestations, pain-induced arrhythmias, and the double product of heart
rate and blood pressure at the time of the anginal chest pain.

Significance and Intervention
Anginal attacks in general, although not indicative of infarction, can be considered as
forerunners of more progressive impairment and/or more severe changes within the
myocardial wall. Thus, the therapeutic approach to myocardial ischemia is the correction
of the imbalance between oxygen supply, substrate delivery, and demands placed upon
the heart (14, 23, 24). Pharmacologic agents such as B-adrenergic blockers and vasodilators are often employed for purposes of providing greater coronary blood flow.
Substrate transport, according to Heng and Corday (14), can likewise be enhanced by
the agent hyaluronidase.

TRANSMURAL INFARCTION

Disparity between supply and demand of myocardial nutrients may render that muscle
ineffective as the main force responsible for organ and tissue perfusion. Circulatory
deficits may occur subendocardially, subepicardially, and/or transmurally. It is not the

intent of the authors to write a treatise on myocardial infarction and sequelae, for the market abounds in numerous excellent texts related to the subject. The aim, however, is to develop in as simplistic a sequence as possible the schematic representation of hemodynamic alterations and subsequent clinical manifestations associated particularly with a transmural infarction.

Electrocardiographically, the changes associated with an underperfused myocardium are reflected by T wave inversion, signifying ischemia, ST segment elevation depicting an injury pattern, and the presence of a pathological Q wave reflective of necrosis and death of tissue (25, 26) (Fig. 10-3).

Changes identified in leads overlying the involved myocardial area are designated as indicative changes, while leads in the position opposite to the area will reveal reciprocal changes (27). For example, a person who has sustained an acute inferior (diaphragmatic) myocardial infarction, will exhibit indicative changes predominantly in leads II, III and aV_F and reciprocal changes in leads I, aV_L, and the chest leads (Fig. 10-4). In an anterior

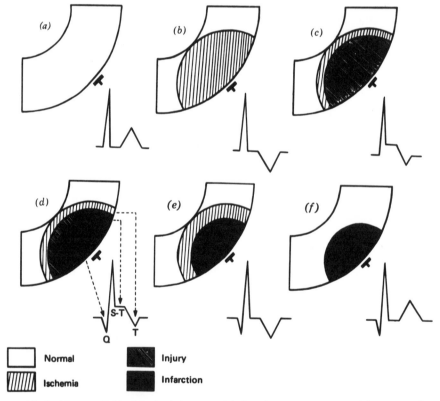

Figure 10-3. Myocardial ischemia, injury, and infarction, to compare with a normal myocardium. During acute myocardial infarction, the electrocardiogram discloses all three stages, including ischemia (outer layer), injury (middle layer), and necrosis (center) as shown in diagram (*d*). (*a*) normal myocardium; (*b*) myocardial ischemia; (*c*) myocardial injury and ischemia; (*d*) myocardial ischemia, injury, and necrosis (acute myocardial infarction); (*e*) subacute myocardial infarction; (*f*) old myocardial infarction. (Reproduced with permission from Chung EK: *Electrocardiography: Practical Applications With Vectorial Principles.* Hagerstown, Md, Harper & Row Pub Inc, 1974.)

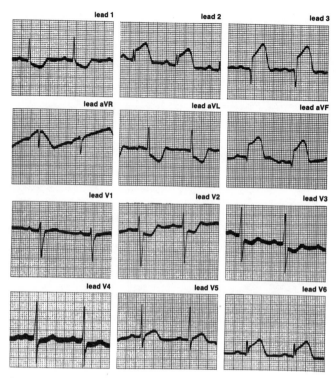

Figure 10-4. Acute inferolateral myocardial infarction. (Reproduced with permission from Warner Lambert Pharmaceutical Div, Warner Lambert Co, Morris Plains, NJ.)

myocardial infarction, indicative changes are reflected in leads I, aV_L, and the chest leads V_1 through V_6 and reciprocal changes will be evident in leads II, III, aV_F. Poor R wave progression across the precordial leads suggests an old anterior myocardial infarction (28) (Fig. 10-5).

A relatively tall R wave in lead V_1 is the only electrocardiographic criterion associated with a posterior myocardial infarction (29) (Fig. 10-6).

Although generally all types of arrhythmias may be observed in association with a myocardial infarction, most patients develop either a tachyarrhythmia or a bradyarrhythmia. Premature ventricular contractions tend to occur in approximately 80% of the patients, the various forms of atrial tachycardia are seen in 25% of the myocardial infarction patients, and at least 25% develop some form of atrioventricular conduction blocks.

Genesis of Arrhythmias

The exact etiology of arrhythmias in a patient with a myocardial infarction is currently a matter of conjecture. Various hypothesis have been explored and factors which have received widespread attention are schematically outlined in Table 10-3.

Hypoxia/Ischemia

The degree of excitability of cardiac muscle fibers is altered by the process of ischemia. This could range initially from a process of hyperexcitability to hypoexcitability and as a result could contribute to the genesis of arrhythmias after myocardial infarction.

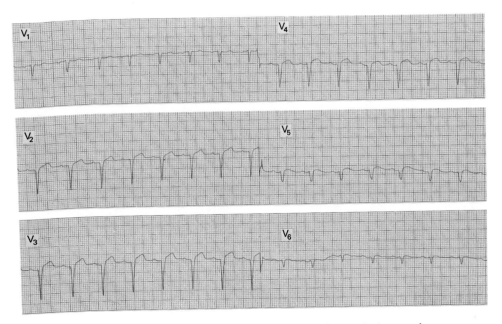

Figure 10-5. Anterior myocardial infarction showing evolutionary change.

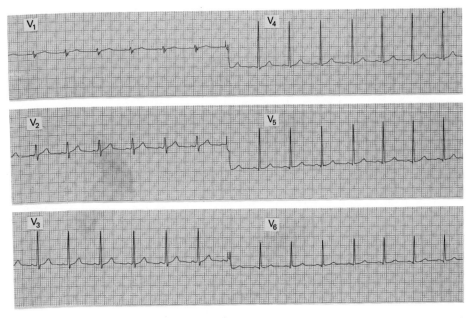

Figure 10-6. Sinus tachycardia. There are changes compatible with a true posterior myocardial infarction.

Table 10–3. Arrhythmogenic Factors in Myocardial Infarction

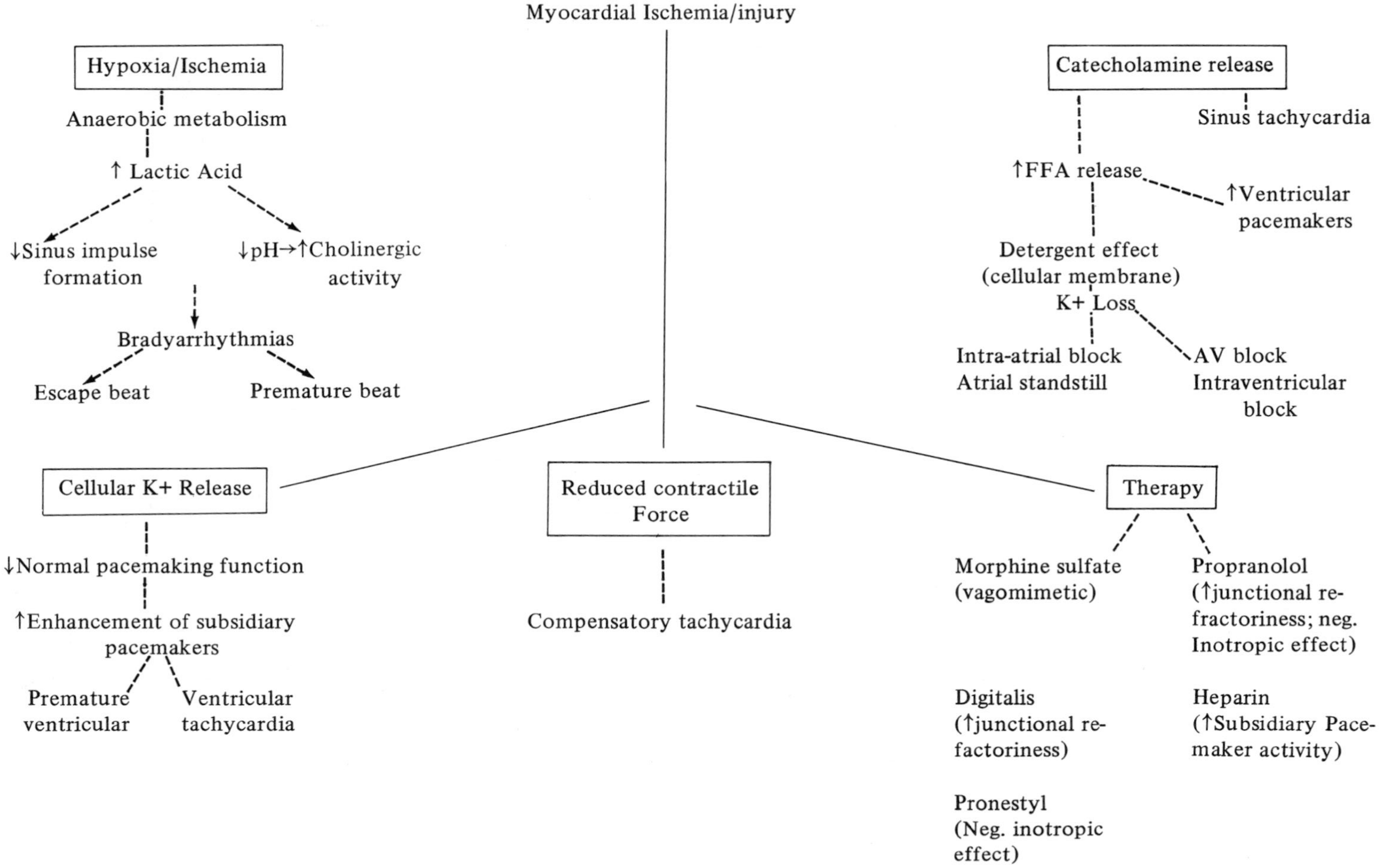

Myocardial Ischemia/injury

Hypoxia/Ischemia

Anaerobic metabolism

↑ Lactic Acid → ↓pH→↑Cholinergic activity

↓Sinus impulse formation

Bradyarrhythmias → Premature beat

Escape beat

Cellular K+ Release

↓Normal pacemaking function

↑Enhancement of subsidiary pacemakers → Ventricular tachycardia

Premature ventricular

Catecholamine release

Sinus tachycardia

↑Ventricular pacemakers

↑FFA release

Detergent effect (cellular membrane) K+ Loss

AV block

Intraventricular block

Intra-atrial block

Atrial standstill

Reduced contractile Force

Compensatory tachycardia

Therapy

Morphine sulfate (vagomimetic)

Propranolol (↑junctional re-fractoriness; neg. Inotropic effect)

Heparin (↑Subsidiary Pace-maker activity)

Digitalis (↑junctional re-factoriness)

Pronestyl (Neg. inotropic effect)

185

The direct effect on the electrical properties of the myocardium in the presence of ischemia is thought to be related to the following:

1. Increased automaticity of the Purkinje fibers by an increase in diastolic depolarization, thus predisposing the heart to enhanced automaticity with subsequent vulnerability to ectopy.
2. A decrease in conduction velocity secondary to a decrease in the resting membrane potential, resulting in impairment of dominant pacemaking action.
3. Alterations in the action potential and/or refractory period of myocardial cells, predisposing ischemic muscle to reentry (30).

End-product accumulation consequential to infarcted and/or ischemic muscle, predisposes the heart to metabolic alterations. Thus, it is not unusual for the surrounding area of compromised circulation to become acidotic in nature. The mechanism of acidosis is probably related to the leaking of metabolites through the affected myocardial wall, hence producing a medium with a lowered pH level. Several effects occur as a result of an acidotic pH (31, 32):

1. Impulse formation within the SA node is depressed.
2. Subservient pacemaking sites are activated and usurpation of pacemaking function becomes evident.
3. By the process of reentry, an ectopic rhythm becomes established.

In addition, acidosis has a direct effect upon neural structures (adrenergic and cholinergic fibers). Initially, there is a predominant effect upon the cholinergic nerve fibers, which produces profound vagal effects. The presence of continued acidotic medium can in time produce loss of neural function within the region of the conducting tissue. Supression of neural influence can likewise enhance ectopic foci, which if more rapid than the sinoatrial impulse, can become pacemakers of the heart.

Acidosis can likewise contribute indirectly to the enlargement of infarct size by altering the intracellular enzymatic system.

Another interesting finding with a continuous drop in pH is the fact that the medium can now mimic the action of increased levels of serum potassium; that is, it may cause the heart to cease to beat as the myocardial muscle becomes progressively quiescent.

The process of depolarization and repolarization are equally affected by metabolite accumulation within contiguous tissue of the infarction and hence predispose the individual to ectopy. It is possible that as the ectopic impulse conducts to the surrounding tissue, it may meet islets that are still in a state of refractoriness and hence conduct more slowly through the area. Emergence of the delayed activity can in fact reenter refractory-free tissue and again stimulate it to perpetuate a state facilitating ectopy.

Altered Electrophysiology
Subsequent to myocardial injury and healing, the return of excitability is not uniform. The function of the sinoatrial node may thus be depressed (predisposing to escape and usurpation), and/or impulse conduction may become disorganized again, enhancing a mechanism by default. Uneven recovery of myocardial tissue further facilitates the circuitous movement and ectopy.

Intracellular Potassium Loss
In the presence of a myocardial infarction, the intracellular and extracellular potassium ratio is disturbed. Injured cells release the potassium ion to the extracellular spaces, thus producing a pool or outer covering over contiguous tissue. Local reabsorption of potassium

then may take place and lead to shortening of the refractory period and a decrease in the resting membrane potential of involved tissue. Enhanced excitability initially ensues, only to be followed by loss of cellular excitability with further increments in the extracellular potassium ion gain. The mechanism responsible for the hyperexcitability and subsequent depression of latent pacemaking cells is thought to be due to an excessive depolarization phase (33).

Catecholamines

The excessive amount of catecholamine release secondary to increased sympathetic tone resulting from fear, anxiety, pain, and/or stress is thought to play a proarrhythmic role (34). Catecholamines enhance automaticity and can indirectly produce a bradycardiac effect by the following mechanism. With a sudden rise in serum norepinephrine, peripheral vascular resistance is increased, resulting in a sudden elevation of blood pressure. The baroreceptors (aortic-carotid), sensing the acute rise of blood pressure and subsequent stretch of aortic arch and carotid sinus receptor sites stimulate the cardioinhibitory center in the medulla, and reflex slowing of the heart ensues. Epinephrine, likewise, has a positive inotropic effect upon the heart muscle, thus requiring greater myocardial oxygen consumption (32).

Another interesting role in which catecholamines are involved is that of accelerating the release of free fatty acids from adipose tissue. In the presence of acutely elevated plasma levels of free fatty acids, there tends to be a rise in cellular uptake of the unbound acids by the myocardium, which during hypoxic conditions can lead to cardiac arrhythmias (32, 35, 36, 37). Several postulations have been offered about how the FFA causes arrhythmias:

1. Noradrenalin causes an acute mobilization of lipids from adipose tissue, resulting in an increase in the metabolic rate of the body and greater oxygen utilization. Vagal tone may be increased, resulting in a suppressant effect upon the sinoatrial and atrioventricular nodes. Enhanced activity of a lower latent pacemaker will ensue.
2. The unbound FFA has a detergent effect upon the cellular membrane as well as on the enzymatic system, thereby producing electrical instability (32).

Decreased Contractility

Not all patients who have sustained an acute myocardial infarction will experience symptoms relative to decreased myocardial contractility. Those who do would probably be placed in class II of Killip's classification of myocardial infarctions. These are the individuals in whom some degree of left ventricular dysfunction is present, resulting in clinical manifestations such as an S_3 gallop, pulmonary rales, and radiographic evidence of pulmonary venous congestion. It is in this group of patients that cardiac output falls, LVED pressure increases, and arterial blood pressure initially increases with sympathetic discharge and then subsequently falls; coronary filling is further compromised, increasing the degree of myocardial ischemia (38).

In an effort to sustain tissue perfusion, the compensatory mechanism of sinus tachycardia ensues. Cardiac ventricular filling time is curtailed with the rapid rate and myocardial oxygen consumption is increased. Thus, as with other compensatory mechanisms, a price must be paid, one that takes its toll on the failing cardiac pump.

Sustained tachycardia in the absence of sympathetic stimulation occurs in approximately 35% of patients with an acute myocardial infarction. If it persists over several days, it could suggest extension of the infarcted area, impending congestive heart failure, and/or cardiogenic shock as well as pulmonary embolization.

Medications

Drugs as a part of the medical treatment may play a proarrhythmic role in the genesis of arrhythmias complicating an acute myocardial infarction. For purposes of this discussion, only the drugs which have a proarrhythmic effect will be considered. Chapter 11 is devoted to the effect of cardiac drugs on the transmembrane action potential.

Digitalis, a drug of choice in many of the supraventricular tachyarrhythmias, increases the refractory period of the atrioventricular junction, and in so doing permits subsidiary pacemaking cells to control the heart (33).

Morphine sulfate, often given for relief of pain, has a vagomimetic effect and as such can induce enhanced automaticity of subsidiary pacemakers.

Pronestyl, employed for long-term suppression of ventricular arrhythmias, has a negative inotropic effect and may contribute to inadequate cardiac output. Compensatory sinus tachycardia responds to a decrease in stroke volume.

Propranolol increases refractoriness of the atrioventricular junction and as such may induce bradyarrhythmias.

Heparin, used primarily to decrease propagation of a thrombus, has been implicated in the increase of free fatty acid levels. It does so by activating the lipoprotein lipase, which subsequently liberates unbound fatty acid. The proarrhythmic role of heparin is the same as that of increased levels of free fatty acid, that is, enhancement of subsidiary pacemakers (39).

Specificity of Rhythmic Disturbances

Certain arrhythmias and/or conduction problems have a predilection for specific infarction sites (Table 10-4).

Bradyarrhythmias, in the form of sinus bradycardia and/or atrioventricular block, are more commonly seen with an inferior wall myocardial infarction than perhaps with other sites of infarction. During the early phase of infarction (within the first four hours) an 8% to 30% incidence of sinus bradycardia has been reported in a number of studies,

Table 10-4. Rhythmic Disturbances Associated with Myocardial Infarction

Inferior Myocardial Infarction	Anterior Myocardial Infarction
Bradyarrhythmias	Supraventricular
Bradycardia	Sinus tachycardia
Atrioventricular blocks	Paroxysmal atrial tachycardia
1st-degree block	Atrial Flutter
2nd-degree block (Mobitz I)	Atrial Fibrillation
3rd-degree block (transient)	Atrioventricular blocks
Ventricular	Mobitz II
Escape PVCs	Complete heart block
Ventricular tachycardia	Hemiblocks
Sick Sinus Syndrome	Ventricular
Inappropriate sinus bradycardia	Tachycardia
Sinus arrest with or without	Fibrillation
escape rhythm	
Bradycardia-tachycardia	
Chronic atrial fibrillation with	
slow ventricular response	

whereas during the remainder of the patient's hospitalization the percentage of brady-cardic episodes varied from 9% to 45%. Although the extent of myocardial damage in an inferior wall infarction is relatively limited and the prognosis favorable, in most instances the involvement of the atrioventricular node and His bundle has greater significance. Both structures are normally served by a branch of the right coronary artery (40).

Perhaps the greatest significance associated with sinus bradycardia in ischemic hearts is the fact that hypotension frequently coexists with the arrhythmia. The hypotensive state may occur as a result of vagal influence and/or peripheral vasodilation. Myocardial ischemia can be increased during hypotension, thus contributing to a greater degree of infarcted tissue.

Extremely slow heart rates predispose the myocardium to escape rhythms, both by the process of usurpation and/or default (26).

Interference with impulse conduction, whether at the level of the atrioventricular junction or at the fascicular level, occurs in approximately 15% of persons who have sustained myocardial infarction. Atrioventricular blocks, second and third degree, gen-erally occur within a short period of time after the onset of symptoms, but can be seen any time during the patient's hospitalization (41, 42).

These conduction blocks are more frequently associated with the inferior wall in-farctions, since in 92% of the populace, the AV nodal artery branches off the parent right coronary vessel. The blocks associated with this type of infarction are generally transient and are due to edema and/or ischemia rather than necrosis of the AV junctional tissue. The transient nature of the block may be related to cellular loss of K, alterations in membrane permeability, or to leukocytic infiltration of the junctional tissue.

The implication of the lymphatic vessels in conduction disturbances is currently under study. It has been found that in canine hearts some of the subendocardial lymphatic vessels are distributed across the region of the right bundle branch. Lymphatic vessels within the inferior border of the myocardium extend across the septum, then behind the right bundle branch, and on toward the atrioventricular junction. In light of these findings, lymphatic vessels probably can serve as vehicles in conveying materials released at distal ischemic and/or infarcted areas to the vicinity of the conduction fibers (43).

Consequences of bradyarrhythmias, irrespective of their genesis, are twofold:

1. A fixed stroke volume
2. Predisposition to ectopy

Normally, the heart, because of its myocardial reserve, can compensate for very slow rates by an increase in diastolic filling and stroke volume. In the presence of a myocardial in-farction, the myocardial reserve may be diminished; hence compensation is ineffective (38).

A less frequently encountered group of dysrhythmias, but perhaps far more prognostic in the elderly patient, is that of the sick sinus syndrome. The term, being collective, encompasses disorders of atrial impulse formation and conduction. Included in this group of rhythm disturbances are inappropriate sinus bradycardia, sinus arrest with or without escape rhythms, and chronic atrial fibrillation with a very slow ventricular response, as well as bouts of supraventricular tachyarrhythmias coexistent with the underlying rhythm disturbances.

The exact mechanism underlying the sick sinus syndrome is unknown. Several ex-planations have been offered for its occurrence (44):

1. Depression of sinus impulse formation due to pacemaker cell death or replacement by fibrous tissue.

2. Presence of defective pacemaker cells.

3. Failure of an impulse to be conducted to the surrounding atrial tissue.

4. Reentry—as the sinus impulse traverses the atria, instead of continuing antegrade to the junctional tissue and ventricular musculature, the impulse reenters the sinoatrial tissue and perpetuates a circuitous movement.

5. The coexistence of several of the mechanisms described.

The most common rhythm disturbances seen with an anterior myocardial wall infarction are sinus tachycardia, atrial fibrillation, atrial flutter, the severe types of second- and third-degree blocks (Mobitz II second-degree AV block, hemiblocks, and complete heart block), ventricular tachycardia, and fibrillation (45).

A third of the persons who have had conditions diagnosed as an anterior myocardial infarction do experience bouts of sinus tachycardia. Fear, anxiety, and stress are commonly implicated in the genesis of sinus tachycardia. Nonetheless, the rapid rate may also suggest that the heart has become significantly compromised.

In 6% to 15% of these patients atrial fibrillation develops. This may be related to a compromised blood supply to the SA node, pericarditis, congestive heart failure, and/or cardiogenic shock. When present, the ventricular rate is irregularly irregular, usually at 120 to 200 beats per minute. Hence cardiac output has a tendency to fall. A consequence of atrial fibrillation is the loss of atrial transport, which can in fact impair cardiac output by as much as a third of the normal volume. Hypotension, angina, and congestive heart failure may ensue. An elevated end-diastolic left ventricular pressure resulting from failure of a poorly contractile heart to empty its contents predisposes the patient to the chaotic rhythm (46).

Atrial flutter has been known to occur in 4% of patients with an acute anterior myocardial infarction (47). It is most commonly associated with a regular rhythm at a ventricular rate of 150 beats per minute. Occasionally varying degrees of AV block with an irregular rhythm may be present. Because of the more rapid ventricular response associated with atrial flutter, there may be greater impairment of ventricular function.

Conduction disturbances are less commonly implicated in the presence of an anterior myocardial wall infarction, but when present they do carry a poor prognosis. The reason for the graver prognostic association is related to several factors:

1. There is more extensive area of ventricular involvement with encroachment into the septum (48).

2. Mobitz II block is associated with necrosis rather than edema/ischemia of junctional tissue and is permanent (49).

3. There is a lack of progression from lesser to more severe degrees of block; it may occur suddenly.

4. The beat by default (escape) produces a much slower rhythm (48).

5. The block is usually distal to the His bundle; therefore an interventricular conduction defect (hemiblock) is commonly present (40).

The presence of an isolated anterior hemiblock or an extreme leftward axis of the heart does not indicate impending cardiac standstill. Nonetheless, when these findings are associated with block of the other fascicle and/or conduction defects, in the presence of an acute myocardial infarction, there is greater significance associated with the findings (50, 51) (see Chap. 8).

During the first few days after an acute myocardial infarction, 85% of patients develop either unifocal or multifocal premature ventricular contractions. The mechanism for their origin is associated with ischemic myocardial tissue and/or is secondary to extremely slow rates of bradyarrhythmias.

Isolated extrasystolic beats by themselves may not affect cardiac output but are nonetheless harbingers of more lethal arrhythmias. According to Lown (52), ventricular extrasystoles become more significant when they occur in succession and/or originate from different foci within the ventricular wall. In addition, VPCs become troublesome in the presence of a QR′/QT ratio of less than 0.85 second or when they interrupt the T wave (see Chap. 9).

Sustained ventricular tachycardia and fibrillation do reduce cardiac output and therefore must be identified and treated as soon as possible. In the presence of cardiogenic shock, the basis for the bursts of ventricular tachycardia is a metabolic acidosis. Therapy then is directed toward correction of the acidotic condition and the use of pressor agents to raise the blood pressure in abolishing the bouts of tachycardia (25).

Ventricular tachycardia may likewise occur secondary to an excessive intake of digitalis.

Clinical Spectrum

The adverse hemodynamic effects of rhythm disturbances associated with an acute myocardial infarction are related to the mechanisms producing a very slow rhythm, a very fast rhythm, loss of atrial transport, and consequently a loss of sequential atrioventricular contraction. Ventricular function is impaired in varying degrees by all types of rhythm disturbances. Clinical manifestations become evident when the coping mechanisms of the body begin to fail as a result of myocardial insult. The greater the surface of myocardial involvement, the higher is the incidence of coping mechanism failure as reflected in the schematic representation in Table 10-5.

The recognition of arrhythmia becomes more meaningful when one is able to correlate the hemodynamic alterations produced by an infarcted myocardial wall with that of the symptomology evident in the clinical setting. This is especially true of the patient who has sustained a massive myocardial infarction and whose very survival and/or recovery is contingent upon early recognition and intervention (53).

Table 10-5. Failure of Adaptive Mechanisms

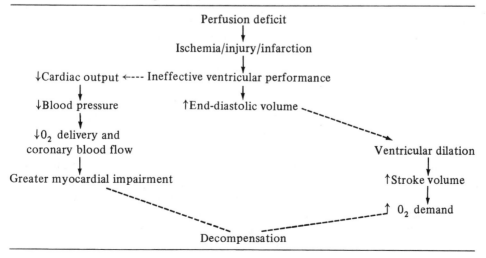

Bradyarrhythmia initially may enhance increased diastolic filling, and therefore cardiac output is not always decreased. Nonetheless, with rates below a critical level, stroke output may be severely compromised. Extremely slow heart rates may further compromise circulation by predisposing the heart to mechanisms of escape or enhanced automaticity. As a result, lower pacemaking sites assume control of heart action. Consequently serious ventricular arrhythmias and ventricular standstill can accompany bradycardia in the presence of an acute myocardial infarction (54).

In addition to the presence of bradycardia, the patient who has sustained an acute diaphragmatic myocardial infarction may become nauseated, and vomit, may be diaphoretic, and/or may salivate excessively. The mechanism involved in the clinical manifestations is thought to be attributed to the presence of autonomic ganglionic fibers having receptor properties. Afferent fiber stimuli are relayed to the atrioventricular junctional region, where excessive discharge of vagal fibers may occur. Peripheral cyanosis, if present, is usually due to a high extraction of oxygen by organs/tissues secondary to inadequate or sluggish circulation.

In association with an acute anterior myocardial infarction, unconsciousness is commonly related to the presence of atrioventricular block, whereas symptoms are minimal when the block is caused by an inferior myocardial infarction.

Varying degrees of organ dysfunction may be attributed to critically slow heart rates, as depicted in the schematic representation (Table 10-6).

The significance of tachyarrhythmias lies in their encroachment upon diastolic filling. The heart can put out only what it receives, and consequently cardiac output usually declines in the presence of rapid cardiac rates. Associated findings with hypotension are a cold and clammy skin; diaphoresis; sensorial changes, as well as a complaint of weakness; shortness of breath; a racing heart; precordial discomfort; and, if cerebral circulation is markedly reduced, syncopal attacks particularly in an upright position (55).

Hemodynamic alterations associated with atrial fibrillation are related to a loss of atrial transport—an insignificant consequence in hearts with adequate cardiac reserve; yet in the presence of decompensation, loss of the added volume during normal atrial contribution may severely limit stroke volume (Table 10-7).

Cyclic ventricular responses to a fibrillating atrium expose heart action to unpatterned rapid and slow rhythms. A ventricular rate of 180 beats per minute, although tolerated in hearts with adequate cardiac reserve, can prove lethal to individuals who have associated coronary underperfusion secondary to occlusive lesions (Table 10-6).

There is some degree of ventricular function impairment in conjunction with the various types of arrhythmias. Yet in the presence of an acute myocardial infarction, these rhythm disturbances can cause hemodynamic deterioration to the point of loss of cardiac reserve and subsequent failure.

Since the majority of myocardial infarctions involve the left ventricle, most of the discussion has been related to transmural infarction of the left heart chamber. Nonetheless, atrial and right ventricular infarctions do occur occasionally. The electrocardiographic features associated with atrial infarction are related to changes in sympathetic tone, to heart failure, and/or to structural changes in the atrial chamber. A downward displacement of the PR and ST segments is attributed to sympathetic stimulation. Ventricular failure or atrial overload would affect the mean electrical axis. The configuration of the P wave may be altered secondary to infarct changes within the atrial wall. Cardiac arrhythmias frequently associated with atrial infarction are the atrial dysrhythmias as well as sinoatrial and atrioventricular conduction disturbances.

Electrocardiographically, right ventricular infarction would undoubtedly reflect evidence of an inferior myocardial infarction, since most of the right ventricle is perfused by way of the right coronary artery. Atrioventricular conduction disturbances could occur for the same reason. Clinically, venous engorgement and hypotension may become evident in the presence of right ventricular infarction.

MYOCARDIAL HYPERTROPHY

Pathogenesis

Cardiac hypertrophy is one of the essential compensatory mechanisms employed by the heart to maintain an adequate cardiac output. It signifies an increase in the size, that is, the diameter of each muscle fiber, as well as an increase in the weight of the heart (56).

Ventricular Hypertrophy

In the strictest sense, hypertrophy is generally considered to be a response to pressure overload or the increased resistance to ejection. However, hypertrophy will develop as a response to volume overload or dilation if it persists for a prolonged period (56). Volume overloading of a ventricle affects its preload state or the length of the muscle fiber at the beginning of systolic ejection. Preload is reflected by the ventricular end-diastolic volume and pressure and is determined by venous return for the most part (57). Characteristically, an increase in the preload is the result of an overfilling of the ventricle and is known as diastolic overloading. Pressure overloading a ventricle affects its afterload state or the force the ventricle must overcome during systole. Afterload is determined largely by the systemic vascular resistance (SVR) (57). An increase in the afterload results in a systolic overloading of the ventricle.

Metabolic functions of the myocardium are normally performed almost entirely under aerobic conditions. The oxidation of fatty acid and carbohydrate substrates normally produces sufficient amounts of adenosine triphosphate (ATP) needed for cardiac contraction. When the heart is subjected to a constantly elevated preload or afterload, another slower mechanism produces an increase in mitochondria. With an increase in the number of functioning mitochondria, the cell's ability to synthesize ATP (adenosine triphosphate) is also increased and it thus serves as a compensatory mechanism to overload states of pressure or volume (58). Recent investigations have determined that the number of mitochondria increase during the early stages of altered preload or afterload; however, during the chronic stage the fractional volume of mitochondria was found to be normal or decreased (59).

An increase in the total RNA (ribonucleic acid), as well as an increased ratio of RNA to DNA (desoxyribonucleic acid), has been found to explain the enhanced size of the cardiac cell in hypertrophy. This supports the belief that the cytoplasm of the myocardial cell, more specifically the RNA fraction, regulates the development of cardiac hypertrophy (60). Although hypertrophy has its compensatory value, it is not without detrimental effects as well. Normally one capillary carries blood to each muscle fiber, and with hypertrophy this 1:1 ratio is not changed (61). A progressive ischemia thus develops as the fibers enlarge, often leading to the production of angina pectoris. Ischemia is further produced since the distance for oxygen diffusion from capillaries to muscle fibers is lengthened. Heart failure usually follows hypertrophy if it is extreme (62).

Table 10–6. Sequelae of Bradyarrhythmia

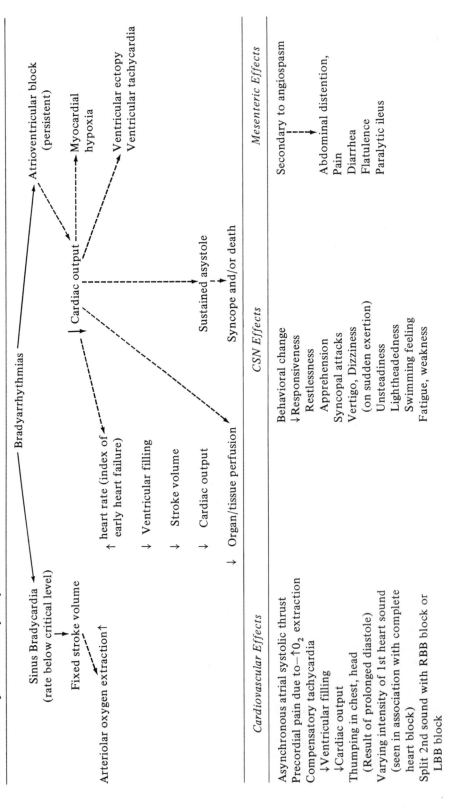

Bradyarrhythmias

Sinus Bradycardia
(rate below critical level)

Fixed stroke volume

Arteriolar oxygen extraction↑

Atrioventricular block
(persistent)

↓ Cardiac output

Myocardial
hypoxia

Ventricular ectopy
Ventricular tachycardia

Sustained asystole
Syncope and/or death

↑ heart rate (index of
early heart failure)

↓ Ventricular filling

↓ Stroke volume

↓ Cardiac output

↓ Organ/tissue perfusion

Secondary to angiospasm

Mesenteric Effects

Abdominal distention,
Pain
Diarrhea
Flatulence
Paralytic ileus

CSN Effects

Behavioral change
↓Responsiveness
Restlessness
Apprehension
Syncopal attacks
Vertigo, Dizziness
(on sudden exertion)
Unsteadiness
Lightheadedness
Swimming feeling
Fatigue, weakness

Cardiovascular Effects

Asynchronous atrial systolic thrust
Precordial pain due to—↑O$_2$ extraction
Compensatory tachycardia
↓Ventricular filling
↓Cardiac output
Thumping in chest, head
(Result of prolonged diastole)
Varying intensity of 1st heart sound
(seen in association with complete
heart block)
Split 2nd sound with RBB block or
LBB block

Peripheral Effects	Pulmonary Effects	Renal Effects
Neck vein pulsation	Dyspnea due to:	No change or if bradycardia and/heart block is prolonged
Diastolic pressure (prolonged diastolic phase)	1. Inability to increase cardiac output with exercise	
Skin: pale, cold, clammy, diaphoresis (Compensatory mechanism of vasoconstriction)		↓Blood flow
Pulse initially fast then decreasing with bradycardia, 50–60/min	2. Anxiety	→ Oliguria
Complete heart block, 30–40/min	3. Left ventricular failure	→ Proteinuria
Pulse volume bounding (second to stroke volume)		
"Waterhammer pulse" (rapid rise and fall) Secondary to ejection of large amount of blood into the low resistance vessels		

195

Table 10–7. Hemodynamic Effects of Supraventricular Tachyarrhythmias

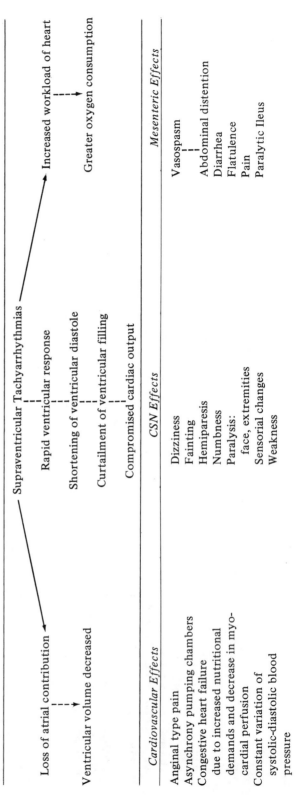

Diaphoresis
"Fluttering of heart"
Precordial thumping
Varying intensity of first
 heart sound

Peripheral Effects	Pulmonary Effects	Renal Effects
Cold, clammy skin	Dyspnea	Increased renal vascular resistance
Cyanotic hue to extremities	Pulmonary congestion	(Homeostatic effort to divert blood to brain, heart)
Diaphoresis	Pulmonary edema	↑Urine volume
Irregular pulse		(Ischemic tubular Impairment of reabsorptive process)
Jugular venous engorgement		↑Urine frequency
Pulse deficit		
"Thumping in head"		Oliguria
"Vascular collapse"		

197

Cardiac hypertrophy for all practical purposes is a postmortem diagnosis based on histologic and gross examination, weight, and measurement of chamber walls. The normal adult male's heart weight is 0.43% of his body weight as opposed to 0.40% in the adult female. This percentage is based on muscular development; therefore, obese persons have a smaller percentage of heart to body weight than those with good muscular development. The heart is usually considered to be hypertrophied if it is heavier than 375 g in an adult female or heavier than 400 g in an adult male (60). The left ventricle is considered hypertrophied if the thickness of its wall, measured midway between the apex and the mitral valve, exceeds 12 mm. If the right ventricular chamber, midway between the apex and pulmonic valve, exceeds 4 mm, it is then considered to be hypertrophied as well (60).

Although hypertrophy is basically diagnosed postmortem, the electrocardiogram, as well as the chest roentgenogram and cardiac angiograph, are additional diagnostic tools that can offer some value in the diagnosis. The precordial leads are by far the best leads to use since they are closer to the ventricles; but valuable information can also be obtained from the standard limb leads. Leads V_{5-6}, as well as leads I and aV_L, overlie the left ventricle and see it with a positive pole. They will be the key leads to use in the assessment of LVH (left ventricular hypertrophy). Lead V_1 also is used to give reciprocal findings since it overlies the right ventricle. The same leads are used in the assessment of RVH (right ventricular hypertrophy), with more emphasis placed on the right precordial leads V_{1-2}. The left ventricle is three times thicker than the right; in addition the left ventricle has an electrical potential approximately 10 times greater than the right ventricle (63). The left ventricle for these reasons dominates the appearance of the QRS complex during ventricular depolarization. This normal left ventricular dominance is further exaggerated in LVH.

Electrocardiographic Features

Normally ventricular depolarization begins when the midportion of the septum is activated from the left to right (see Chap. 3). With leads V_{5-6} this septal activation is shown as leaving the positive poles and is recorded as a small septal Q wave (Fig. 10-7). In LVH this initial septal activation is unchanged and Q waves are still inscribed. However, in marked LVH, this small Q wave may be lost, producing an incomplete left bundle branch block. Sodi-Pallares has found that approximately 90% of patients with the so-called "first-degree" left bundle branch block (incomplete left bundle branch block) have LVH (64). Septal depolarization is reversed in this instance, traveling from right to left, which accounts for the loss of Q waves in V_{5-6} as well as loss of R waves in V_{1-2}. The S wave in V_{1-2}, as well as the R wave in V_{5-6}, will show an increased amplitude, reflecting the thickened ventricle. The intrinsicoid deflection, as previously described in Chapter 4, accounts for the time it takes the electrical stimulus to travel from endocardium to epicardium. A thickened left ventricle will cause a prolongation of the normal intrinsicoid deflection as recorded in V_{5-6} (65). Additionally, the duration of ventricular depolarization is lengthened to account for a wider QRS interval. A shift of the mean QRS axis to the left may develop; however, some investigators have reported a left axis deviation in less than 50% of cases of LVH (63).

Left anterior hemiblock shifts the axis markedly leftward and may mimic or mask the signs of LVH. An improvement in the interpretation of LVH in the presence of LAH (left anterior hemiblock) has been shown by also adding the depth of the S wave in lead V_5 or 6 to the usual sum of waves (66).

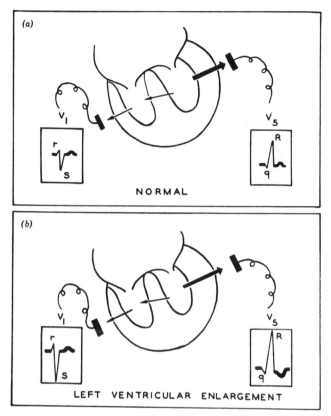

Figure 10-7. Schematic representation of the ECG changes seen with LVH. (Reproduced with permission from Lipman BS, Massie E, Kleiger RE: *Clinical Scalar Electrocardiography*, 6th edition. Copyright © 1972 by Year Book Medical Publishers, Inc., Chicago.)

When LVH is the result of a systolic overload, a so-called "strain pattern" is produced in leads V_{5-6} (Fig. 10-8). The typical strain pattern is present when there is ST segment depression that has a convex appearance along with an inverted T wave (63) (Fig. 10-9). This ST and T wave alteration is considered a secondary change (see Chap. 4) and may be the result of myocardial ischemia and a slowing of intraventricular conduction. The strain pattern is more prevalent in those people who have had LVH for some time.

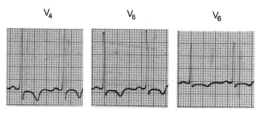

Figure 10-8. The strain pattern associated with LVH is best seen in the left precordial leads. The appearance of ST segment depression with a convex shape and inverted T waves are the characteristic findings in a strain pattern.

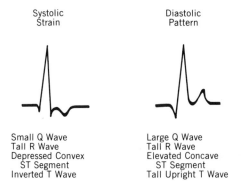

Figure 10-9. Comparative changes found with systolic and diastolic strain patterns.

The strain pattern may become more marked if the left ventricle dilates and is followed by failure. Left ventricular hypertrophy produced by systolic overloading is clinically seen in those with systemic hypertension, aortic stenosis, and coarctation of the aorta (63). When the left ventricle hypertrophies as a result of diastolic overloading, the T wave becomes upright and very tall and pointed over the left precordial leads. This pattern may be seen clinically in patients with aortic insufficiency, mitral insufficiency, ventricular septal defect, and patent ductus arteriosus, all of which produce diastolic overloading (63). The Q waves in V_{5-6} tend to be deeper and the R waves taller in diastolic over-loading as opposed to systolic overloading of the left ventricle. Additionally, the ST segment may be somewhat elevated with a slight concave appearance along with the tall, upright waves (63) (Fig. 10-9). Left ventricular hypertrophy is a fairly frequent finding (66%) in patients with alcoholic cardiomyopathy (67). Whether the LVH is the result of primary systolic or diastolic overloading has not been specified.

Several different criteria have been proposed for the ECG diagnosis of LVH, but the most precise is probably the Estes criteria. Others have modified the original 13-point system to include only 10 points (68, 69). The point system for LVH is shown in Table 10-8.

Table 10-8. Estes Criteria for LVH

1. R or S wave in limb lead of 20 mm or more	
S in V_1, V_2, or V_3: 25 mm or more	
R in V_4, V_5, or V_6: 25 mm or more	3
2. Any ST segment shift without digitalis	3
Strain pattern with digitalis	1
3. Axis deviation of $-15°$ or more	2
4. Intrinsicoid deflection in V_{5-6}	
of 0.04 second or more	1
5. QRS duration of 0.09 second or more	1
	10

LVH = 5 points
LVH (probably) = 4 points

Voltage criteria alone are used by some in the ECG diagnosis of LVH. If an R wave in aV_L is greater than 13 mm or an R wave in V_{5-6} is greater than 27 mm, or if an S wave in V_1 is combined with an R wave in V_{5-6} to equal 35 mm or more, LVH is present (65) (Fig. 10-10).

The right ventricle is as thick or is possibly one-third thicker than the left ventricle at birth, which accounts for the normal appearance of tall R waves in the right precordial leads in the newborn. Gradually during the first months of life this right ventricular predominance diminishes owing to a systemic vascular resistance that is higher than the pulmonary vascular   resistance. Approximately 50% of newborns exhibit a complete reversal of R/S progression in the precordial leads. If this reversal of R/S progression

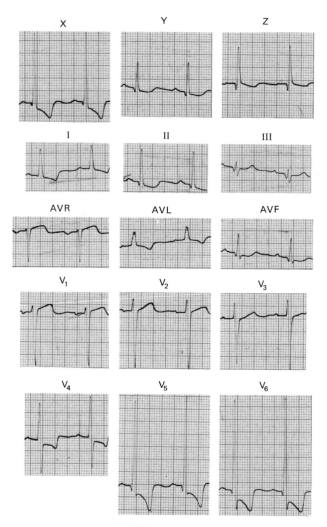

Figure 10-10. Striking changes of LVH were recorded from a patient with valvular aortic stenosis. A total of 9 points is calculated from the Estes scoring system. The changes in voltage, ST and T waves (patient was not receiving digitalis), intrinsicoid deflection, and QRS width comprise the 9-point total.

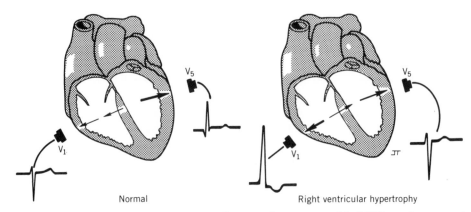

Figure 10-11. Changes in the electrocardiogram that occur with RVH are best seen in the right precordial leads.

persists after one month of life, then the presence of RVH (right ventricular hypertrophy) is likely. The adult right ventricle likewise is one-third the size and has one-tenth the electrical potential of the left ventricle. The right ventricle therefore must have a significant amount of hypertrophy before RVH becomes evident on the electrocardiogram (Fig. 10-11). The presence of mild to moderate RVH is frequently not seen on the electrocardiogram because (*1*) the right ventricle predominates in the infant and (*2*) the left ventricle predominates in the adult. Likewise a tall R wave in V_1 is not diagnostic of RVH but may be seen with other abnormalities (Table 10-9).

The mean QRS forces are directed anteriorly and rightward in RVH, owing to the location of the right ventricle. This shift of the mean QRS vector produces a right axis deviation and is considered a key factor in the recognition of RVH (63). A rightward axis unfortunately is not produced entirely by RVH but is also seen in left posterior hemiblock, inferior wall myocardial infarction, and chronic cor pulmonale. The R:S ratio in V_1 (see Chap. 4) gradually changes as the right ventricle thickens. This abnormal R:S ratio (greater than 1.0) accounts for the "tall" R wave in the right precordial leads (69). The R wave amplitude in V_1 correlates rather poorly with the degree of right ventricular hypertrophy, and so more significance is given to the progressive change from the right to the left precordial leads. In RVH the normal R wave progression across the precordial leads tends to be reversed, and prominent S waves appearing in V_{5-6} produce a clockwise rotation (see Chap. 3) (Fig. 10-12). The deep S waves can also be seen in leads I and aV_L. Very tall R waves tend to be present in states which affect right ventricular afterload, that is, pure valvular pulmonic stenosis (Table 10-10).

The thickness of the right ventricle, even when it is hypertrophied, usually does not exceed that of the left; therefore the QRS width is seldom prolonged. Some authorities (63, 64) have found that RSR' pattern with normal QRS duration (incomplete RBBB)

Table 10-9. Clinical Settings Producing Tall R Waves in V_1

True posterior myocardial infarction
Right ventricular hypertrophy
Type A Wolff-Parkinson-White syndrome
Right bundle branch block

I   II   III

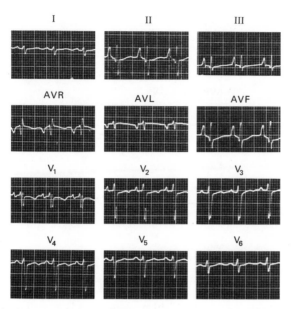

AVR   AVL   AVF

V_1 V_2 V_3

V_4 V_5 V_6

Figure 10-12. Clockwise rotation of the QRS complex (transition zone is lead V_6) accompanies RVH and right atrial enlargement.

to be commonly found in RVH produced by an increased preload or diastolic overloading state. The RSR′ pattern is frequently seen in patients with atrial septal defects. Sometimes it is impossible to distinguish RVH from incomplete RBBB. The RSR′ pattern in V_1 is thought to be the result of hypertrophy of the basal proportions of the right ventricle. Other authorities (69) have found the presence of an RSR′ in V_1 in mitral stenosis, which is primarily an increased afterload state. An interesting but often puzzling finding in some cases of RVH is the appearance of Q waves in V_{1-3} (Fig. 10-13). Septal activation is not disturbed and still begins at midseptum, from which it proceeds from left to right in RVH as it does normally. However, as the right ventricle enlarges and rotates on its longitudinal axis (see Chap. 3) in a clockwise fashion, so does the septum. The right side of the septum now becomes more anterior and slightly leftward, whereas the left side of the septum faces just opposite, more posterior, and to the right. The

Table 10-10. Clinical Settings Producing Right Ventricular Hypertrophy

Increased Preload	*Increased Afterload*
(diastolic overload)	(systolic overload)
Atrial septal defect	Mitral stenosis
Tricuspid insufficiency	Tetralogy of fallot
	Chronic obstructive lung disease
	Pulmonary hypertension

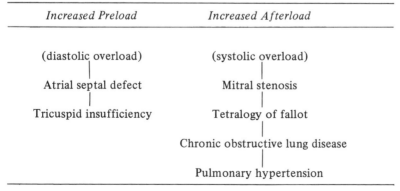

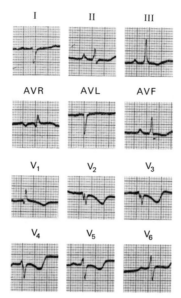

Figure 10-13. Q waves are seen in the right precordial leads as well as deep S waves are seen in leads I, aV_L, and V_{4-6}. Right axis deviation also is present in this ECG of RVH.

normal septal activation still proceeds from left to right, but is seen by the recording leads as traveling just opposite or right to left owing to the masked rotation (64). The presence of Q waves in V_{1-3} may mimic an anteroseptal myocardial infarction in those instances.

Additional criteria of RVH to be looked for on the ECG is the appearance of a prolonged intrinsicoid deflection time in V_1 of 0.035 second or more (64). The QRS width seldom prolongs in RVH as opposed to LVH, owing to the normally smaller-sized right ventricle. The ST segment and T wave in V_1 may have a typical strain pattern found in V_{5-6} with LVH, but it is usually not a prominent finding. Other variant findings in RVH are the presence of deep S waves in the three standard limb leads, or the S_1, S_2, S_3 pattern; prominent Q waves in leads II, III, and aV_F (simulating an inferior myocardial infarction), along with a typical strain pattern in these same leads; and an upright T wave in V_1 in an infant after one or two days of life (69). The key findings in RVH are summarized in Table 10-11).

Biventricular hypertrophy is rather difficult to assess on the electrocardiogram because the hypertrophied walls with their increased electrical forces in both the right and left

Table 10-11. Key Findings in Right Ventricular Hypertrophy

1. Right-axis deviation
2. Delayed intrinsicoid deflection in V_{1-2} of 0.035 second or more
3. Tall R waves (R:S ration of 1.0 or more) in V_1
4. Deep S waves in V_{5-6}, I or aV_L (or reversal of the normal precordial pattern)
5. Strain pattern in V_{1-3}
6. Normal QRS duration

ventricles may cancel each other out and produce a relatively normal tracing. Two of the most helpful findings on the ECG are: (*1*) a left axis deviation in the limb leads with a pattern of RVH in the precordial leads and (*2*) the opposite picture of right axis deviation in the limb leads with a pattern of LVH in the precordial leads (63). The Katz-Wachtel sign, which consists of an equiphasic QRS (RS pattern) complex in the middle left precordial leads, is another finding indicative of biventricular hypertrophy and is often seen in patients with a ventricular septal defect (64).

Atrial Hypertrophy

Atrial hypertrophy is even more difficult to interpret from the electrocardiogram than ventricular hypertrophy, primarily owing to the relatively small size of the P wave. There is a fair amount of evidence pointing out the poor correlation between chamber size of the atria and ECG findings. The typical pattern of P pulmonale thought to be the result of right atrial enlargement has been found in those persons with a normal-sized atrium but who instead had an acute myocardial infarction (70) or angina pectoris without infarction (71). Similarly, data illustrating the presence of P mitrale on the ECG do not always correlate with left atrial enlargement (72). It must not be forgotten, however, that ECGs that show the typical findings of left or right atrial enlargement have been made for persons who indeed have chamber enlargement.

Clinically, enlargement of the left atrial chamber has been traditionally thought to influence the production of atrial arrhythmias, primarily atrial fibrillation. Hemodynamically, atrial fibrillation causes two problems: (*1*) in those persons who have a fast ventricular response cardiac output is compromised and (*2*) the formation of thrombi in the atrial chambers occurs owing to stasis of flow and may produce peripheral embolic episodes. Studies conducted by Probst (73) have demonstrated that an enlarged left atrium is not uniformly present in those persons with atrial fibrillation. Therefore, when one interprets atrial hypertrophy on the basis of ECG findings, it is not an absolute correlation.

The atrial chambers are considered to be thin-walled structures, which, unlike their ventricular counterparts, lack a highly specialized conduction system. Normally atrial depolarization begins at the level of the junction of the superior vena cava (SVC) with the right atrium (RA) and proceeds inferiorly (toward the feet) and anteriorly (toward the front). This direction of depolarization accounts for the tall, upright P waves seen in leads II, aV_F, and possibly III. The first half of the P wave represents right atrial depolarization and the second half represents depolarization of the left atrium (74).

Electrocardiographic Features

The normal P wave axis in the frontal plane is $0°$ to $+90°$. Usually, shifts in the P wave axis to the right do not exceed $+90°$ in persons with right atrial enlargement; and likewise, leftward axis shifts do not usually exceed $0°$ in persons with left atrial enlargement. The following ECG components must be evaluated in the assessment of atrial hypertrophy or enlargement:

1. Mean P wave axis (normal $0°$ to $+90°$) (see Chap 3).
2. P wave amplitude in leads II, III, or aV_F (normal 2.5 mm).
3. P wave width in lead II (normal is 0.11 second or less).
4. Presence of notching of P waves (usually best seen in leads II, V_1 and V_{5-6}) (Fig. 10-14).

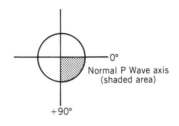

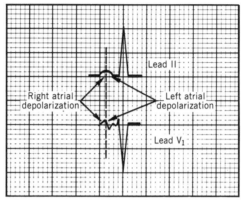

Normal P Wave Width = .11 sec or less
Normal P Wave Height = <2.5 mm

Figure 10-14. The criteria for the normal P wave includes measurements of the width, height, and axis. (Reproduced with permission from Chung EK: *Electrocardiography: Practical Applications with Vectorial Principles.* Copyright © 1974 by Harper and Row Publishers, Inc., Hagerstown, Maryland.)

Enlargement of the right atrium may be seen whenever there is a pressure or a volume overload imposed upon it. This characteristically produces very tall (2.5 mm) peaked P waves in leads II, III, and aV_F. The normal spread of atrial activation (inferiorly and anteriorly) is exaggerated, which accounts for these tall P waves. This has a tendency to shift the P wave axis toward the right. This P wave configuration has been termed P pulmonale, P tricuspidale, or P congenitale, and is seen in the clinical settings of tricuspid stenosis, pulmonic stenosis, cor pulmonale, chronic obstructive pulmonary disease, and various congenital heart defects (75, 76) (Fig. 10-15).

Pulmonale that produces tall, peaked P waves in the inferior leads as well as in V_1 and a P wave axis of +70° or more may be seen in those patients with chronic lung disease (75). Similarly, patients with congenital heart defects may produce tall, notched P waves with a P wave axis not quite as far rightward (+30°-+45°). This has been termed P congenitale. The right atrium may so enlarge in these persons that it extends across the front of the heart and to the left, which may produce a negative P wave in V_1. This falsely produces the ECG appearance of the left atrial enlargement (75). P congenitale is commonly present in patients with cyanotic forms of congenital heart defects, but it may also be seen in those patients with pulmonic stenosis (75). Right atrial depolarization is seen in the first half of the P wave, and this portion may peak larger in patients who have tricuspid valve disease. This notched P wave in which the first peak is the taller of the two has been termed P tricuspidale (76). The ECG criteria of tall P waves in V_1

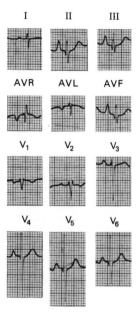

Figure 10-15. Tall P waves (4 mm in lead II) are seen in this ECG recorded from a 45-year-old woman. Right-axis deviation of the QRS is also present.

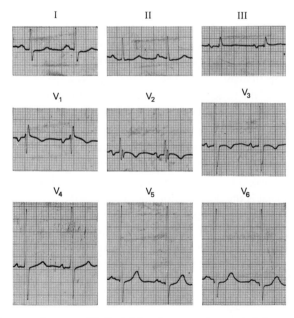

Figure 10-16. P wave changes of left atrial enlargement recorded from a 36-year-old man with mitral stenosis and insufficiency. The P waves have the typical M shape of P mitrale. A deep negative component of the P wave is seen in leads III and V_1. (See text on next page.)

as well as tall, peaked P waves in leads II and III with a P wave axis of +60° or greater are fairly specific for right atrial enlargement; however, they are not very sensitive criteria (77).

Left atrial enlargement is produced by pressure or volume overload of the left atrium and is clinically seen in patients with mitral stenosis or insufficiency and congestive heart failure due to left ventricular disease. Lead V^1 is the most reliable source for ECG evidence of left atrial enlargement. The P wave becomes more noticeably diaphasic in this lead than normal, and the terminal part of the P wave becomes large and negative. Morris (78) proposed a very specific set of criteria for the diagnosis of left atrial enlargement on the basis of lead V_1. His criteria include (1) the P wave in V_1 usually has an initial positive deflection and a terminal negative deflection and (2) an algebraic product of the terminal force of the P wave is calculated by multiplying the duration (in seconds) by the magnitude (in millimeters) of the terminal part of V_1 under standard conditions.

Additional criteria for left atrial enlargement include a P-wave duration of 0.12 second or more as well as notching of the P wave, termed P mitrale, often seen with mitral valve disease (Fig. 10–16). The interval between the notches of the P wave becomes significant if it exceeds 0.04 second (75).

Enlargement of both right and left atrial chambers, biatrial hypertrophy, is most often present in individuals with cardiomyopathies and various forms of congenital heart defects. Since the right atrium is enlarged, a tall P wave is present and is usually 3 mm or more wide. Likewise, a broad P wave of 0.12 second or more is present owing to the enlarged left atrium (79).

REVIEW QUESTIONS

1. Mr. Lewis, a 45-year-old executive of an oil company experienced an inferior myocardial infarction with resultant idioventricular episodes that were increasing in frequency. Which leads are suggestive of this type of myocardial infarction?

2. During her assessment of a patient, Miss Jony, a staff nurse in the coronary care unit, detected what she thought was a newly developed systolic murmur in the anterior area of the chest of the patient, who had been admitted to the unit three days before. Which conditions could possibly produce this mumur?

3. What is the significance of the persistence of ST-segment elevation?

4. A sustained episode of sinus tachycardia when associated with a myocardial infarction is said to be of grave significance. What does the presence of the tachycardia imply?

5. Occasionally, to break a tachycardic episode, measures are taken to raise the patient's blood pressure. What is the rationale for this plan of care?

6. A 58-year-old maintenance worker was admitted to the cardiology ward after experiencing severe chest pain a few hours before admission. Upon admission, his pulse rate was palpated at 46 beats per minute. The order "place in Trendelenburg position" was given. What is the rationale in the use of the Trendelenburg position as opposed to the administration of atropine?

REFERENCES

1. Matthews MB: Clinical diagnosis, in Julian D (ed): *Angina Pectoris.* Edinburgh, Churchill Livingstone, 1977, p 53.

2. Sodeman WA, Sodeman WA Jr: *Pathologic Physiology*, ed 4. Philadelphia, WB Saunders Co, 1968, p 468.

3. Hurst JW, Logue JB, Walter PF: in Hurst, Logue, Schlant, Wenyer (eds): *The Heart, Arteries and Veins*. New York, McGraw-Hill Book Co, 1978, p 1174.

4. Fulton M, Julian DG: Unstable angina, in Julian D (ed): *Angina Pectoris*. Edinburgh, Churchill Livingstone, 1977, p 70.

5. Shine KI, Kattus AA, Tillisch JH: Pathophysiology of myocardial infarction. *Ann Int Med* 87:79, 1977.

6. Corday E, Irving DW: *Disturbances of Heart Rate, Rhythm and Conduction*, Philadelphia, WB Saunders Co, 1962, p 63.

7. Eliot RS, Holsinger JW: The potential role of the subendocardium in the pathogenesis of myocardial infarction. *Heart Lung* 1:358, 1972.

8. Prakash R, Chhablan R: Immunoreactive serum insulin and growth hormone reponses in patients with preinfarction angina and acute myocardial infarction. *Chest* 65:412, 1974.

9. Philips GB: Relationship between serum sex hormones and glucogen, insulin and lipid abnormalities in men with myocardial infarction. *Proc Natl Acad Sci USA* 74:1732, 1977.

10. Lanecki J, Ceremusqnski L, Rogala H, et al: Relationship between the blood glucogen, growth hormone and glucose levels in myocardial infarction. *Pol Med Sc Hist Bull* 15:62, 1976.

11. Silber EN, Katz LN: *Heart Disease,* New York, Macmillan Inc, 1975, p 57.

12. Fowler NO; *Cardiac Diagnosis and Treatment*, ed 2. Hagerstown, Md, Harper & Row Pub Inc, 1976, p 17.

13. Gorlin R, Herman WV: Physiology of the coronary circulation, in Hurst JW and Logue RB (ed): *The Heart*. New York, McGraw-Hill Book Co, 1978, p 101.

14. Heng MK, Corday E: Interventions to reduce myocardial infarct size. *Practical Cardiol* 3:48, 1977.

15. Ross J: Effects of afterload or impedance on the heart: afterload reduction in the treatment of cardiac failure. *Cardiovasc Med* 2:1115, 1977.

16. Sodeman WA, Sodeman WA Jr: *Pathologic Physiology,* ed 4. Philadelphia, WB Saunders Co, 1968, p 340.

17. Pitt B: Hemodynamic feedback mechanisms during acute myocardial ischemia, in Maseri A, Klassen GA, Lesch M (eds): *Primary and Secondary Angina Pectoris*. New York, Grune & Stratton Inc, 1978, p 336.

18. Karliner JS: The differential diagnosis of angina pectoris. *Practical Cardiol* 2:18, 1976.

19. Falicev RE: Unstable angina pectoris. *Hosp Med* 10:8, 1974.

20. d'Hemecourt A, Deter R: Possible physiological basis for locally induced "spasm" of large coronary arteries, in Maseri A, Klassen G, Lesch M (eds): *Primary and Secondary Angina Pectoris*. New York, Grune & Stratton Inc, 1978, p 177.

21. Johnson AD: Prinzmetal's variant angina: current concepts and management. *Practical Cardiol* 3:18, 1977.

22. Bassenge E, Holtz J, Restorff W: What is the physiological significance of sympathetic coronary innervation? in Maseri A, Klassen GA, Lesch M (eds): *Primary and Secondary Angina Pectoris*. New York, Grune & Stratton Inc, 1978, p 212.

23. Gelfand ML: Medical management of angina pectoris. *Primary Cardiol* 1:29, 1975.

24. Humphries JO: Selection of therapy for angina pectoris: medical versus surgical. *Cardiovasc. Med* 2:1097, 1977.

25. Chung EK: *Electrocardiography: Practical Applications with Vectorial Principles*. Hagerstown, Md, Harper & Row Pub Inc, 1974, p 109.

26. Schamroth L: *The Disorders of Cardiac Rhythm*. Oxford, Blackwell Scientific Publications, 1971, p 409.

27. Marriott, HJL: *Practical Electrocardiography*, ed 5. Baltimore, Williams & Wilkins Co, 1972, p 228.

28. Williams R, Cohn P, Vokonas P, Young E, Herman M, Gorlin R: Electrocardiographic, arteriographic and ventriculographic correlations in transmural infarction. *Am J Cardiol* 31:596, 1973. 1973.

29. Goldman MJ: *Principles of Clinical Electrocardiography*, ed 9. Los Altos, Calif, Lange Medical Publications, 1976, p 156.

30. Han J: Mechanism of ventricular arrhythmias associated with myocardial infarction. *Am J Cardiol* 24:802, 1969.

31. Surawicz B: Electrolytes and the electrocardiogram. *Postgrad Med* 55:129, 1974.

32. Kurien VA, Oliver MF: A metabolic cause for arrhythmias during acute myocardial hypoxia. *Lancet* 23:813, 1969.

33. Shapiro W: Correlative studies of serum digitalis and the arrhythmias of digitalis intoxication. *A J Cardiol* 41:852, 1978.

34. Vohra J: Beta-adrenergic blockade in arrhythmias of acute myocardial infarction. *Heart Lung* 2:662, 1973.

35. Henderson AH, Sonnenblick EH: Effect of free fatty acids on the hypoxic heart. *Lancet* 18:1179, 1970.

36. Nelson PG: Free fatty acids and cardiac arrhythmias. *Lancet* 30:783, 1970.

37. Rutenberg HL, Soloff LA: Serum-free fatty acids and arrhythmias after acute myocardial infarction. *Lancet* 1:198, 1970.

38. Killip T: Management of arrhythmias in acute myocardial infarction. *Hosp Pract* 7:131, 1972.

39. Kurien VA, Oliver MF, Yates PA: Free fatty acids, heparin, and arrhythmias during experimental myocardial infarction. *Lancet* 23:185, 1969.

40. Gupta PK, Lichstein E, Chadda MO: Heart block complicating acute inferior wall myocardial infarction. *Chest* 69: 599, 1976.

41. Stock E: Arrhythmias after myocardial infarction. *Am Heart J* 75:435, 1968.

42. D'Ambrosio U, Czarnecki SW: Treatment of arrhythmias in acute myocardial infarction. *Hosp Med* 7:141, 1971.

43. Bradham RR, Parker EF, Barrington BA, Webb CM, Stallworth JM: The cardiac lymphatics. *Ann Surg* 171:902, 1970.

44. Walter PF: The sick sinus syndrome. *Med Times* 107:84, 1979.

45. Winslow EH, Powell AH: Sick sinus syndrome. *Am J Nurs* 76:1262, 1972.

46. Cristal N, Peterburg I, Szwarcberg J: Atrial fibrillation in the acute phase of myocardial infarction. *Chest* 70:8, 1976.

47. Liberthson RR, Salesbury KW, Hutter AM, De Sanctis: Atrial tachyarrhythmias in acute myocardial infarction. *Am J of Med* 60:956, 1976.

48. Chamberlin O, Leinbach R: Electrical pacing in heart block complicating acute myocardial infarction. *Br Heart* 1:70, 1970.

49. Goldman MJ: *Principles of Clinical Electrocardiography*, ed 9. Los Altos, Calif, Lange Medical Publications, 1976, p 23.

50. Kincaid DT, Botti RE: Significance of isolated left anterior hemiblock and left axis deviation during acute myocardial infarction. *Am J Cardiol* 30:797, 1972.

51. Lie KI, Liem KL, Schuilenburg RM, David GK, Durrer O: Early identification of patients developing late in-hospital ventricular fibrillation after discharge from the coronary care unit. *Am J Cardiol* 41:674, 1978.

52. Lown B, Fakhro AM, Hood WB, Thorn GW: Coronary care unit. *JAMA* 199: 188, 1967.

53. Mayer GG, Kaelin PB: Arrhythmias and cardiac output. *Am J Nurs* 72:1597, 1972.

54. Stuckey J: Atropine in bradycardia in the coronary care unit and elsewhere. *Heart Lung* 2:666, 1973.

55. McIntosh HD, Morris JJ: Hemodynamic consequences of arrhythmias. *Prog Cardiovasc Dis* 8:352, 1966.

56. Sodeman WA Jr, Sodeman WA: Hypertrophy and dilatation of the heart, in *Pathologic Physiology: Mechanisms of Disease,* ed 5. Philadelphia, WB Saunders Co, 1974, p 386.

57. Chatterjee K: Chronic congestive heart failure and vasodilator therapy. *J Contin Ed Cardiol* 6:17, 1978.

58. Rabinowitz M, Zak R: Mitochondria and cardiac hypertrophy. *Circ Res* 36:367, 1975.

59. Hatt PY: Cellular changes in mechanically overloaded heart. *Basic Res Cardiol* 72:198, 1977.

60. Friedberg CK: Enlargement of the heart, in *Diseases of the Heart,* ed 3. Philadelphia, WB Saunders Co, 1966, p 160.

61. Smith C: Cardiovascular lesions. Part I. *Hosp Med* 9:100, 1973.

62. Rothe CF: Cardiodynamics, in Selkurt EE (ed): *Physiology,* ed 3. Boston, Little Brown & Co, 1971, p 395.

63. Chung EK: *Electrocardiography: Practical Applications with Vectorial Principles.* Hagerstown, Md, Harper & Row Pub Inc, 1974, p 62.

64. Lipman BS, Massie E, Kleiger RE: *Clinical Scalar Electrocardiography,* ed 6. Chicago, Year Book Medical Pub Inc, 1972, p 93.

65. Goldman MJ: *Principles of Clinical Electrocardiography*, ed 10. Los Altos, Calif, Lange Medical Publications, 1979, p 85.

66. Bozzi G, Gifini A: Left anterior hemiblock and electrocardiographic diagnosis of left ventricular hypertrophy. *Adv Cardiol* 16:495, 1976.

67. Bashour TT, Fahdul H, Cheng TO: Electrocardiographic abnormalities in alcoholic cardiomyopathy: A study of 65 patients. *Chest* 68:24, 1975.

68. Romhilt DW, Estes EH: A point score system for the ECG diagnosis of left ventricular hypertrophy. *Am Heart J* 75:752, 1968.

69. Marriott HJL: *Practical Electrocardiography*, ed 6. Baltimore, Williams & Wilkins Co, 1977, p 50.

70. Grossman JJ, Delman AJ: Serial P wave changes in acute myocardial infarction. *Am Heart J* 77:336, 1969.

71. Gross D: Electrocardiographic characteristics of P pulmonale waves of coronary origin. *Am Heart J* 73:453, 1967.

72. Saunders JL, Calatayud JB, et al: Evaluation of ECG criteria for P wave abnormalities. *Am Heart J* 74:757, 1967.

73. Probst P, Goldschlager N: Left atrial size and atrial fibrillation in mitral stenosis. Factors influencing their relationship. *Circulation* 48:1282, 1973.

74. Levine HD: Clinical electrocardiography, in Levine SA (ed): *Clinical Heart Disease,* ed 5. Philadelphia, WB Saunders Co, 1958, p 405.

75. Marriott HJL: *Practical Electrocardiography*, ed 6. Baltimore, Williams & Wilkins Co, 1977, p 51.

76. Gamboa R et al: The electrocardiogram in tricuspid atresia and pulmonary atresia with intact ventricular septum. *Circulation* 34:24, 1966.

77. Estes EH Jr: Electrocardiography and vectorcardiography, in Hurst JW, Logue RB (ed): *The Heart, Arteries, and Veins.* New York, McGraw-Hill Book Co, 1966, p 130.

78. Morris JJ Jr, Estes EH Jr et al: P wave analysis in valvular heart disease. *Circulation* 29:242, 1964.

79. Chung EK: *Electrocardiography: Practical Applications with Vectorial Principles.* Hagerstown, Md, Harper & Row Pub Inc, 1974, p 60.

11
Antiarrhythmic Therapy

The prevention and treatment of cardiac arrhythmias requires a comprehensive evaluation of the patient. This evaluation should include the patient's past and present medical history as well as the signs and symptoms produced by the arrhythmia. Extraneous factors are frequently the source of cardiac arrhythmias and a thorough search must be undertaken to expose them. Hyperthyroidism, acid-base and electrolyte abnormalities, congestive heart failure, and drugs (digitalis at toxic levels, antihistamines, amphetamines) are among extraneous factors responsible for arrhythmias. Their elimination is usually the main, if not the only, treatment necessary. The etiology of arrhythmias may be subdivided into three categories: (1) abnormality of automaticity (impulse formation), (2) abnormality of impulse conduction, and (3) a combination of 1 and 2. (1). Automaticity (rate of pacemaker discharge) is controlled by three factors: (1) rate of spontaneous diastolic depolarization, (2) value of maximum diastolic potential, and (3) threshold potential (see Chap. 2, Figs. 2-12 and 2-13). When the sinus rate becomes abnormally slow or irregular, an ectopic automatic focus may become the dominant pacemaker. This rhythm is considered to be a passive or a default rhythm, and the normal sinus rhythm can usually be restored by increasing the automaticity of the sinus node with agents such as atropine and catecholamines. These agents enhance impulse formation by increasing the slope of phase-4 diastolic depolarization. If the sinus node function is depressed from the tachycardia-bradycardia syndrome (sick sinus syndrome), therapeutic interventions directed toward increasing the automacity of the SA node are frequently not satisfactory (1).

Abnormalities of impulse conduction (slowing or blockage) that produce arrhythmias include (1) sinoatrial block, (2) atrioventricular block, (3) His bundle block, (4) bundle branch block, and (5) Purkinje fiber block (1). Unidirectional block and associated reentry (Chap. 6) are well known as the cause of many arrhythmias. The conduction of an impulse is related to the resting potential. When the resting potential is decreased (less negative value than normal), conduction is impaired; and conversely, when the resting potential is increased (more negative value than normal), conduction is improved. Reentrant arrhythmias may be abolished, therefore, by improving conduction in a depressed area or by further depressing conduction to the point of complete block (2).

CLASSIFICATION OF DRUGS

Classification of antiarrhythmic drugs based on conduction, action potential duration, and responsiveness of the cardiac fiber was proposed in 1971 by Hoffman and Bigger (3).

The division of antiarrhythmic drugs into two groups was then made: (*1*) those that depressed conduction and responsiveness and (*2*) those that improved conduction and responsiveness. This classification of only two groups was not generally accepted, and Vaughn Williams proposed four classes of antiarrhythmic drugs (4). This classification is based on the drug's ability to (*1*) decrease the amplitude of the action potential and the maximum rate of rise of phase O, (*2*) produce sympathetic blockade, and (*3*) increase the duration of the action potential or modify the inward calcium current during depolarization (5). Newer antiarrhythmic agents have once again necessitated a revision of the classification. Singh and Hauswirth in 1974 (6) and Josephson (7) in a later study have subdivided the drugs into five groups (Table 11-1).

The group I drugs act primarily by decreasing the membrane conductance of sodium (Na^+) (8). Automaticity, therefore, is decreased, since the rate of spontaneous diastolic depolarization (phase 4) is decreased and threshold potential is increased (made less negative). The velocity of phase 0 is slowed and the duration of the effective refractory period is prolonged. Conduction velocity is slowed on these two accounts (Fig. 11-1). Quinidine, procainamide, and disopyramide are similar in their effects with a few exceptions. Quinidine has been shown to shorten the effective refractory period of the AV node and to enhance conduction through that node (9) (Fig. 11-2). Disopyramide has less effect on the AV node than quinidine (10). Group I drugs have the ability to interrupt the reentry circuit because of their effect on conduction velocity. However, group I drugs work equally as well on arrhythmias owing to the automaticity of both the ventricular and supraventricular types (Table 11-2). Problems encountered with the use of quinidine include: (*1*) intolerance due to gastrointestinal reactions (diarrhea, nausea, and vomiting), (*2*) skin eruptions and rash, (*3*) drug fever, and (*4*) visual and aural complaints of cinchonism (12). Procainamide can produce a systemic lupus-like syndrome with long-term administration (12). Complications of the group I drugs include asystole and conduction delays (Table 11-3).

Group II drugs suppress automaticity by depression of spontaneous diastolic depolariza-

Table 11-1. Classification of Antiarrhythmic Drugs

Group	Drugs	Primary Mechanism
Group I	Quinidine Procainamide Disopyramide Antazoline Ajmaline	Increases (lengthens) refractory period and reduces conduction velocity. Decreases rate of spontaneous diastolic depolarization and increases threshold potential.
Group II	Lidocaine Diphenylhydantoin Tocainide Aprindine Mexiletine	Shortens refractory period and increases conduction velocity. Decreases rate of spontaneous diastolic depolarization and increases threshold potential.
Group III	Propranolol Practolol	Antiadrenergic (beta blocking) effect.
Group IV	Bretylium tosylate Amiodarone	Primary action is antiadrenergic effect with little direct membrane effect.
Group V	Verapamil	Primary action is directed toward decreasing the slow inward Ca^{2+} current.

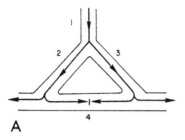

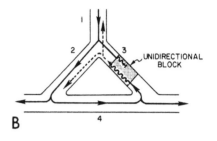

PRODUCTION OF BIDIRECTIONAL BLOCK (GROUP I,Ⅲ,Ⅴ)   ABOLITION OF UNIDIRECTIONAL BLOCK (GROUP Ⅱ)

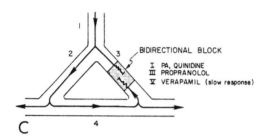

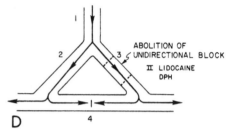

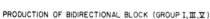

Figure 11-1. The effect of antidysrhythmic drugs on reentry. In (*a*) the normal situation is shown where an impulse traversing the central Purkinje fiber (1) spreads into two branches of the Purkinje fiber (2 and 3) and activates the ventricular tissue (4). In (*b*) a segment showing unidirectional antegrade block and slow retrograde conduction is established in one limb of the Purkinje fiber bifurcation (3) as a result of ischemia or other injury. The impulse descending from the central Purkinje branch finds itself blocked proximally by the area of unidirectional block in the depressed limb (3). It traverses the other limb, branch 2, normally, however, and enters the ventricular tissue (4), producing a normal QRS complex on the surface electrogram. From the ventricular tissue, it may penetrate depressed limb 3 distally and conduct in a retrograde fashion to the bifurcation. As indicated by the interrupted lines, if limb 2 has recovered its excitability, the impulse may reenter this pathway, thereby once more reaching the ventricular tissue resulting in a premature ventricular depolarization, or it may even travel in a retrograde fashion up the central Purkinje (1). Conceivably, not only a reentrant beat, but a reentrant rhythm, can be established by such a circus movement. In (*c*) the reentrant loop is abolished by group I, V (slow response), and perhaps III agents, converting unidirectional to bidirectional block. In (*d*) the conditions required for reentry are eliminated by group II drugs, thereby abolishing unidirectional block. Similar models of reentry can be postulated in atrial, junctional, and anomalous specialized cardiac tissue as well. (Reproduced with permission from Arnsdorf, MF: Electrophysiologic properties of antidysrhythmic drugs as a rational basis for therapy. *Med Clinics N Am* 60:213, 1976.)

tion (phase 4) (13, 14, 15). Diphenylhydantoin and lidocaine neither prolong the refractory (ERP) period nor depress the excitability of atrial or ventricular muscle or the specialized conduction tissue (16, 13, 14, 15) (Fig. 11-1). Diphenylhydantoin produces a marked increase in the rate of rise of phase 0 in Purkinje fibers, especially when action potential (APD) is shortened with diphenylhydantoin, but the effective refractory period is not decreased in proportion, so that the ERP/APD is increased (15) (Fig. 11-3). This effect, combined with the effect on the rate of rise of phase 0, diminishes the chance of impaired conduction and block and thereby reduces the chance of reentrant arrhythmias.

Table 11-2. Clinical Effectiveness of Antidysrhythmic Agents

	Group I		Group II		Group III
	Quinidine	*Procaine Amide*	*DPH*	*Lidocaine*	*Propranolol*
Supraventricular					
Premature atrial contractions	+++	++++	++	+	++
Paroxysmal atrial tachycardia	++	+++	++	+	+++
Atrial flutter	++	+++	+	+	++[a]
Atrial fibrillation					
Conversion	+++	++++	+	+	++[a]
Maintenance	+++	++++	+	+	++
Junctional premature contractions and tachycardia	+++	+++	+	+	+
Ventricular					
Ventricular premature contractions	+++	+++	+++	+++	+++
Tachycardia	++	+++	+++	+++	+++
Digitalis-induced arrhythmias					
Supraventricular and ventricular	++[b]	++[b]	+++	+++	+++[b]

Source: Reproduced with permission from Arnsdorf, MF: Electrophysiological Properties of Antidysrhythmic Drugs as a Rational Basis for Therapy, *The Medical Clinics of North America* (Philadelphia, WB Saunders Co, 1976).

Response: ++++ excellent; +++ good; ++ fair; + poor.

[a]Propranolol effectively decreases the ventricular response to atrial flutter and fibrillation by decreasing conduction through the atrioventricular node.

[b]Although effective in supressing digitalis-induced dysrhythmias, these drugs may in themselves produce conduction problems and combined with their antiautomatic effects may eventuate in atrioventricular dissociation and asystole.

Table 11-3. Bioelectric Complications and Other Selected Undesirable Effects of the Antidysrhythmic Drugs

	Group I Quinidine Procaine Amide	Group II Lidocaine Diphenylhydantoin	Group III Propranolol
Electrocardiography			
PR interval	↑ ↔ ↓	↓ ↔	↔ ↑
QRS duration	↑	↓	↑
QTc	↑	↓	↔ ↓
His Bundle			
Atrial-His time	↓ ↔ ↑ (pts c IVCD)	↔	↔ ↑
His-ventricle time	↔ ↑	↔	↔
Selected undesirable effects			
Cardiac	Ventricular tachycardia Ventricular fibrillation Asystole Pacemaker suppression "Atropine-like" effect	Asystole Pacemaker suppression	Asystole Pacemaker suppression Atrioventricular nodal block May aggravate or produce heart failure
Blood pressure cardiac output	Marked decrease	Some decrease	Marked decrease

Left ventricular and diastolic pressure	May increase	Unchanged or slight increase	May increase
Central nervous system	Quinidine: Cinchonism	Lidocaine: Convulsions, Respiratory arrest, Mental confusion; Diphenylhydantoin: Cerebellar signs, Coma convulsions	
Other	Quinidine: Thrombocytopenia, Hemolysis, Hypersensitivity, Gastrointestinal; Procaine amide: Lupus syndrome, Agranulocytosis, Gastrointestinal	Diphenylhydantoin: Megaloblastic anemia and lymphoma-like syndrome with chronic therapy, Anticoagulants interfere with metabolism	Bronchospasm, May mask symptoms of insulin overdose

Source: Reproduced with permission from Arnsdorf MF: Electrophysiological properties of antidysrhythmic drugs as a rational basis for therapy (*Med Clinics N Am* 60:213, 1976).

↔ = no change; ↑ = increase; ↓ = decrease

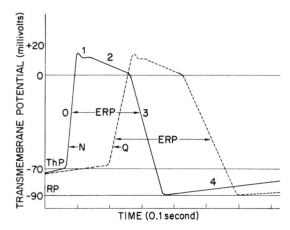

Figure 11-2. Effects of quinidine on transmembrane potential of isolated Purkinje fiber. The solid line (N) depicts the transmembrane potential of a hypothetical spontaneously activation, normal Purkinje fiber in vitro during the phases (0–4) of the cardiac cycle; the dash line (Q) shows its modification by a low concentration of quinidine. Automaticity is suppressed by a decrease in the rate of spontaneous depolarization from the resting potential (RP) during diastole (phase 4) and an increase in the threshold potential (ThP). The rate of depolarization during phase 0 is reduced; the effective refractory period (ERP), action-potential duration (APD), and ERP/APD are increased. At therapeutic concentrations of quinidine in situ, automaticity at ectopic sites would be expected to be completely suppressed; the above pattern would be modified further by the vagal blocking action of quinidine, which would result in an increase in heart rate and other changes. (Reproduced with permission from Goodman LS, Gilman A [eds] : *The Pharmacological Basis of Therapeutics,* 5th edition. Copyright © by Macmillan Publishing Co., Inc., New York.)

Group II drugs, primarily, exert their influence by increasing the membrane conductance of potassium (8). These drugs are relatively ineffective against supraventricular arrhythmias but are effective against ventricular arrhythmias of both the automatic and reentry types (Table 11-2). Tocainide, Mexilentine and Aprindine are lidocaine-like drugs that are currently available on an experimental basis in the United States. Mexiletine (17, 18) can be given orally or intravenously for the treatment of acute and chronic ventricular arrhythmias. Tocainide is similar to Mexiletine; however, it does not appear to have as many side effects (17, 19, 20). Aprindine has been used to suppress both supraventricular and ventricular arrhythmias that do not respond to conventional drug therapy. One must be on the alert for the development of agranulocytosis with the use of this drug (21, 22, 23). Lidocaine toxicity may produce central nervous system manifestations (seizures).

Group III drugs consist entirely of the β-adrenergic blocking agents. Propranolol is the most commonly used beta blocker. Other β-adrenergic blocking agents include: practolol, sotalol, timolol, pindolol, and metoprolol. Currently, metoprolol (Lopressor) is the only one of these β-adrenergic blocking agents available in the United States. Their precise mode of action in the treatment of cardiac arrhythmias remains unclear. Two main effects of beta blocking agents are: (*1*) β-adrenergic blockade (see Chap. 1), and (*2*) membrane-stabilizing activity (24). Propranolol is useful in controlling arrhythmias caused by reentry and increased automaticity (Fig. 11-1). Increased catecholamine levels, which enhance automaticity, are seen in such clinical states as halothane anesthesia,

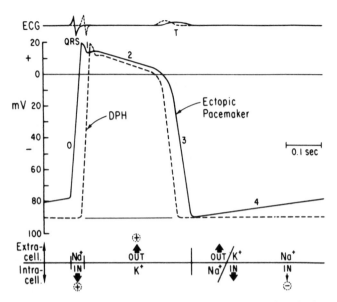

Figure 11-3. Diagrammatic representation of transmembrane electrical potential (middle), electrocardiogram (top), and transmembrane cation movements (bottom) of a spontaneously depolarizing conductive fiber in the atrial, junctional or ventricular myocardium (solid line) and following administration of diphenylhydantoin (DPH: broken line).
Top: QRS wave occurs at time of depolarization and T wave during the final phase of repolarization. Middle: 0 = depolarization; 1, 2, and 3 = phases of repolarization; 4 = resting period exhibiting diastolic depolarization prior to quinidine; mV = millivolts. Bottom: The horizontal line represents the cell membrane; the arrows indicate the transmembrane flux of sodium (Na+) and potassium (K+) ions during depolarization, repolarization, and the resting period. At the onset of the resting period is shown the active exit (↑) of Na+ extracellularly (extracell.), accompanied by active entrance (↓) of K+ intracellularly (intracell.). During the remainder of the resting period, diastolic depolarization takes place with passive Na+ movement into the cell. The sizes of the arrows are directly related to large or small movement of cations. (Reproduced with permission from Dreifus, LS, Likoff W [eds]: *Cardiac Arrhythmias.* Copyright © 1973 by Grune & Stratton, Inc., New York.)

myocardial infarction, and pheochromocytoma. However, beta blocking agents may be effective in treating arrhythmias other than those related to catecholamines. Beta blocking agents may exert their antiarrhythmic effect by their membrane-stabilizing action. This mechanism is referred to as a quinidine-like action and is characterized by a decrease in the rate of rise of the action potential (25). The concentrations of propranolol needed to produce this effect are extremely high; therefore, the main factor in the antiarrhythmic effect of these drugs is beta blockade (26, 27). A decrease in the rate of discharge of the SA node and ectopic pacemakers and an increase in the effective refractory period of the AV node has been demonstrated (28, 29). Propranolol is more effective in the treatment of supraventricular, rather than ventricular, arrhythmias (30). The slowing of atrioventricular conduction by propranolol is effective in the treatment of atrial fibrillation and flutter. The effect that propranolol has on ventricular tachyarrhythmias is variable, unless those arrhythmias are the result of digitalis or catecholamines, which respond

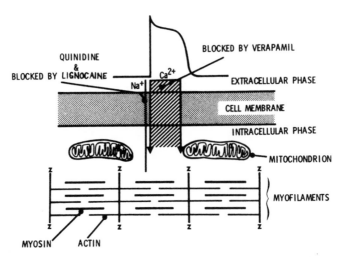

Figure 11-4. Schematic representation of the interaction of quinidine and lignocaine with the inward-flowing Na+ current. This current flows during the rapid depolarization phase of the action potential. Verapamil interacts with the inward Ca^{2+} current. (Reproduced with permission from Krikler DM, Goodwin JF [eds]: *Cardiac Arrhythmias: The Modern Electrophysiologic Approach.* Copyright © 1975 by W. B. Saunders Co., Ltd., London.)

favorably to beta blockade (31). Side effects of propranolol include bronchoconstriction, congestive heart failure, hypotension, AV block, and asystole (32).

Group IV drugs include bretylium tosylate and Amiodarone and act primarily by their antiadrenergic effects (33). Bretylium has been found to increase the electrical ventricular-fibrillation threshold more than lidocaine, procainamide, propranolol, quinidine, or diphenylhydantoin (34). Its primary use has been for the treatment of ventricular arrhythmias refractory to most forms of therapy. It has the unique advantages of augmenting myocardial contractility and increasing automaticity and conduction velocity. These actions would make bretylium tosylate even more valuable in treating patients with heart failure and/or heart block (35, 36, 37). Bretylium is available only in the parenteral form and side effects include postural hypotension, diarrhea, nausea, and vomiting (38). Amiodarone is not available in the United States.

The group-V category consists of verapamil. This drug blocks the slow inward calcium current (Fig. 11-4), thereby decreasing conduction velocity in depolarized tissue (8). Reentrant circuits, dependent on the slow response, are thought to be interrupted with verapamil (Fig. 11-1). It has been effective against both supraventricular and ventricular arrhythmias and is currently available on an experimental basis in the United States.

DIGITALIS

Digitalis is the drug of choice in the treatment of heart failure, and it has several additional uses as an antiarrhythmic agent. The resting membrane potential is reduced (made less negative) by digitalis, causing an increased excitability of the atrial and ventricular specialized conduction fibers (39). The rate of rise of phase 0 is reduced, which in turn prolongs depolarization and depresses conduction (40). Spontaneous diastolic depolariza-

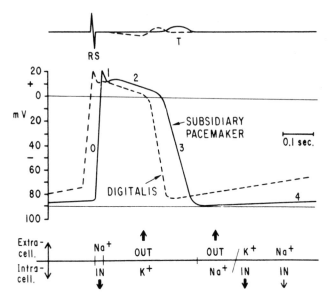

Figure 11-5. Diagrammatic representation of the transmembrane electrical potential (middle panel), unipolar electrocardiogram (top panel), and transmembrane cation movements (bottom panel) of a spontaneously depolarizing conductive fiber in the atrial or ventricular myocardium (solid line) and after administration of digitalis (broken line). The effects of digitalis on ST segment depression and QT interval shortening are shown by the broken line in the top panel. Upper panel: RS wave occurs at time of depolarization and T wave during the final phase of repolarization. Middle panel: 0 = depolarization; 1, 2, and 3 = phases of repolarization; 4 = resting period exhibiting diastolic depolarization before administration of quinidine; mV = millivolts. Bottom panel: the horizontal line represents the cell membrane; the arrows indicate the transmembrane flux of sodium (Na+) and potassium (K+) ions during depolarization, repolarization, and resting period. At the onset of the resting period is shown the active exit (↑) of Na+ extracellularly (extracell.), accompanied by active entrance (↓) of K+ intracellularly (intracell.); during the remainder of the resting period, diastolic depolarization takes place with passive Na+ movement into the cell. The sizes of the arrows are directly related to large or small movement of cations. (Reproduced with permission from Mason DT et al: Current concepts and treatment of digitalis toxicity. *Am J Cardiol* 27:546, 1971.)

tion (phase 4) is enhanced, resulting in an increase in automaticity (39) (Fig. 11-5). The fact that the refractory period of the AV node is prolonged is the major way of slowing the ventricular response in atrial fibrillation and flutter. This prolongation of the AV nodal refractory time is evident on the electrocardiogram as a prolonged PR interval. In contrast to this, the refractory period of the atrial and ventricular myocardium is shortened by digitalis (40) and results in a shortened QT interval.

Digitalis has a positive inotropic effect, which is most likely brought about through the inhibition of the enzyme ATPase (adenosine triphosphatase). The main energy source for the regulation of intracellular sodium and potassium is adenosine triphosphate (ATP). The enzyme ATPase is involved in the breakdown of ATP, and digitalis inhibits ATPase and results in an increased intracellular sodium and decreased potassium concentration (41).

Digitalis may be used in the treatment of reentrant arrhythmias since intra-atrial conduction is enhanced, thereby interrupting the reentry circuit.

As many as 20% of all patients receiving digitalis will experience digitalis toxicity (42). Disorders of the gastrointestinal tract (nausea, vomiting, anorexia) are the most common side effects; however, digitalis is also capable of producing any kind of arrhythmia. Digitalis intoxication may be precipitated by hypokalemia, hypercalcemia, hypoxia, and catecholamines (43). Recently, it was found that the administration of quinidine increased the serum digoxin level in the first few days after it was administered (44, 45).

REVIEW QUESTIONS

1. What are the differences and similarities between class I drugs and class II drugs?
2. Explain the effects of beta blockade with propranolol. Why is this drug contraindicated in patients with congestive heart failure?
3. How does diphenylhydantoin alter the action potential curve? Why is this drug effective in the treatment of digitalis-induced arrhythmias?

REFERENCES

1. Hoffman BF, Rosen MR, Wit AL: Electrophysiology and pharmacology of cardiac arrhythmias. III. The causes and treatment of cardiac arrhythmias. Part A *Am Heart J* 89:115, 1975.
2. Coltart J: Anti-arrhythmic therapy: physiological basis and practical methods, in Krikler DM, Goodwin JF (ed): *Cardiac Arrhythmias: The Modern Electrophysiological Approach*. London, WB Saunders Co Ltd, 1975, p 224.
3. Hoffman BF, Bigger JT: Antiarrhythmic drugs, in DiPalma JR (ed): *Drill's Pharmacology in Medicine*, ed 4. New York, McGraw-Hill Book Co, 1971, p 824.
4. Baughn Williams EM: Classification of antiarrhythmic drugs, in Sandøe E, Flensted-Jensen E, Olesen KH (ed): *Symposium on Cardiac Arrhythmias*. Sweden, Astra, 1977, p 449.
5. Singh BN, Vaughn Williams EM: Fourth class of antidysrythmic action? Effect of verapamil on ouabain toxicity, on atrial and ventricular intracellular potentials and on other features of cardiac function. *Cardiovasc Res* 6:109, 1972.
6. Singh BN, Hauswirth O: Comparative mechanisms of action of antiarrhythmic drugs. *Am Heart J* 87:367, 1974.
7. Josephson ME: Update of quinidine, procainamide, disopyramide, and verapmil. *Hosp Formulary* 42:896, 1978.
8. Arnsdorf MF: Electrophysiological properties of antidysrhythmic drugs as a rational basis for therapy, in Resnekov L (ed): *The Medical Clinics of North America*. Philadelphia, WB Saunders Co, 1976, p 213.
9. Freedman DD, Goldschlager N: The electrocardiology of quinidine. *Practical Cardiol* 5:27, 1978.
10. Mathur P: Cardiovascular effects of a new antiarrhythmic agent, disopyramide phosphate. *Am Heart J* 84:764, 1972.
11. Bassett AL, Hoffman BF: Antiarrhythmic drugs: electrophysiological actions, in Elliott HW, Okun R, Dreisbach RH (ed): *Ann Rev Pharmacol* vol II, Palo Alto, Calif, Annual Reviews Inc, 1971, p 143.
12. White BB: Antiarrhythmic therapeutic agents, in *Therapy in Acute Coronary Care*. Chicago, Year Book Medical Pub Inc, 1971, p 67.
13. Helfant RH, Lau SH, et al: Effects of diphenylhydantoin on atrioventricular conduction in man. *Circulation* 36:686, 1967.
14. Rosati R, Alexander JA, et al: Influence of diphenylhydantoin on electrophysiological properties of the canine heart. *Circ Res* 21:757, 1967.

15. Bigger T, Bassett AL, Hoffman BF: Electrophysiological effects of diphenylhydantoin on canine Purkinje fibers. *Circ Res* 22:221, 1968.

16. Bigger JT Jr, Heissenbuttel RH: The use of procaine amide and lidocaine in the treatment of cardiac arrhythmias. *Progr Cardiovasc Dis* 11:515, 1969.

17. Morgan J, Kupersmith J: Pharmacology and clinical use of newer antiarrhythmic agents. *Practical Cardiol* 5:89, 1979.

18. Danilo P Jr: Mexiletine. *Am Heart J* 97:399, 1979.

19. Danilo P Jr: Tocainide. *Am Heart J* 97:259, 1979.

20. Engler R, Ryan W et al: Assessment of long-term antiarrhythmic therapy: studies on the long-term efficacy and toxicity of Tocainide. *Am J Cardiol* 43:612, 1979.

21. Zipes DP, Gaum EW et al: Aprinidine for treatment of supraventricular tachycardias with particular application to Wolff-Parkinson-White syndrome. *Am J Cardiol* 40:586, 1977.

22. Fasola AF, Noble RJ, Zipes DP: Treatment of recurrent ventricular tachycardia and fibrillation with aprinidine. *Am J Cardiol* 39:903, 1977.

23. Van Leeuwen R, Meyboom RHB: Agranulocytosis and aprindine. *Lancet* 2:1137, 1976.

24. Frishman W, Silverman R: Clinical pharmacology the new beta-adrenergic blocking drugs. Part 2. Physiologic and metabolic effects. *Am Heart J* 97:797, 1979.

25. Levy JV, Richards V: Inotropic and chronotropic effects of a series of β-adrenergic blocking drugs: some structure activity relationships. *Proc Soc Exp Biol Med* 122:373, 1966.

26. Coltart DJ, Gibson DG, Shand DG: Plasma propranolol levels associated with supression of ventricular ectopic beats. *Br Med J* 1:490, 1971.

27. Shand DG: Pharmacokinetic properties of beta-adrenergic blocking drugs. *Drugs* 7:39, 1974.

28. Smithen CS, Balcon R, Sowton E: Use of bundle of His potentials to assess changes in atrioventricular conduction produced by a series of beta-adrenergic blocking agents. *Br Heart J* 33:955, 1971.

29. Seides SF, Josephson ME et al: The electrophysiology of propranolol in man. *Am Heart J* 88:733, 1974.

30. Frishman W. Silverman R: Clinical pharmacology of the new beta-adrenergic blocking drugs. Part 3. Comparative clinical experience and new therapeutic applications. *Am Heart J* 98:119, 1979.

31. Ahlquist RP: Present state of alpha and beta adrenergic drugs III. Beta blocking agents. *Am Heart J* 93:117, 1977.

32. Winkel RA, Harrison DC: Beta blockers in the treatment of acute arrhythmias. *Heart Lung* 6:62, 1977.

33. Koch-Weser J: Bretylium. *N Engl J Med* 300:473, 1979.

34. Bacaner M: Quantitative comparison of bretylium with other antifibrillatory drugs. *Am J Cardiol* 21:504, 1968.

35. Amsterdam EA, Spann JF et al: Characterization of the positive effect of bretylium tosylate, a unique property of antiarrhythmic agent (abstr). *Am J Cardiol* 25:81, 1970.

36. Wit AL, Steiner C, Damato AM: Microelectrode studies in the effects of bretylium tosylate on Purkinje fibers and ventricular muscle (abstr). *Circulation* 60(Suppl 3): 217, 1969.

37. Watanabe Y, Josipovic V, Dreifus LS: Electrophysiological mechanisms of bretylium tosylate (abstr). *Circulation* 38(Suppl 6):202, 1968.

38. Day HW, Bacaner M: Use of bretylium tosylate in the management of acute myocardial infarction. *Am J Cardiol* 27:177, 1977.

39. Wollenberger A, Halle W: Action of cardiac glycosides on automaticity and contractile activity in single cardiac muscle cells grown in vitro. *Proc First Int Pharmacol Meeting*, vol 3, Oxford, Pergamon, 1963, p 87.

40. Moe GK, Mendez R: The action of several cardiac glycosides on conduction velocity and ventricular excitability in dog heart. *Circulation* 4:729, 1951.

41. Cooksey JD, Dunn M, Massie E: Digitalis antiarrhythmic drugs and electrolyte imbalance, in *Clinical Vectorcardiography and Electrocardiography*. Chicago, Year Book Medical Pub Inc, 1977, p 621.

42. Fisch C, Knoebel SB: Recognition and therapy of digitalis toxicity. *Progr Cardiovasc Dis* 13:71, 1970.

43. Mason DT, Zelis R, et al: Current concepts and treatment of digitalis toxicity. *Am J Cardiol* 27:546, 1971.

44. Leahey EB Jr, Reiffel JA, et al: A drug interaction between quinidine and digoxin. *JAMA* 240: 533, 1978.

45. Leahey EB Jr, Reiffel JA, et al: Enhanced cardiac effect of digoxin during quinidine treatment. *Arch Intern Med* 139:519, 1979.

12
Electrolyte Imbalance and Arrhythmias

Cellular activity of the body is optimal when the fluid and electrolytes within and around the cells remain relatively constant in composition and volume. This optimal environment is maintained despite the fact that variations do occur in body-fluid intake and output. Within this text it is appropriate not to consider the various regulatory mechanisms of the body that ensure the constancy of body fluids and electrolytes but rather to consider the effects electrolyte imbalance may have upon the heart. In this chapter, only the electrolytes that have a major effect upon cardiac activity will be considered, namely, potassium, calcium, magnesium, and sodium. Electrolytes in general are implicated in four physiological functions of the body: maintenance of body-water distribution, osmotic pressure, acid-base balance, and neuromuscular irritability. Imbalance of electrolyte levels may thus disturb the environment of body function.

POTASSIUM

The normal serum potassium range is 3.5 to 5.0 mEq/liter (1). Changes in one or the other direction of the range may or may not be associated with electrocardiographic changes, and thus other parameters must be observed. The body store of potassium in an average adult male weighing 70 kg is approximately 3500 mEq. Most of the potassium is contained within the cells, whereas less than 2% may be found extracellularly. The heart is very sensitive to variations in potassium levels (2).

Hyperkalemia

Hyperkalemia, according to Cohen (3), may be defined as a serum potassium concentration in excess of 5.5 mEq/liter. The most common conditions leading to potassium excess are renal failure, diabetes mellitus, tissue destruction, tranfusion by large amounts of bank blood, high doses of penicillin, therapy with diuretic drugs such as spironolactone, and excessive dietary intake of potassium-containing foods in the presence of poorly functioning kidneys (4). Therefore the nurse and the other members of the health team should counsel the patient with a compromised renal system to avoid foods high in potassium. Robinson (5) identifies the potassium content, in milligrams per 100 grams, of some of the most common foodstuffs of the American diet:

Bacon (Canadian)	432
Banana	320
Beans (lima)	612
Bran	1070
Bread (whole wheat)	273
Chili powder	1000
Cocoa	1522
Coffee (instant)	3256
Milk (dry, nonfat)	1725
Molasses (blackstrap)	2927
Orange juice (fresh)	200
Potato chips	1130
Potatoes (French fried)	853
Tea	4530
Wheat	1121

Hyperkalemia can occur from a considerably small increase in body potassium. The level of potassium is maintained primarily by renal excretion. Therefore hyperkalemia is most likely due to the impairment of renal excretory mechanisms or an alteration of the factors maintaining the normal transcellular gradient of potassium (3).

Action on the Cardiac Cell

Hyperkalemia has a direct effect upon the action potential of the cardiac cell (3, 6) by decreasing the resting-membrane potential as well as the rate of rise of phase 0 of the action-potential curve (Fig. 12-1). This produces a slowing of the intraventricular conduction. A widening of the QRS complex can produce disturbance in the transmission of impulse at various levels of the specialized conduction tissue. Therefore the sinoatrial, atrioventricular, and intraventricular conduction tissue may be affected by hyperkalemia (7). The tall, peaked T waves result from changes that occur in the downslope of the action potential curve or an alteration of the repolarization process. Changes on the electrocardiogram may not become evident with serum potassium levels of 6 mEq/liter (8). Beyond this level, gradations of effects may become manifest. A symmetrically tall T wave is the earliest electrocardiographic change associated with hyperkalemia. Fowler (8, 9) describes the most hyperkalemic progressive changes—widening of the QRS complex, prolongation of the PR interval, and depression of atrial activity—with levels of serum potassium above 7 mEq/liter. At very high levels, ventricular conduction time increases enough to produce merging of the QRS complex with the elevated T wave. Cardiac standstill may then ensue. This last event is a result of the very high levels of potassium that impede sodium and calcium influx into the cardiac cell, an essential factor for repolarization (2). The excitability, conduction, and rhythm of cardiac muscle are affected by changes in levels of extracellular potassium (1).

Clinical features include weakness, hypotension, impaired cerebral function secondary to extreme bradycardia resulting from dysfunction of sinoatrial activity (5, 10), paresthesias of the scalp and face, weakness and numbness of the arms and legs, flaccid paralysis, abdominal distention, and diarrhea.

Therapy

When hyperkalemia occurs suddenly—as may be found with metabolic acidosis, acute renal failure, or intravenous infusion of potassium—and rhythm disturbances are evident,

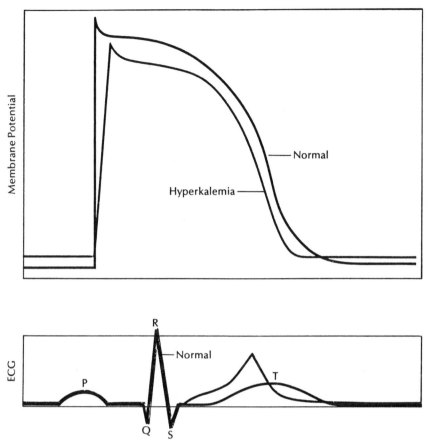

Figure 12-1. Effects of hyperkalemia on action potential in cardiac muscle cell include slowing of action potential and reduction in its amplitude; since repolarization is accelerated, duration of potential is also reduced. Initial effect on ECG is usually peaking of T wave as shown. More severe effects include widening of QRS and lengthening of PR interval. (By A Miller from Cohen JJ. Disorders of potassium imbalance. *Hosp Practice* 14:1, 1979. Reproduced with permission.)

emergency treatment is directed toward the restoration of normal transcellular distribution (7). This can be accomplished by the administration of calcium or sodium, by transporting potassium into the cell with solutions of glucose and insulin, by alkalinizing the extracellular fluid with sodium bicarbonate, and/or by the removal of potassium from the body. Potassium removal may be accomplished by the use of diuretics, by hemodialysis or peritoneal dialysis, or by cation resin exchange. Sodium bicarbonate rapidly diminishes the level of potassium, whereas calcium acts as a potassium antagonist.

Hypokalemia

Normally losses of excess potassium ions occur as a result of the regulatory function of the distal renal tubule, which senses the need for excretion or retention of potassium. In addition, at the distal tubule in the presence of aldosterone there is an ionic exchange of sodium for potassium. A greater-than-normal potassium intake stimulates the aldosterone mechanism, resulting in greater excretion of potassium. Other normal losses are through the gastrointestinal system and sweat loss.

The most common causes of potassium depletion are related to inadequate intake, such as may occur in anorexia nervosa; loss secondary to renal contribution, as may be associated with primary aldosteronism; heavy ingestion of licorice; diuretic therapy; chronic interstitial nephritis; gastrointestinal losses due to diarrhea, vomiting, and fistulae; losses due to intracellular shifts of potassium under conditions in which the pH level may be altered, as is associated with alkalosis. In this situation, potassium moves into the cell as the hydrogen ions move into the extracellular space to neutralize the effects of alkalosis. The transference maintains electrical neutrality. A rather interesting aspect related to licorice ingestion is that the main ingredient of licorice is glycyrrhizic acid, a potent mineralocorticoid-like substance. Ingestion of products containing licorice as a base can result in stimulation of pseudoaldosteronism and subsequent hypokalemia (11). In old persons, inactivity can lead to cellular breakdown and subsequent potassium loss (12). The significance of hypokalemia lies in its effect on the heart, on metabolic function, and on neuromuscular and renal function. In the patient taking digitalis, hypokalemia can potentiate the action of digitalis. According to Cohen (7), a plausible explanation for a greater propensity toward digitalis intoxication in the presence of a low potassium level may be related to the intracellular and extracellular transference of potassium.

Clinical Manifestations
An extremely low potassium level diminishes neuromuscular activity (1, 5). Therefore the patient may have a paralytic ileus as a result of diminished motility and/or propulsive action of the intestinal tract (11). Muscular weakness and diminished deep tendon reflexes are early manifestations that initially involve the limb muscles and later the muscles of the trunk and respiratory system (7). In addition, disorientation, confusion, and memory impairment may result from a low potassium level.

Electrocardiographic Features
Fowler (8) describes the difficulties in identifying electrocardiographic changes associated with hypokalemia in the presence of sinus tachycardia with rates above 120 beats per minute; when there is evidence of bundle branch block and left ventricular hypertrophy; and during digitalis therapy as well as hypoxic states. With levels of serum potassium slightly below 3 mEq/liter, only a small number of persons may have electrocardiographic changes; whereas in the presence of potassium levels below 2 mEq/liter, more than 80% of subjects do have associated electrocardiographic changes. The most frequently observed changes are related to a shortening of the plateau phase 2 and a lengthening of phase 3 of the action potential (Fig. 12-2). This results in a shortening and depression of the ST segment, in low amplitude or diphasic T waves, and in the appearance of U waves (7). McGurn (2) hypothesizes that the U wave is due to attempts at retrograde depolarization. As the U wave becomes prominent and there is flattening of the T wave, the pattern may simulate a prolonged QT interval. However, upon analysis of the wave form, there actually is a QU interval (11). Dysrhythmias commonly associated with hypokalemia are premature atrial and ventricular beats, reflecting irritability. The influx of intracellular sodium with diminished potassium content may account for the increased irritability of cardiac muscle (2). The incidence of cardiac irritability is enhanced when the patient is receiving digitalis, since digitalis tends to force potassium out of the intracellular into the extracellular compartment, where it may be excreted by the kidney (12).

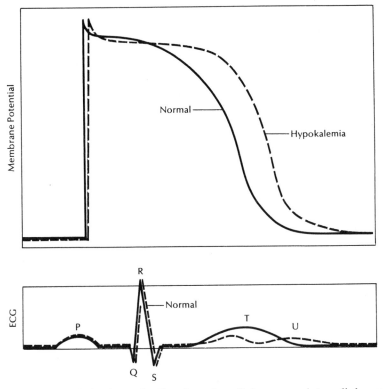

Figure 12-2. In hypokalemia, reduction in extracellular versus intracellular concentration of potassium widens the differential between the resting membrane potential and the excitation potential (top), impeding impulse formation and propagation. Slowed rate of repolarization apparent in the ECG can set the stage for asynchrony and arrhythmias. (By A. Miller from Cohen JJ. Disorders of potassium imbalance. *Hosp Practice* 14:1, 1979. Reproduced with permission.)

Therapy

Therapy for depleted stores of potassium is directed toward the correction of the underlying cause. If the condition is due to the use of diuretics for the management of cardiac edema and/or systemic hypertension, potassium supplements are usually prescribed.

CALCIUM

The role of calcium is varied. Without the calcium ion, the excitation-coupling mechanism for cardiac contraction would not occur. (See Chap. 2 for further discussion of cardiac muscle contraction.) In addition to cardiac activity, calcium plays a role in providing a framework for bones and teeth; is an essential factor for normal blood clotting; is essential for neuromuscular irritability; maintains integrity of the cell membrane; and has enzymatic properties. Body calcium requirements vary according to need. Normally the dietary intake of calcium is absorbed by the jejunum in the presence of a vitamin D complex. The absorbed calcium is transported in the blood to storage sites in the skeletal parts of the body (13). The normal serum calcium level is 9 to 11 mg/100 ml (14).

Changes in the level of calcium may result in hypercalcemia or hypocalcemia. One of the mechanisms involved in maintaining normal calcium levels is the feedback mechanism between calcium and the parathyroid gland. As serum calcium decreases, parathyroid hormone secretion increases, which in turn stimulates the gastrointestinal mucosa to absorb a larger quantity of calcium. The parathyroid hormone likewise promotes renal tubular reabsorption of calcium. Both parathyroid hormone and vitamin D cause removal of calcium from bone. Calcitonin, the thyroid hormone secretion, also maintains a regulatory function on the calcium level by decreasing its rate of removal from bone (14).

Hypocalcemia

Calcium levels can be decreased in a variety of settings: after a parathyroidectomy or a total thyroidectomy; during necrotizing pancreatitis; with chronic renal insufficiency; with hypoalbuminemia; after prolonged continuous suctioning; during shock states; and with multiple transfusions of large amounts of citrated blood. It may also occur as a sequel to the malabsorption syndrome and to antibiotic therapy with mithramycin (13). During pancreatitis, enzymes are released that eventually cause formation of free fatty acids. The acids combine with serum ionizable calcium to form soaps. This condition ultimately leads to the lowering of serum calcium (14). Approximately 50% of serum calcium is bound to serum albumin. Conditions associated with hypoalbuminemia, therefore, are indirectly implicated in the genesis of hypocalcemia. During shock states associated with hypoperfusion, calcium shifts into the cell with sodium, creating a deficit in the extracellular compartment. The pH of the blood has a direct bearing on calcium. During an alkalotic state, calcium ionizes poorly, whereas in acidosis an increase in the ionization of calcium occurs. With decreased levels of calcium, cellular membrane pore gates remain open, thus accounting for the increased cellular permeability. As a consequence, there is greater stimulation of the central and peripheral nervous system. In patients who are on digitalis, and who may be receiving repeated transfusion for other conditions, the hypocalcemia associated with the transfusions may reduce the effect of digitalis, and therefore the patient should be observed for signs of cardiac decompensation.

Clinical Manifestations

As a result of the hyperactivation of the nervous system, rapid contractions occur both in skeletal and smooth muscle. There is likewise some pain associated with the rapidly contracting muscle. Hence the person may experience muscle and abdominal cramps or tetanic convulsions. Laryngospasm may occur, and accounts for the deaths attributable to hypocalcemia. Other clinical features associated with hypocalcemia are stridor, dyspnea, tingling of distal phalanges, and/or carpopedal spasm (16). Several simple tests that may be done at the bedside of the patient to identify the presence of hypocalcemia are the Trousseau and Chvostek tests. In the former, Tripp (15, 16) suggests that a blood pressure cuff be applied and inflated slightly higher than the systolic value. After a period of time, if the test is positive for tetany, carpal spasm with contraction primarily of the thumb and fingers and loss of ability to open the hand will be observed. Chvostek's test is done for the detection of hyperexcitability of muscles. By tapping on the facial nerve just anterior to the ear, the muscles at the angle of the mouth on the same side will contract if the test is positive for hyperexcitabilitly as associated with hvpocalcemia (15).

Electrocardiographic Features

Increased irritability of cardiac muscle can predispose the heart to ectopic rhythm (14). During states of hypocalcemia, usually beginning with levels below 7 to 8 mg, the plateau phase of the action membrane is prolonged but the downslope of the curve is not affected. This results in prolongation of the ST segment and subsequent QT interval (17, 18).

Therapy

In acute situations, calcium chloride and/or calcium gluconate may be given. However, after the acute state, therapy is directed to a correction of the underlying cause for hypocalcemia.

Hypercalcemia

Hypercalcemia may be due to various pathophysiologic states. However, the two principal causes are malignancy and hyperparathyroidism (19). Other conditions associated with hypercalcemia are prolonged immobilization, renal failure, diuretic therapy, and/or serum phosphate depletion. In regard to cellular membrane permeability, an excess in calcium ions may block the entrance of sodium into the cell. Normally, it is thought that calcium lining the cell membrane acts as portal of entry for the sodium ion. Diuretic therapy, especially the thiazines, may at times cause increases in serum calcium. One of the factors contributing to the hypercalcemia is an increase in the proportion of albumin-bound calcium, which may be attributed to saline diuresis and to the failure of the kidney to excrete calcium. Depletion of serum phosphate secondary to frequent ingestion of aluminum hydroxide may induce hypercalcemia. The mechanism involved is thought to be due to the increased availability of calcium for absorption from the intestinal tract as well as from bone in the presence of hypophosphatemia (20).

Clinical Manifestations

Since many organ systems are affected by elevated levels of serum calcium, the signs and symptoms vary. Symptoms of gastrointestinal system involvement are nausea, vomiting, anorexia, and atony of the gastrointestinal tract. Symptoms associated with central nervous system involvement are drowsiness, depression, apathy, syncope, hallucinations, and in extreme cases, coma. Renal function may become impaired, as evidenced by polyuria and polydipsia, which reflect a loss of concentrating power. Renal calculi can also occur (16). Since a consequence of hypercalcemia is decreased muscular contractility, resulting from blockage of sodium entrance sites, hypercalcemia may shorten mechanical and electrical systole (13, 1). The plateau phase is shortened, the QT interval is shortened, and heart block can occur. Hypercalcemia, through its action on mechanical systole, may enhance the effect of digitalis.

Therapy

Therapy involves the elimination of calcium ions. This may be accomplished through the use of diuretics such as furosemide (Lasix) or ethacrynic acid (Edecrine); adequate hydration; an assessment of the voiding pattern; frequent changes of the position of the bedridden patient to prevent stasis of urine, which generally occurs in the supine position; and chelating (binding) agents which form complexes with calcium that had not been reabsorbed by the renal tubules.

MAGNESIUM

Cardiac homeostasis is maintained in the presence of magnesium (21). It is thought to influence adenosine triphosphate breakdown in providing the energy for movement of actin toward the middle of the myosin filament. Another area of the cation involvement is in the glycogenesis of cardiac muscle fibers (1). The normal serum magnesium concentration is 1.5 to 2.5 mEq/liter. About 35% of magnesium is bound to protein. A high concentration of magnesium is found in cardiac muscle.

Hypermagnesium may occur in the presence of renal insufficiency and after ingestion of antacids such as Maalox and Gelusil, which contain the absorbable form of the cation (2). Hypomagnesemia is usually the result of excessive diuretic therapy. It can also be found in diabetic acidosis, chronic alcoholism, malnutrition, and excessive gastrointestinal suctioning as well as sometimes after parathyroidectomy (21, 13).

Clinical Manifestations

Features associated with hypomagnesemia are related to hyperirritability of the nervous system. Thus it is not unusual to observe jerking and coarse and asterixis-like movements of the hands of the individual. Disorientation and seizures may also occur, as can tetany, hypertension, tachycardia, and changes in vasomotion. Since hypermagnesemia causes depression of the nervous system, it is not unusual to note diminished levels of excitability as well as confusion. Hypotension occurs secondary to the vasodilatory effect of the vessels brought about by blocking of sympathetic nerve fibers (13). Muscle weakness is a common finding, and if severe, can lead to the death of the person as a result of decreased ventilatory capabilities.

Electrocardiographic Features

The electrocardiographic changes associated with early magnesium deficiency, consist of a tall, peaked T wave and a normal QT interval. The T wave differs somewhat from that reflective of hyperkalemia in that it is not as narrow as is seen with potassium excess. A prolonged state of magnesium deficiency results in a prolongation of the PR interval, a widening of the QRS complex, depression of the ST segment, and decreased voltage of the T wave (21, 22, 6). The majority of electrocardiographic changes have been associated with hypermagnesemia. With elevated levels of magnesium, a cardioinhibitory effect occurs, both PR interval and QRS duration are prolonged, third-degree heart block may become evident; and terminally, cardiac arrest ensues as the level of serum magnesium increases (13, 23).

Therapy

A deficit in the magnesium concentration in the body requires replacement therapy by intravenous fluids containing magnesium. A hypermagnesemic state may require restoration of renal function by hemodialysis. Calcium, a magnesium antagonist, may likewise be given (1).

SODIUM

Although sodium disturbances are not reflected electrocardiographically, the ion may be viewed as "friend" and/or "foe." In the absence of sodium, the excitation-contraction coupling mechanism is impaired, whereas in the presence of an elevated serum sodium level, the electrolyte precipitates the formation of edema (29, 25). Sodium is the major cation of the extracellular fluid and is essential for the maintenance of osmotic pressure and water balance. It maintains a regulatory effect on the intracellular and extracellular electrolyte composition (5).

Hyponatremia; Hypernatremia

Losses of sodium occur in association with excessive diuretic therapy, from gastrointestinal sources, with adrenocortical hormone deficiency, and/or in conjunction with

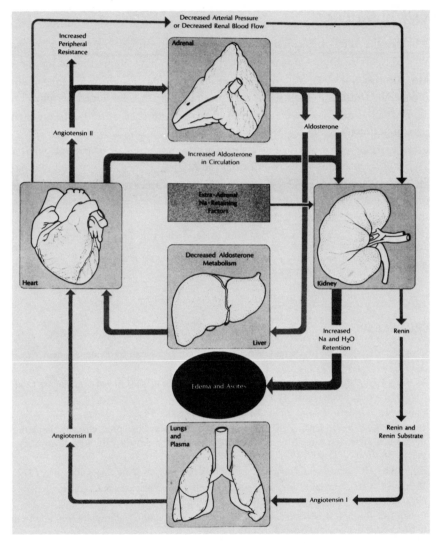

Figure 12-3. This schematic representation of factors leading to salt and water retention in congestive failure is arranged with the starting point at the cardiac defect that results in decreased renal perfusion pressure and renal plasma flow. This triggers renin release and activates the angiotensin-aldosterone system. In addition to direct effects on the kidney, alterations are present in circulatory dynamics in the liver and the periphery. The role of extraadrenal Na-retaining factors is also indicated. (Reproduced with permission from Davis JO, Braunwald E [ed]. Mechanisms of salt and water retention in cardiac failure, in *The Myocardium: Failure and Infarction.* New York, HP Pub Co Inc, 1974.) (See text on next page.)

excessive perspiration (5). Serum sodium gain usually is a result of water loss without concomitant loss of sodium (hypernatremia). Excessive intake of sodium-containing foodstuffs may contribute to an increase in total serum sodium. Increases in sodium content likewise occur as a consequence of cardiac and/or renal failure and may enhance the occurrence of edema (25) (Fig. 12-3).

REVIEW QUESTIONS

1. What is the role of magnesium in the excitation-contraction coupling mechanism?
2. What effect do hypokalemia and hyperkalemia have upon the action potential?
3. Mrs. Minton, a 48-year-old college professor, sustained a right ventricular myocardial infarction. During the course of her hospital stay, she developed peripheral edema.
   a. What physical forces were involved in the transference of fluid into the interstitial compartment?
   b. In carrying out a physical assessment in the nonambulatory patient, what area of the body is usually reflective of fluid retention?
4. Mr. Jones has just received a dose of Lasix. In the process of diuresis what electrolyte predominantly is lost to the body? What clinical manifestations usually accompany the deficiency of such an electrolyte?
5. How does the T wave of hyperkalemia differ from the T wave associated with hypermagnesemia?
6. What are the clinical manifestations of each?

REFERENCES

1. Trunkey DD: Review of current concepts in fluid and electrolyte management. *Heart Lung* 4:117, 1975.
2. McGurn WC: Cardiac effects of electrolyte disturbance, in Kintzel (ed): *Advanced Concepts in Clinical Nursing*. Philadelphia, JB Lippincott Co, 1977, p 332.
3. Cohen JJ: Disorders of potassium imbalance. *Hosp Practice* 14:124, 1979.
4. Chawla KK, Cruz J, Kramer NE, Towne WD: Electrocardiographic changes simulating acute myocardial infarction caused by hyperkalemia: report of a patient with normal coronary arteriograms. *Am Heart J* 95:637, 1978.
5. Robinson CH: *Normal and Therapeutic Nutrition,* ed 14. New York, Macmillan Inc, 1972, p 670.
6. Blomquist CG: Principles of electrocardiography, in Willerson and Sanders (eds): *Clinical Cardiology*. New York, Grune & Stratton Inc, 197, p 325.
7. Cohen HC, Rosen KM, Pick A: Disorders of impulse conduction and impulse formation caused by hyperkalemia in man. *Am Heart J* 89:501, 1975.
8. Fowler NO: *Cardiac Diagnosis and Treatment,* ed 2. Hagerstown, Md, Harper & Row Pub Inc, 1976, p 1023.
9. Rushmer RF: *Cardiovascular Dynamics,* ed 3. Philadelphia, WB Saunders Co, 1970, p 414.
10. Kee JL: The critically ill patient and possible fluid and electrolyte imbalances. *Nursing 72* 2:10, 1972.
11. Johnston JM, Kem DC: Differential diagnosis of hypokalemia. *Practical Cardiol* 3:21, 1977.
12. Kee JL: Fluid imbalance in elderly patients. *Nursing 73* 73:37, 1973.
13. Bergersen BS: *Pharmacology in Nursing.* St. Louis, CV Mosby Co, 1976, p 421.

14. Corday E, Irving DW: *Disturbances of Heart Rate, Rhythm and Conduction.* Philadelphia, WB Saunders Co, 1962, p 272.

15. Tripp A: Hyper and hypocalcemia. *Am J Nursing* 76:1143, 1976.

16. Recker RR, Saville PD: Hypercalcemia and hypocalcemia in clinical practice. *Hosp Med* 15:82, 1979.

17. Fowler NO: *Cardiac Diagnosis and Treatment,* ed 2. Hagerstown, Md, Harper & Row Pub Inc, 1976, p 1128.

18. Blomquist CG: Principles of electrocardiography, in Willerson and Sanders (eds): *Clinical Cardiology.* New York, Grune & Stratton Inc, 1977, p 362.

19. Dailey GW, Deffos LJ: Differential diagnosis of hypercalcemia. *Hosp Med* 11:30, 1975.

20. Nugent CA: Answers to questions on the differential diagnosis of hypercalcemia. *Hosp Med* 14:106, 1978.

21. Burch GE, Giles TD: The importance of magnesium deficiency in cardiovascular disease. *Am Heart J* 94:649, 1977.

22. Fowler NO: *Cardiac Diagnosis and Treatment,* ed 2. Hagerstown, Md, Harper & Row Pub Inc, 1976, p 1028.

23. Crouch JE, McClintic JR: *Human Anatomy and Physiology.* New York, John Wiley & Sons Inc, 1971, p 319.

24. Berne RM, Levy MN: *Cardiovascular Physiology.* St. Louis, CV Mosby Co, 1977, p 30.

25. Davis JO: Mechanisms of salt and water retention in cardiac failure, in Braunwald (ed): *The Myocardium: Failure and Infarction.* New York, HP Pub Co Inc, 1975, p 80.

13
Miscellaneous Electrocardiographic Changes

PERICARDITIS

The pericardium, unlike the myocardium, does not produce electrical activity that can be detected by the conventional electrocardiogram. Abnormalities of the electrocardiogram can develop, however, when the pericardium becomes diseased. The typical ECG finding in acute pericarditis is diffuse ST segment elevation (Fig. 13-1). This ST segment abnormality is actually an indirect effect of the spread of the inflammation from the pericardium to the subepicardial layer of the heart (1). A superficial myocarditis develops and produces a zone of injury, accounting for the appearance of the ST segment elevation (2). In pericarditis, the ST segment elevation usually appears in all the leads except lead aV_R. Abnormal Q waves do not develop since the injury is superficial. The absence of Q waves as well as the diffuse nature of the ST segment elevation is helpful in the differentiation of an acute myocardial infarction. The typical ST segment in pericarditis has an upward concave appearance as opposed to the upward convex ST segment in acute myocardial infarction (Fig. 13-2). After the ST segment returns to the baseline, the T waves become inverted symmetrically. Both the T wave and the ST segment abnormalities usually have resolved by four to eight weeks (3).

If the pericarditis is associated with effusion, the amplitude of the QRS complex may be reduced. This voltage change is presumably due to the short-circuiting of the electric currents in the heart through the accumulated pericardial fluid. Low voltage of the QRS complex is not pathognomonic of pericarditis with pericardial effusion and can be seen in several clinical conditions: chronic constrictive pericarditis, chronic obstructive lung disease, pleural effusion, amyloidosis, and scleroderma (2). Arrhythmias are uncommon in acute pericarditis (4); however, the heart rate is usually rapid (greater than 100 beats per minute) when the inflammatory process is at its peak (1) (Fig. 13-3).

Abnormalities in the electrocardiogram in chronic constrictive pericarditis do not change and are nonprogressive and usually consist of T wave inversion and low voltage (5). Atrial arrhythmias, especially atrial fibrillation and flutter, are common in constrictive pericarditis (6). Total electrical alternans is pathognomonic of cardiac tamponade and usually is seen in patients with effusion due to malignancy (7).

The causes of pericarditis are numerous and include infections (bacterial, tuberculosis, fungus, viral), neoplasms, myocardial infarction, postthoracotomy syndrome, and con-

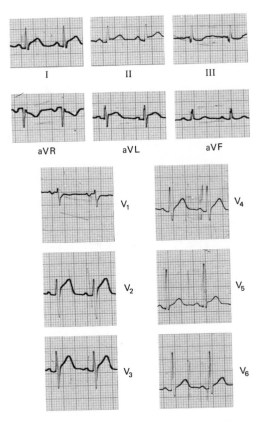

Figure 13-1. Widespread ST segment elevation is present in this tracing from a 29-year-old man with acute pericarditis.

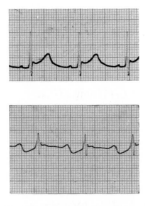

Figure 13-2. Comparison of the ST segment elevations seen with pericarditis and myocardial infarction. Top: Concave ST segment elevation in pericarditis. Bottom: Convex ST segment elevation in myocardial infarction.

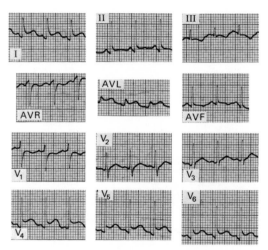

Figure 13-3. Rapid sinus tachycardia frequently accompanies the acute phase of pericarditis. This ECG was recorded from an 18-year-old girl with idiopathic pericarditis.

nective tissue diseases (rheumatoid disease, lupus erythematosus). Chest pain is most often the major symptom. The chest pain may be intensified by deep inspiration, hiccoughs, and a recumbent position. The pain mimics chest pain due to an acute myocardial infarction; however, the evolutionary ECG changes that accompany an acute myocardial infarction will be absent in pericarditis.

ACUTE COR PULMONALE; PULMONARY EMBOLISM

The electrocardiogram is usually not a very sensitive means of detecting pulmonary embolism and may have a normal reading in the presence of severe massive pulmonary embolism (8, 9) (Table 13-1). However, the electrocardiogram is valuable in excluding cardiac disease (10). The pattern associated with pulmonary embolism may resemble an inferior myocardial infarction, further complicating the clinical picture. The electrocardiographic changes in acute cor pulmonale usually develop quite rapidly, and they may persist for minutes, hours, or days (5) (Table 13-2).

The $S_1 Q_3$ pattern (S wave in lead I and Q wave in Lead III) has been described by McGinn and his associates (3) as a typical feature of acute cor pulmonale. The ST segment becomes elevated, and a small inverted T wave in lead III accompanies the Q wave. Lead I develops an S wave and ST segment depression. These changes resemble the reciprocal changes of an inferior myocardial infarction. Careful attention must be given to lead II, for its pattern is similar to lead I rather than lead III, which is not true with a true inferior infarction (Fig. 13-4). Lead aV_F also is helpful because it does not show an abnormal Q wave. A right bundle branch block pattern may develop transiently and is thought to be the result of acute right ventricular dilatation. The production of a clock-

Table 13-1. Frequency of ECG Changes in Patients with Acute Pulmonary Embolism

	Cutforth (13) 50 cases (% of cases)	Weber (14) 60 cases (% of cases)	Szucs (15) 50 cases (% of cases)	Stein (16) 90 cases (% of cases)
S_1Q_3 or $S_1Q_3T_3$	28	27		12
Right axis shift		18	15	7
Right bundle branch block	14	25		15
Incomplete			8	6
Complete				9
T inversion in right precordial leads	46	10		42[a]
Clockwise rotation	60	17		7
Left axis shift		17		7
QR in V_1				
ST changes	18			26[a]
Depression leads I or III		18		
Elevation lead III		28		16[a]
ST, T changes in V_5, V_6	12	10		
P pulmonale	68	28		6
Sinus tachycardia	14	48		
Atrial arrhythmias		38	19	
Atrial fibrillation		10		
Atrial flutter		12		
Atrial tachycardia		2		
First-degree AV block		8		1
No significant abnormality	24	20		13

Source: Reproduced with permission from Chou TC: *Electrocardiography in Clinical Practice* Copyright ©1979, Grune and Stratton, Inc., New York.

[a]Leads not specified.

Table 13-2. Electrocardiographic Changes Associated with Acute Cor Pulmonale (Pulmonary Embolism)

---

1. $S_1 Q_3$ pattern
2. Transient right bundle branch block pattern
3. Inverted T waves and/or ST segment elevation in the right precordial leads
4. Tendency to right axis deviation and clockwise rotation in the precordial leads

---

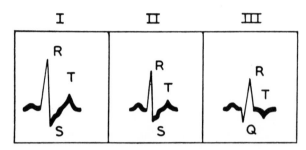

Figure 13-4. The $S_1 Q_3$ pattern of acute cor pulmonale (pulmonary embolism). Note the depressed ST segment with "staircase ascent" in leads I and II. Lead III superficially resembles diaphragmatic infarction with a prominent Q wave and symmetrically inverted T wave, although the ST segment is isoelectric. (Reproduced with permission from Lipman BS, Massie E, Kleiger RE: *Clinical Scalar Electrocardiography*, 6th edition. Copyright © 1972 by Year Book Medical Publishers, Inc., Chicago.)

wise rotation and a shift in the frontal plane axis to the right probably is due to acute dilatation of the chambers of the right side of the heart (3) (Fig. 13-5).

CHRONIC COR PULMONALE

Cor pulmonale (pulmonary heart disease) is an abnormality of the right ventricle that is a result of primary lung disease. The electrocardiographic diagnosis of cor pulmonale in the past was usually centered around the appearance of right ventricular hypertrophy (RVH). The clinical correlation of documented cor pulmonale with the electrocardiogram picture of RVH, however, was found in less than 30% of patients (11). The reason the RVH picture is absent from the majority of electrocardiograms is that actual hypertrophy of the right ventricle is a late manifestation of chronic cor pulmonale (1). The characteristic findings of chronic cor pulmonale on the electrocardiogram are listed in Table 13-3. Tall, peaked P waves are seen best in leads II, III, and aV_F and are thought to be due to enlargement of the right atrium. The frontal plane axis of the P wave is generally between +60° to +90°. Hypertrophy and anterior rotation of the right ventricle produce an rS complex across the precordium (clockwise rotation) as well as a right axis deviation in the frontal plane. Low voltage of the QRS complex is often seen in the precordial leads, presumably owing to the hyperinflated lungs, which hamper the spread of the electrical current to the body surface (12) (Fig. 13-6).

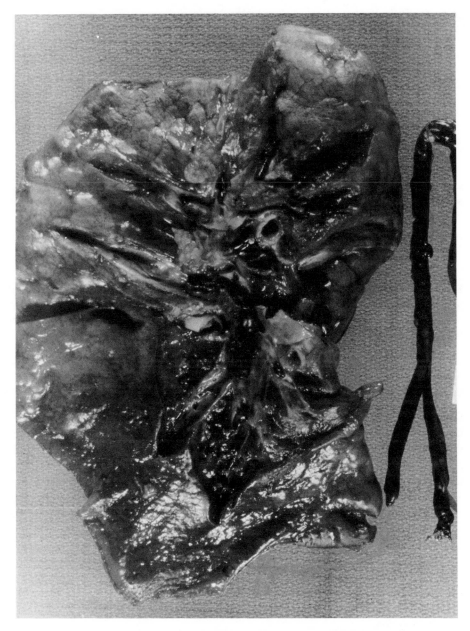

Figure 13-5. Venous thrombosis, seen on the right, produced multiple pulmonary emboli in this patient, who exhibited none of the ECG findings for pulmonary embolism.

Table 13-3. Electrocardiographic Changes of Chronic Cor Pulmonale

1. P-pulmonale pattern of right atrial enlargement
2. Right axis deviation
3. rS pattern in V_1-V_6 (clockwise rotation)
4. RVH (appears late)
5. Low voltage QRS complexes

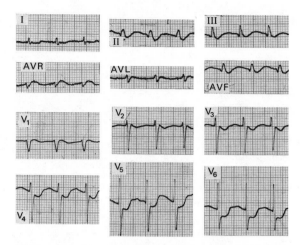

Figure 13-6. Low QRS voltage in the limb leads as well as a clockwise rotation in the precordial leads is present. Junctional tachycardia is also present in this ECG, which was recorded from a man suffering from chronic cor pulmonale. At autopsy, extensive pulmonary atherosclerosis and right ventricular hypertrophy were found.

CARDIOGENIC SHOCK

Dysrhythmias are usually a consequence of the electrical instability of the heart or of failure of the heart as a pump, resulting in underperfusion of body tissues and a state of shock. Cardiogenic shock may occur secondary to loss of myocardial muscle and is present with an extensive myocaridal infarction or possibly after cardiac surgery. A treatise on the subject of cardiogenic shock is beyond the scope of this text, and there are numerous excellent references that cover the topic exclusively. For purposes of this chapter, the aspects of cardiogenic shock that will be covered are those that ultimately will influence nursing intervention in shock of cardiac origin.

Cardiogenic shock as a clinical syndrome denotes the presence of arterial hypotension and signs of inadequate tissue perfusion. Hypotension exists when the systolic blood pressure is less than 90 mmHg in a previously normotensive person and/or when the pressure is 30 mmHg lower than a previously documented level (17, 18). Signs of inadequate tissue perfusion are manifested by a cool, moist skin; oliguria; cyanosis; and mental confusion.

Pepine and associates (19) identify two types of cardiogenic shock. One type is associated with a reduction in the filling of the ventricle without direct involvement of the myocardium. This can occur with acute cardiac tamponade, atrioventricular valve stenosis, and atrial myxoma. The second type of shock is due to restricted ventricular emptying. Conditions associated with the latter are acute myocardial infarction; presence of a left ventricular aneurysm; previous myocardial infarctions; acute mitral and aortic insufficiency; as well as aortic and pulmonic stenosis.

Tissue hypoperfusion in the first type of cardiogenic shock (cardiac filling restricted) is a result of a sequence of events. A reduction of ventricular volume limits stretching of myocardial fibers and affects the force of myocardial fiber contraction or shortening (Starling's law of the heart). Since the heart can put out only what it receives, stroke volume is diminished. Physiological compensatory mechanisms respond in an effort to maintain adequate arterial pressure by tachycardia, increased resistance, and increased contractility, which occurs secondary to intrinsic catecholamine stimulation. After a period of time, the compensatory mechanisms begin to fail, leading to hypoperfusion of body tissues. In the second type of cardiogenic shock (inadequate emptying of the ventricles), residual left ventricular volume increases as does the end-diastolic pressure. It thus becomes more difficult for the left atrium to empty, a factor that further curtails cardiac output. Litwak (20) describes this series of events as a major curtailment of the capability of the left ventricle to eject its content, and ascribes it to a combination of pathophysiologic derangements associated with a myocardial infarction. First, a segment of the ventricle does not contract. This is particularly true when at least 40% of the transmural left myocardium is affected by acute necrosis, as is commonly found in cardiogenic shock. The second factor contributing to loss of left ventricular function is the presence of an acute left to right shunt produced by a ventricular septal defect. In addition, strain on the left ventricular performance can likewise occur when severe mitral insufficiency results from infarction-related papillary muscle rupture.

Under normal conditions and during basal states, shortening of myocardial fibers and hence stroke volume are regulated by four major factors: preload (muscle fiber length before onset of contraction, Frank-Starling mechanism), afterload (the impedance to left ventricular ejection), inotropic state (contractility) of the myocardium, and frequency of contraction.

According to Kones (17) preload is a function of stress of the wall of the myocardium as well as the end-diastolic volume. It has a direct effect upon the force, speed, and extent of muscle fiber shortening, thereby influencing stroke volume. In cardiogenic shock, left ventricular end-diastolic pressure is usually elevated.

Afterload may be defined as the force or load imposed on the myocardial fibers during the ejection phase of the cardiac cycle (17). Frequently, measurements of the arterial blood pressure or vascular resistance are used in the gross determination of afterload. Reduction of the load against which the heart contracts usually results in a more effective stroke volume (18).

The main mechanisms regulating contractility, or the inotropic state of the myocardium, are sympathetic nerve activity as well as the amount of norepinephrine that may be released at the nerve fiber ending. Contractility can also be influenced by pharmacologic agents such as isoproterenol and digitalis, which enhance inotropism of the heart; whereas acidosis, hypoxia, and anesthetic agents have negative inotropic effect upon the heart action (21).

In the presence of end-diastolic volume that is held constant, aortic flow tends to increase as the frequency of contractions increases. However, in extremely rapid or slow rates, cardiac output may become reduced (22). The regulatory factors of stroke volume and cardiac performance likewise determine cardiac oxygen consumption. Preload has the least effect on oxygen consumption.

Depressed ventricular function as is associated with cardiogenic shock directly affects the factors influencing stroke volume. Left ventricular filling pressure as reflected in the pulmonary wedge pressure is usually elevated (>18 mmHg). Loss of segmental contraction results in incomplete emptying of the ventricle and hence increase in residual volume. As a compensatory mechanism to maintain adequate arterial perfusion pressure, peripheral resistance is increased. The peripheral resistance has a direct bearing upon afterload. The impediment to ventricular emptying is thus increased.

The physiological response to reduced cardiac output is tachycardia, which partially restores the declining volume. However, in cardiogenic shock the reflex tachycardia shortens the filling time of the ventricles as well as increases myocardial oxygen demands.

To understand how derangement of left ventricular function contributes to hypoperfusion of tissue, the principle of transmembrane capillary transference based on Starling's law of the capillaries must be reviewed. Normally, several forces influence the delivery of nutrients and oxygen to body cells and remove waste products of metabolism. The two physical forces are hydrostatic pressure (blood pressure) and osmotic pressure (protein content). Hydrostatic pressure exerts a pushing force, while osmotic pressure maintains a drawing or retaining force (23). According to Bern and Levy (24), several variables influence hydrostatic pressure. They are arterial and venous pressures, precapillary and postcapillary resistances, and the type of cell. A rise in either arterial or venous pressures increases the hydrostatic pressure, whereas a reduction in any of the pressures decreases the hydrostatic pressure. Osmotic (colloid, oncotic) pressure is influenced by the presence of plasma proteins and electrolytes.

Filtration and absorption are among several forces influencing cellular nutrition, which may vary according to the metabolic needs of the body. A representative example (using arbitrary figures) for the process involved in substrate and waste product exchange is schematically represented in Table 13-4. Movement of substrates and metabolic products across the capillary membrane occur as a result of an existent gradient between the effective hydrostatic and osmotic pressures. In the presence of cardiogenic shock, the hydrostatic pressure at the arterial end of the capillary membrane is markedly reduced. As a result, the nutritional flow of blood to the tissues is inadequate to meet the changing needs of the body, and shock ensues.

The clinical counterparts of left ventricular failure, diminished cardiac output, arterial hypotension, and vasoconstriction associated with cardiogenic shock are the presence of S_3 and/or S_4 heart sound; altered sensorium; urine output less than 20 ml per hour; tachycardia; thready pulse; systolic pressure less than 90 mmHg, or 30 mmHg lower than the previously recorded level; and cold, clammy skin. The third heart sound, according

Table 13-4. Transference of Fluid Across Cell Membrane

Blood		Interstitial Fluid
Arterial End of the Capillary		
Hydrostatic pressure: 35 mmHg	Capillary Wall	Hydrostatic pressure: 4 mmHg
Effective hydrostatic pressure: 31 mmHg ⟶		
Osmotic pressure: 25 mmHg		Osmotic pressure: 2 mmHg
Effective osmotic pressure: 23 mmHg ⟵		
Determinant pressure: EHP – EOP = 8 mmHg		
Venous End of the Capillary		
Hydrostatic pressure: 15 mmHg	Capillary Wall	Hydrostatic pressure: 1 mmHg
Effective hydrostatic pressure: 14 mmHg ⟶		
Osmotic pressure: 25 mmHg		Osmotic pressure: 3 mmHg
Effective osmotic pressure: 22 mmHg ⟵		
Determinant pressure: EHP – EOP = 8 mmHg		

to Kuhn (25), is the best clinical indicator that pulmonary capillary pressure is elevated. Although the clinical appearance of patients in cardiogenic shock is similar, Kuhn (25) is of the opinion that the hemodynamic patterns responsible for the manifestations of shock may differ.

The mechanism associated with the physical signs of cold skin and oliguria usually suggests the presence of maximal systemic vasoconstriction. This may be true in some patients; however, it has been found that systemic peripheral resistance does not consistently increase. Therefore regional vasoconstriction must take place (25).

The hypotensive state seen with shock of cardiac origin may not be related to the precipitous drop in cardiac output, as generally thought, but rather may be attributed to the effect of shock on the peripheral vasculature. According to Kuhn (25), experimental occlusion of a coronary artery and/or acute distension of the left ventricle have been found to evoke a reflex mediated by the vagus nerve. The response to the reflex results in peripheral vasodilation. The same sequence of events, Kuhn feels, may likewise be responsible for the genesis of hypotension in cardiogenic shock. As was mentioned in Chapter 1, there is increasing evidence that vagal fibers, according to Braunwald (26), may likewise extend to ventricular muscle.

The electrocardiographic findings are related to the type and location of the myocardial infarction. A detailed discussion of myocardial infarction is found in Chapter 10. Schiedt and associates (27) found a similarity in the distribution of infarcts (anterior-inferior). Although the number of subendocardial infarctions as evidenced by changes in the ST-T waves was small, shock developed in six of eleven patients in Schiedt's series. Although dysrhythmias are a common finding and have been considered as precipitating causes of cardiogenic shock, many are secondary to the shock state. These are thought to be a consequence of altered flow to the myocardium and/or to alterations in metabolism. In Schiedt's series, the presence of atrioventricular block and sinus tachycardia as secondary dysrhythmias were associated with a higher mortality rate than were sinus bradycardia, atrial fibrillation, junctional and ventricular rhythm, and/or tachycardia (27).

Killip (18), citing the results of a study, relates the incidence of arrhythmias to the severity of infarction. Generally, all patients experiencing cardiogenic shock had some type of arrhythmia. There was a greater incidence (94%) of life-threatening arrhythmias in this group of patients than in the group with myocardial infarction without cardiogenic shock (45%). There was a higher incidence of atrioventricular block and ventricular fibrillation in the group of patients with cardiogenic shock.

The incidence of cardiogenic shock as a sequel to myocardial infarction is about 15%. It occurs more commonly with an extensive anterior myocardial infarction than with an inferior myocardial infarction. The mortality rate associated with cardiogenic shock in this setting is approximately 80% to 90% (19).

Schiedt and associates (28), in an attempt to identify factors that might predict which patient admitted to the hospital after sustaining a myocardial infarction might experience cardiogenic shock, explored a number of variables. The following were considered: cardiac rhythm, drugs administered, age of patient, time interval between time of infarction and admission to hospital, location of myocardial infarction, and past medical history. Although data from the study did reveal that there was a higher incidence of cardiogenic shock associated with an acute myocardial infarction when it was superimposed upon residual tissue of an old infarction, additional findings were that the patient in whom shock develops is the older patient. The clinical observations analyzed in the study, however, failed to identify the patient who is more prone to cardiogenic shock.

Therapy in the management of patients experiencing cardiogenic shock, according to Shine and associates (29), should be directed toward: optimizing the ratio of supply and demand, provision for adequate blood oxygen content, reduction of afterload, augmenting preload, and improving the contractile force of the ventricle. Such objectives can be accomplished through the use of volume expansion, if left ventricular filling pressure is less than 24 mmHg (29); diuretic therapy; and vasodilating agents such as sodium nitroprusside, nitroglycerin, inotropic agents, and/or mechanical support of the failing circulation. The use of vasodilating agents, while decreasing afterload, will indirectly decrease myocardial oxygen demand. The nitrates are considered to be potent vasodilators of both arteries and veins. If venous capacitance is increased, a greater pooling of blood occurs, which results in less venous return to the heart and a decrease in the size of the left ventricle. The reduction of the left ventricular chamber implies reduced wall tension and therefore a decrease in myocardial oxygen consumption (30).

The goal of intra-aortic balloon counterpulsation, according to Ross (21), is two-fold. First, systolic aortic pressure is reduced, which favors an increase in cardiac output; and second, the diastolic aortic pressure is increased. The latter therefore provides for better coronary perfusion pressure.

The intra-aortic balloon counterpulsation device is inserted by way of a femoral arteriotomy and is positioned distal to the left subclavian artery and proximal to the renal arteries. Inflation and deflation of the balloon are correlated with the electrocardiogram, which is part of the monitoring device on the external pump. Inflation corresponds to the tip of the T wave (onset of diastole). During this time the aorta is partially obstructed, causing blood displacement distally to the extremities and proximally to the major branches of the aortic arch and toward the coronary arteries. This phase of intra-aortic balloon counterpulsation, according to Frazee and Nail (31), increases oxygenation of the myocardium and augments perfusion of organs. Balloon deflation is planned to occur just before the onset of ventricular systole. This corresponds to the ending, or downslope, of the P wave. During this phase of the mechanical support of circulation, end diastolic and systolic arterial pressures are reduced (20). Hence, the left ventricle does not contract against as high a systemic vascular resistance, which decreases the workload and myocardial oxygen consumption of the ischemic myocardium.

Although intra-aortic balloon counterpulsation does frequently improve the hemodynamic status of cardiovascular system during cardiogenic shock, Litwak (20) explains that many of the patients are intra-aortic balloon counterpulsation—dependent and therefore cannot be weaned off the device.

In Kuhn's opinion (25), the reason for the high mortality rate, even with the use of the circulatory support device among patients in cardiogenic shock, is related to the profound damage of the myocardium during the development of shock. He thus advises the use of the intra-aortic balloon counterpulsation in preshock states in order that shock may be prevented. According to Kuhn (25), there are various stages of development in the dysfunction of the left ventricle that are associated with a recent or an old infarction. Thus if the ischemic myocardial tissue can be preserved, there will be less necrosis. Gutovitz and associates (32), in a study of 15 patients, attempted to determine by laboratory values of plasma MB creatine kinase whether the extensive myocardial injury associated with cardiogenic shock was the result of a progressive rather than a primary massive insult. The results of their findings were compatible with the concept that continuing release of MB creatine kinase into the blood-stream of patients experiencing cardiogenic shock reflects a vicious cycle of progressing myocardial injury, compromise of cardiac function, exacerbation of ischemia, and continuance of myocardial damage. They, too, advocate intervention before cardiogenic shock becomes apparent.

In view of the fact that problems inherent with the use of intra-aortic balloon counterpulsation still exist, Takamoto and associates (33) advocate the concomitant use of the intra-aortic balloon counterpulsation and venoarterial bypass (right atrium–femoral artery) in situations where perfusion pressure has dropped profoundly and the counterpulsation device was not effective.

The literature abounds in excellent references detailed in the nursing management of patients experiencing cardiogenic shock. For this reason, in this text, the "how to care for the patient" general discussion has been omitted. The nurse does have a definitive role in the methods of intervening in the pathology associated with circulatory compromise. Nursing intervention, as outlined by McGurn (34), includes the assessment of vital signs or parameters; emotional support of the patient; and judgement in determining whether the patient's condition warrants the physician's reevaluation of the clinical status and/or therapeutic plan of care.

CARDIAC TAMPONADE

Cardiac tamponade, as defined by Baines and Beattle (35), is the embarrassment of cardiac function resulting from an increase in the intrapericardial pressure. A pressure rise within the pericardium can occur in association with diverse factors. Tew and associates (36) have described cardiac tamponade as secondary to nonhemorrhagic pericardial fluid as a complication of Dressler's syndrome. Hochberg (37) reported an incident of delayed onset (the fifth day after the operation) of cardiac tamponade that was associated with prophylactic anticoagulant therapy after coronary artery bypass surgery. A rare form of tamponade (chylopericardium) was described by Hargus (38). The tamponade occurred after a Blalock-Taussig palliative procedure to relieve the circulatory derangement of tricuspid atresia with severe infundibular stenosis. More commonly, cardiac tamponade occurs as a result of trauma to the chest or upper abdomen, with effusions, and with malignancy; and it may occasionally be iatrogenic. The latter may be associated with cardiac catheterization procedures, insertion of pacemaker wires, and/or with insertion of central venous pressure lines (39, 40).

Normally, the pericardial space contains approximately 20 cubic centimeters of fluid. During disease states, a large amount of fluid can often accumulate in the pericardial space without producing decompensation of the heart. This is true only if the accumulation of fluid has been gradual. With time, the pericardial sac can distend to accommodate the increased volume of pericardial fluid. However, if the filling of the sac is extreme, the pericardium cannot stretch, resulting in compression of the heart. Therefore, if the filling is slow, as much as 2 liters of fluid can be present in the pericardial space without producing abnormal signs or symptoms (35). In time, however, intrapericardial pressure will rise and can affect the filling of the heart. Before decompensation occurs, compensatory mechanisms attempt to maintain adequate perfusion pressures. The physiological responses that attempt to compensate for the cardiac compression are increased peripheral resistance, increased central venous pressure, and tachycardia. Hypotension resulting from a decreased stroke volume causes the release of catecholamines, which have a vasoconstrictive effect on vessels as well as a positive chronotropic effect on the heart.

The increase in peripheral vascular resistance is an attempt to maintain blood pressure despite the fact that the cardiac output is declining. A rise in central venous pressure is secondary to the redistribution of venous blood and a greater return of blood to the heart. The atrioventricular gradient improves, and subsequently there is greater ventricular filling. The stretch of myocardial fibers brings about more effective contractility. Tachycardia partially restores the declining stroke volume. With greater perfusion, the coronary arteries likewise receive more blood (35, 39). Decompensation occurs when filling exceeds ability of the pericardium to stretch.

Arterial and venous pressures ultimately are affected by a high intrapericardial pressure. As the pressure rises, the vena cavae and atria are compressed, which impairs venous return to the heart. As a consequence, venous pressure will rise. In the arterial system, atrial and end-diastolic pressures of the ventricles increase, ventricular filling decreases, stroke volume is reduced, cardiac output falls, and pulmonary and arterial pressures are lowered, resulting in hypoperfusion of tissues and organs.

Shoemaker (40) identifies the following stages in the development of tamponade that influence such clinical manifestations: In stage I blood pressure remains stable as a result of compensatory mechanisms. The pericardial sac probably contains less than 200 cc of fluid. Although the blood pressure remains stable because of compensatory mechanisms, the central venous pressure continues to rise, reaching a level of 15 cm of water. Stage II represents a greater degree of intracardial pressure, as evidenced by the presence of Beck's triad (hypotension, jugular venous distension, muffled heart sounds) and represents the inadequacy of the compensatory mechanisms to counter the effects of the high pressure within the pericardium. Stage III represents further deterioration of circulation and an advanced degree of tamponade. The physiological compensatory mechanisms are unable to maintain perfusion pressure as both arterial and venous pressures fall.

The clinical manifestations vary according to the rate of fluid accumulation. The patient may be anxious and have evidence of cerebral hypoxia, cyanosis, and vasoconstriction, as reflected by pale, cold, moist skin. Beck's triad may be present.

A common finding with tamponade is pulsus paradoxus. Normally when the blood pressure is measured, a slight fall in systolic pressure, pulse pressure, and heart rate occur during inspiration (less than 10 mmHg). In cardiac tamponade, exaggeration of this physical phenomenon occurs. The drop in systolic pressure during inspiration is much greater than 10 mmHg. A method of ascertaining the presence of pulsus paradoxus as identified by Shoemaker (40) is as follows:

1. Deflation of the blood pressure cuff is carried out during normal respiration until the auscultation of first sound.
2. The systolic pressure is noted both on inspiration and expiration.
3. Pulsus paradoxus is said to be present when the difference between inspiratory and expiratory systolic pressure is 15 mmHg.
4. A decline in systolic blood pressure during the inspiratory phase of respiration may also be palpable at the radial pulse.

Nonspecific ST and T wave changes occur. The voltage of the QRS complex as well as the T wave may be low. These phenomena may suggest subepicardial ischemia associated with the intrapericardial pressure (39). Electrical activity within the heart must be detected by the stylus of the galvanometer through a water medium within the pericardial sac. Occasionally, alternating voltage of the P wave, the QRS complex, and the T wave (electrical alternans) may be evident. If present, this is a pathognomonic sign of cardiac tamponade (35, 39). Sharbaro and Brooks (41) ascribe the oscillating motion of the heart that produces the alternate configuration of either a QRS complex or the P wave to the presence of pericardial fluid. In effusion without tamponade, the frequency of heart motion is equivalent to heart rate; however, in effusion with tamponade, the frequency of heart motion is reduced. Diagnosis of cardiac tamponade is usually based on Beck's triad.

Cardiac tamponade, although it does not occur frequently, is however a medical emergency and does require immediate intervention since a rise in intrapericardial pressure impedes cardiac filling to the point of drastically reducing cardiac output necessary for survival. Since there is a direct relationship between intrapericardial pressure and volume, Clark (42) suggests that removal of only a small quantity of fluid from the pericardial sac would result in a dramatic fall in intrapericardial pressure. Removal of the fluid can be accomplished by needle aspiration and/or pericardiotomy for the removal of the clot. When the tamponading effect on the heart has been removed, therapy is directed toward the underlying cause.

REVIEW QUESTIONS

1. Explain how the ECG changes seen with a myocardial infarction may be similar to those seen with acute pericarditis.
2. What does the $S_1 Q_3$ sign refer to?
3. What is the determining factor in producing circulatory compromise when cardiac tamponade occurs?
4. What are the early signs versus the late signs of cardiac tamponade?
5. Cardiogenic shock can occur in any hospitalized population. Which group of patients is more apt to develop cardiogenic shock?
6. Identify the clinical manifestations frequently associated with cardiogenic shock.
7. List the principal goals in the treatment of cardiogenic shock.
8. The presence of pulsus alternans is highly suggestive of which condition?

REFERENCES

1. Spodick DH: Pathogenesis and clinical correlations of the electrocardiographic abnormalities of pericardial disease, in Rios JC (ed): *Clinical Electrocardiographic Correlations*. Philadelphia, FA Davis Co, 1977, p 201.
2. Chou TC: *Electrocardiography in Clinical Practice*, New York, Grune & Stratton Inc, 1979, p 242.
3. Lipman BS, Massie E, Kleiger RE: *Clinical Scalar Electrocardiography*, ed 6. Chicago, Year Book Medical Pub Inc, 1972, p 259.
4. Spodick DH: Arrhythmias during acute pericarditis. A prospective study of 100 consecutive cases. *JAMA* 235:39, 1976.
5. Marriott, HJL: *Practical Electrocardiography*, ed 6. Baltimore, Williams & Wilkins Co, 1977, p 296.
6. Dalton JC, Pearson RJ, White PD: Constrictive pericarditis. A review and long-term follow-up of 78 cases. *Ann Intern Med* 45:445, 1956.
7. Bashour FA, Cochran PW: The association of electrical alternans with pericardial effusion. *Dis Chest* 44:146, 1963.

8. Sleisenger MH, Abdallah PS: The pathogenesis, diagnosis, and treatment of pulmonary embolism. *Calif Med* 114:36, 1971.

9. Fitzmaurice JB, Sasahara, AA: Current concepts of pulmonary embolism. Implications for nursing practice. *Heart Lung* 3:209, 1974.

10. Bloomfield DA: The recognition and management of massive pulmonary embolism. *Heart Lung* 3:241, 1974.

11. Phillips RW: The electrocardiogram in cor pulmonale secondary to pulmonary emphysema. A study of 18 cases proved by autopsy. *Am Heart J* 56:352, 1958.

12. Hartman RB: Pulmonary heart disease. Pathophysiology, diagnostic signs and therapy. *Postgrad Med* 66:58, 1979.

13. Cutforth RH, Oram S: The electrocardiogram in pulmonary embolism. *Br Heart J* 20:41, 1958.

14. Weber DM, Philips JH: A re-evaluation of electrocardiographic changes accompanying acute pulmonary embolism. *Am J Med Sci* 251:381, 1966.

15. Szucs MM, Brooks HL et al: Diagnostic sensitivity of laboratory findings in acute pulmonary embolism. *Ann Intern Med* 74:161, 1971.

16. Stein PD, Dalen JE, et at: The electrocardiogram in acute pulmonary embolism. *Prog Cardiovasc Dis* 17:247, 1975.

17. Kones RJ: *Cardiogenic Shock: Mechanism and Management.* New York, Futura Publishing Co, Inc, 1974, p 3.

18. Killip T: Management of arrhythmias in acute myocardial infarction, in Braunwald, E (ed): *The Myocardium: Failure and Infarction.* New York, HP Pub Co Inc, 1974, p 131.

19. Pepine CJ, Nichols WW, Alexander JA: Guidelines to evaluation and management of shock. *Hosp Med* 15:88, 1979.

20. Litwak RS: Mechanical support of the failing circulation. *Primary Cardiol* 5:32, 1979.

21. Ross J: Effects of afterload or impedance on the heart: afterload reduction in the treatment of cardiac failure. *Cardiovas Med* 2:115, 1977.

22. Ross J: Hemodynamic changes in acute myocardial infarction, in Braunwald, E (ed): *The Myocardium: Failure and Infarction,* New York, HP Pub Co Inc, 1974, p 125.

23. Brobeck JR (ed): *Best and Taylor's Physiological Bases for Medical Practice,* ed 9. Baltimore, The Williams & Wilkins Co, 1973, p 122.

24. Berne RM, Levy MN: *Cardiovascular Physiology,* ed 3. St. Louis, CV Mosby Co, 1977, p 122.

25. Kuhn LA: Management of shock following acute myocardial infarction. *Am Heart J* 95:533, 1978.

26. Braunwald E (ed): *The Myocardium: Failure and Infarction.* New York, HP Pub Co Inc, 1974, p 31.

27. Scheidt S, Killip T: Axioms on cardiogenic shock. *Hosp Med* 6:31, 1970.

28. Scheidt S, Ascheim R, Killip T: Shock after acute myocardial infarction. *Am J Cardiol* 26:557, 1970.

29. Shine KI, Kattus A, Brucker C, Tillisch JH: Pathophysiology of myocardial infarction. *An Internal Med* 87:75, 1977.

30. Abrams J: Current status of long-acting nitrates in clinical medicine. *Practical Cardiol* 3:19, 1977.

31. Frazee S, Nail L: New challenge in cardiac nursing: the intra-aortic balloon. *Heart Lung* 2:528, 1973.

32. Gutovitz AL, Sobel BE, Roberts R: Progressive nature of myocardial injury in selected patients with cardiogenic shock. *Am J Cardiol* 41:469, 1978.

33. Takamoto S, Omoto R, Wambuchi Y, Yokote Y, Kimura S, Kyo S, Furuta S, Oya G, Ono H, Kono T: Hemodynamic effect of the concomitant use of intra-aortic balloon pumping and veno-arterial bypass without oxygen in cardiogenic shock. *Jap Heart J* 19:938, 1978.

34. McGurn WC: The patient in shock: mechanisms of shock, related therapy, nursing goals, and functions, in Kintzel (ed): *Advanced Concepts in Clinical Nursing.* Philadelphia, JB Lippincott Co, 1977, p 378.

35. Baines MS, Beattle EJ: Cardiac tamponade. *Hosp Med* 12:47, 1976.

36. Tew FT, Russell RO, Rackley CE: Cardiac tamponade with nonhemorrhagic pericardial fluid complicating Dressler's syndrome. *Chest* 72:93, 1977.

37. Hochberg MS, Merrill WH, Gruber M, McIntosh CL, Henry WL, Morrow AG: Delayed cardiac tamponade associated with prophylactic anticoagulation in patients undergoing coronary artery bypass. *J Thorac Cardiovas Surg* 75:771, 1978.

38. Hargus EP, Carson SD, McGrath RL, Wolfe RR, Clark D: Chylothorax and chylopericardium tamponade following Blalock-Taussig anastamosis. *J Thorac Cardiovasc Surg* 75:642, 1978.

39. Fowler NO: *Cardiac Diagnosis and Treatment*, ed 2. Hagerstown, Md, Harper & Row Pub Inc, 1976, p 862.

40. Shoemaker WC: Early diagnosis and management of pericardial tamponade. *Hosp Med* 14:7, 1978.

41. Sharbaro JA, Brooks HL: Pericardial effusion and electrical alternans: echocardiographic assessment. *Postgrad Med* 63:109, 1978.

42. Clark WH: Axioms on diseases of the pericardium. *Hosp Med* 13:16, 1977.

14
Artificial Pacemakers

The first successful clinical use of external thoracic pacing for complete heart block was in 1952 by Zoll (1). Weirich and his associates (2) in 1957 reported the use of two stainless steel leads attached to the myocardium and brought through the skin at the time of cardiac surgery. These leads were then connected to an external battery-operated pacemaker. Transvenous endocardial pacing was first reported by Furman and his associates (3) in 1959. The power source was still located externally, but eventually the whole system was successfully implanted in 1960 by Chardock (4).

INDICATIONS FOR ARTIFICIAL PACING

The major indication for the use of pacemakers today is the presence of an inappropriately slow heart rate. Pacemaker therapy is employed if the slow heart rate is the result of an abnormality of impulse formation, impulse conduction, or both. A slow rate is commonly due to complete heart block, marked sinus bradycardia, atrial fibrillation with high-grade atrioventricular block, and tachycardia-bradycardia syndrome (sick sinus syndrome). Controversies exist over the use of artificial pacemakers in the treatment of asymptomatic patients with bifascicular block (RBBB with left anterior or left posterior fascicular block) with or without first-degree AV block (5,6). Some of the newest indications for artificial pacing include the prevention and termination of tachyarrhythmias, both atrial and ventricular. Tachycardias are believed to be the result of enhanced automaticity or reentry, and current electrophysiologic studies through the use of His bundle electrograms may identify the responsible mechanism. Critically timed programmed extrasystoles during His bundle studies can predictably initiate and terminate reentry tachycardias. The introduction of programmed extrasystoles does not induce or terminate tachyarrhythmias due to enhanced automaticity (7).

TYPES OF ARTIFICIAL PACEMAKERS

The types of pacemakers are listed in Table 14-1. The QRS- or ventricular-inhibited pacemaker is by far the most widely used pacemaker today. The QRS-inhibited pacemaker is synchronized with the patient's normally appearing QRS complex and is set to discharge only when the normal beats do not appear. This pacemaker then functions on *demand* when it does not sense the patient's normal QRS complex (Fig. 14-1).

The continuous asynchronous pacemaker stimulates the heart at a constant preset interval regradless of the patient's rhythm. This pacemaker is commonly referred to a

252

Table 14-1. Types of Cardiac Pacemakers

Ventricular	QRS-inhibited (demand)
	QRS-triggered (demand)
	Continuous asynchronous (fixed rate)
	P wave triggered
Atrial	P wave-inhibited
	P wave-triggered
	Continuous asynchronous
	QRS-inhibited
AV	Continuous sequential AV
	QRS-inhibited sequential AV (bifocal demand)

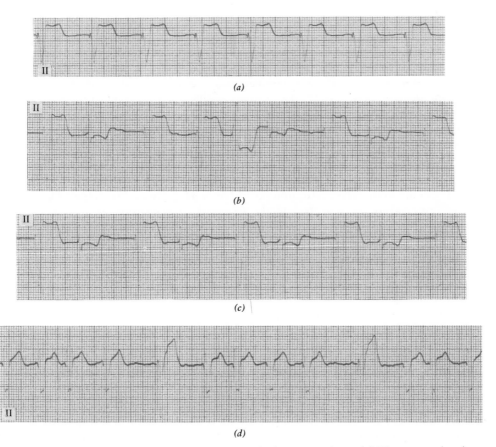

(a)

(b)

(c)

(d)

Figure 14-1. Normal functioning demand ventricular pacemakers. (*a*) The pacemaker is required by the patient for every beat, giving the appearance of a fixed-rate pacemaker. (*b*) The pacemaker senses the patient's premature beat (fifth complex) as well as the other normal beats (narrow QRS). (*c*) Patient's own beats alternate with paced beats, producing a bigeminal type rhythm. (*d*) Atrial fibrillation with two paced beats. This pacemaker was used in the treatment of the tachycardia-bradycardia syndrome (sick-sinus). Note the presence of pacer spikes preceding the wide bizarre QRS complexes.

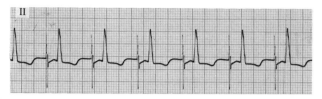

Figure 14-2. Normal functioning atrial pacemaker. The pacer spikes are seen clearly before each QRS complex.

fixed-rate pacemaker and is seldom used today because it has the potential for developing complex arrhythmias since there are two pacemakers competing for control (the artificial pacemaker and the patient's prevailing rhythm).

The QRS-triggered pacemaker senses the patient's QRS complex and activates during the absolute refractory period. The pacemaker spike therefore occurs in the middle of the QRS complex as opposed to appearing before the QRS complex as with the ventricular-inhibited pacemaker. The ventricular-triggered pacemaker is considered a demand pacemaker since actual pacing (capture) will not occur until the patient's own QRS complex fails to appear. The disadvantages of this pacemaker are: (*1*) a constant nonproductive energy drain occurs since the pacemaker fires during every QRS complex, reducing the life of the battery, and (*2*) the constant stimulation distorts the QRS morphology, making it impossible to diagnose other myocardial abnormalities, that is, myocardial infarction (5). The advantage the QRS-triggered pacemaker has is that it cannot be inhibited by electromechanical interference; however, it is used very seldom.

The atrial-triggered pacemaker senses the normal P wave and stimulates the ventricles at a preset interval. Atrial pacemakers are occasionally used in those individuals who need the additional atrial contraction (kick) for an adequate cardiac output (Fig. 14-2). Atrial pacemakers are also used in the treatment of refractory atrial or ventricular arrhythmias. Atrial pacing, regardless of the type used, has its limitations because of the difficulties encountered in maintaining a stable electrode position in the atria.

The AV pacemakers produce atrial and ventricular stimulation and the bifocal-demand pacemaker is the more sophisticated of the two in that both the atrial and ventricular electrodes are capable of sensing as well as capturing on demand.

Electrodes

There are basically two types of electrodes used, unipolar and bipolar. The bipolar lead has both the cathode (negative pole) and anode (positive pole) on the lead itself, as opposed to the unipolar lead, which has the negative pole in the pacing tip and the positive pole in the pulse generator. The unipolar catheter senses intracardiac impulses more easily than the bipolar catheter, owing to the increased distance between the poles. However, the unipolar catheter also detects extracardiac signals, and more easily thus inhibition of the pacemaker can occur (5).

Electrocardiographic Features of Ventricular Pacemakers

1. Pacer spike, which in turn produces a wide, bizarre QRS complex.
2. Fusion beats.

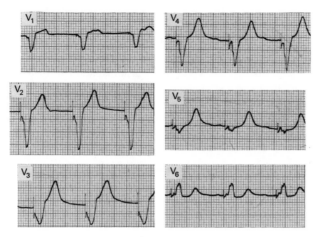

Figure 14-3. Appearance of left bundle branch block produced by a pacemaker located in the right ventricle. (See text on next page.)

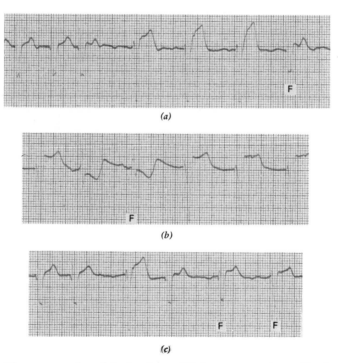

Figure 14-4. Three examples of fusion beats (F) from pacemakers. The fusion beat resembles the paced beat more in (c), while the fusion beats in (a) and (b) are similar to the patient's own beats. (See text on next page.)

If the pacemaker is located in the right ventricle (transvenous pacemaker), the QRS complex stimulates a left bundle branch block pattern since the right ventricle is activated before the left ventricle (Fig. 14-3). A right bundle branch block pattern will be recorded if the pacemaker is located on the left ventricle (epicardial pacemaker). The QRS morphology is important to observe because dislodgement of a transvenous pacemaker can be detected with the ECG tracing. If the transvenous pacer is advertently inserted into the coronary sinus, the ECG recording will show tall R waves across the precordial leads (8). Normally the QRS complex should show a left bundle branch block pattern when the pacemaker is inserted transvenously in the right ventricle, and if a right bundle branch block is seen, perforation of the interventricular septum should be suspected. Fusion beats are commonly found because demand pacemakers operate like a ventricular escape beat (9). (Fig. 14-4).

COMPLICATIONS

Complications of pacemakers include wound infections, perforation of the ventricle, and ventricular tachyarrhythmias during insertion of a transvenous pacemaker. Pacemaker malfunction may be the result of fractures of the leads, dislodgement of the leads, or battery failure (Fig. 14-5). Clinically, hiccoughs often develop when a transvenous pacemaker has perforated the ventricle and paces the diaphragm. Pacemaker malfunction may result in a marked reduction in heart rate, which in turn produces a fall in the patient's cardiac output. A decreased cerebral blood flow may manifest itself in the following ways: syncope, seizures, confusion, and lethargy. Signs and symptoms of cardiac and renal ischemia may likewise develop.

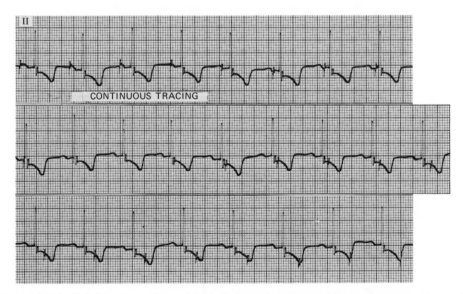

Figure 14-5. Continuous tracing of lead II from a patient with a transvenous demand ventricular pacemaker. Pacemaker malfunction has occurred, as is evident by the fixed-rate firing of the pacemaker. Pacer spikes are seen firing on and near the T wave (vulnerable period), setting the environment for the development of ventricular arrhythmias. The pacemaker has failed to sense the patient's own beats.

REVIEW QUESTIONS

1. What are the differences between a fixed-rate and a demand pacemaker?
2. Describe what a ventricular fusion beat is. Why are pacemakers potent producers of fusion beats?
3. The tracing below is a continuous recording from standard lead II of a 61-year-old male who came to the medical clinic with the chief complaint of having "a slow heart rate." His past history reveals the insertion of an epicardial-demand pacemaker. The etiology of the original problem which necessitated pacemaker insertion is not known at this time. The patient's heart rate on admission was 44 beats per minute. Analyze the effectiveness of the artificial pacemaker activity.

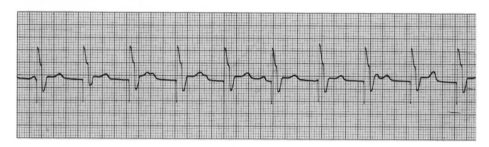

REFERENCES

1. Zoll P: Resuscitation of the heart in ventricular standstill by external electrical stimulation. *N Engl J Med* 247:768, 1952.
2. Weirich W, Gott V, Lillehei C: The treatment of complete heart block by combined use of a myocardial electrode and an artificial pacemaker. *Surg Forum* 8:360, 1957.
3. Furman, S, Schwedel J: An intra-cardiac pacemaker for Stokes–Adams seizures. *N Engl J Med* 261:943, 1959.
4. Chardack W, Gage A, Greatbach W: Correction of complete heart block by self contained and subcutaneously implanted pacemaker. *J Thorac Cardiovasc Surg* 42:814, 1961.
5. Carver J, Spitzer S, Mason D: Pacemaker update–1979. *Practical Cardiol* 5:129, 1979.
6. Dhingra R, Denes P: Prospective observations in patients with chronic bundle branch block and marked H-V prolongation. *Circulation* 53:600, 1976.
7. Fisher, JD, Cohen HL, et al: Cardiac pacing and pacemakers II. Serial electrophysiologic-pharmacologic testing for control of recurrent tachyarrhythmias. *Am Heart J* 93:658, 1977.
8. Lipman BS, Massie E, Kleiger RE: *Clinical Scalar Electrocardiography*, ed 6. Chicago, Year Book Medical Pub Inc, 1972, p 441.
9. Marriott HJL: *Practical Electrocardiography*, ed 6. Baltimore, Williams & Wilkins Co, 1977, p. 228.

Index